Case Studies in Oncology

Case Studies in Oncology

Editor: Zion Allen

AMERICAN
MEDICAL PUBLISHERS
www.americanmedicalpublishers.com

AMERICAN
MEDICAL PUBLISHERS
www.americanmedicalpublishers.com

Cataloging-in-Publication Data

Case studies in oncology / edited by Zion Allen.
p. cm.
Includes bibliographical references and index.
ISBN 979-8-88740-610-7
1. Oncology. 2. Tumors. 3. Cancer. 4. Tumors--Treatment.
5. Cancer--Treatment. I. Allen, Zion.
RC254 .053 2023
616.994--dc23

American Medical Publishers,
41 Flatbush Avenue,
1st Floor, New York,
NY 11217, USA

ISBN 979-8-88740-610-7 (Hardback)

Contents

Preface

Cancer is a disease characterized by the uncontrolled growth and spread of abnormal cells in the body. Oncology is an area of medicine that focuses on the prevention, diagnosis, and treatment of cancer. The field of oncology encompasses several subspecialties, such as surgical oncology, medical oncology and radiation oncology. Surgical oncology deals with surgical procedures to remove cancerous tumors and surrounding tissues, in order to eradicate the disease. Medical oncology focuses on the systemic treatment of cancer, utilizing chemotherapy, targeted therapies, immunotherapies and other medications to combat cancer cells throughout the body. Radiation oncology employs radiation therapy, using high-energy radiation to target and destroy cancer cells in specific areas. This book brings forth some of the most innovative concepts and elucidates the unexplored aspects of oncology. It is appropriate for students seeking detailed information in this area of medicine as well as for experts.

This book is the end result of constructive efforts and intensive research done by experts in this field. The aim of this book is to enlighten the readers with recent information in this area of research. The information provided in this profound book would serve as a valuable reference to students and researchers in this field.

At the end, I would like to thank all the authors for devoting their precious time and providing their valuable contribution to this book. I would also like to express my gratitude to my fellow colleagues who encouraged me throughout the process.

Editor

1

A Case of Stage I Vulvar Squamous Cell Carcinoma with Early Relapse and Rapid Disease Progression

Marta Peri,[1] Antonino Grassadonia,[1] Laura Iezzi,[1] Patrizia Vici,[2] Michele De Tursi,[1] Clara Natoli,[1] Nicola Tinari,[1] and Marinella Zilli[3]

[1]*Medical Oncology Unit, Department of Medical, Oral and Biotechnological Sciences, University "G. D'Annunzio", Chieti, Italy*
[2]*Division of Medical Oncology 2, IRCCS Regina Elena National Cancer Institute, Rome, Italy*
[3]*Medical Oncology Unit, SS Annunziata Hospital, Chieti, Italy*

Correspondence should be addressed to Antonino Grassadonia; grassadonia@unich.it

Academic Editor: Jose I. Mayordomo

Squamous cell carcinoma (SCC) is the most common subtype of vulvar cancer. Locoregional surgery is often curative when the tumor is diagnosed at an early stage. However, the disease can unexpectedly evolve with a dismal prognosis even after an early diagnosis. We report a case of a woman who experienced a rapid, chemorefractory tumor progression after surgery for stage IB vulvar SCC.

1. Introduction

Vulvar cancer is the fourth most common gynecologic cancer after endometrial, ovarian, and cervical cancer, accounting for about 5% of all female genital tract malignancies [1].

The most common histological type of vulvar cancer is squamous cell carcinoma (SCC), which accounts for about 90% of the cases. Two different types of SCC have been described: a keratinizing form and a warty/basaloid form [2]. The former occurs predominantly in postmenopausal women with a background of lichen sclerosus or lichen planus evolving in differentiated vulvar intraepithelial neoplasia (d-VIN) and is associated with poorer prognosis [3, 4]. The latter is more common in younger patients and is related to high-risk papillomavirus (HPV) infection evolving in high-grade squamous intraepithelial lesion (HSIL or VIN3) [3, 5].

Radical local excision with inguinofemoral lymph node dissection currently represents the standard of treatment for women with vulvar cancer [6]. Since surgery is associated with high morbidity, noninvasive methods are commonly utilized to evaluate the extension of disease in the preoperative setting. In particular, magnetic resonance imaging (MRI) is helpful for the assessment of local tumor extension and inguinal lymph node involvement [7].

The dissemination pattern of vulvar carcinoma is mostly lymphogenic, and the inguinofemoral lymph nodes are the primary site of regional spread [8]. Distant spread usually occurs late in the course of the disease. In the absence of distant metastases, the most important prognostic factor is represented by pathologic status of the inguinal nodes, while the size of the primary tumor is less important in defining prognosis [9].

Herein, we describe a case of vulvar carcinoma diagnosed at stage IB FIGO that displayed a very aggressive behavior. The patient experienced early local recurrence and rapid metastatic disease progression causing death just a few months after relapse.

2. Case Presentation

A 70-year-old woman presented at the gynecology unit of our hospital complaining about a painful vulvar lesion in May 2017. She had no significant medical history. Physical examination revealed an exophytic and ulcerative vulvar mass, approximately 4 cm in diameter, localized on the right labium majus at less than 2 cm from the midline, without palpable inguinal lymph nodes bilaterally. An incisional biopsy was performed, and histology revealed an invasive poorly

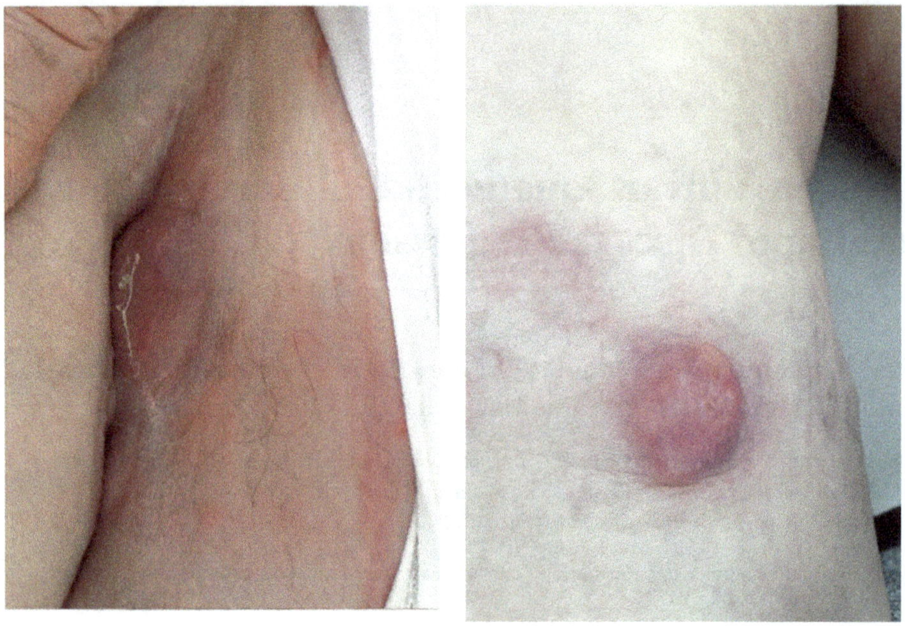

(a) (b)

Figure 1: Cutaneous tumor progression during the first-line chemotherapy. Erythematosus nodules on the skin of the right groin (a) and thigh (b).

differentiated vulvar SCC. A total-body CT scan performed to stage the disease resulted negative for distant metastases.

The patient underwent right hemivulvectomy in order to obtain wide tumor-free pathological margins in June 2017. Concomitant inguinal lymph node dissection was not performed due to the patient's refusal (risk of lymphedema). Histopathologic findings confirmed a poorly differentiated vulvar SCC arising on a background of lichen sclerosus. The size of the invasive SCC lesion was 4.5 cm with a depth of invasion of 2.7 mm and no lymphovascular invasion. All surgical margins of the lesion were tumor-free (more than 1 cm).

She was addressed to our oncology unit in July 2017. We required a disease restaging by abdominal and pelvic MRI scan and chest CT scan. No evidence of distant metastases resulted from the imaging studies. Therefore, we suggested locoregional lymph node dissection in order to define the pathologic stage of the tumor and to plan postoperative adjuvant radiotherapy to the groin just in case of lymph node involvement.

In August 2017, a bilateral inguinofemoral lymph node dissection was performed with all nodes (twelve) resulting negative for metastatic spread on conventional hematoxylin-eosin staining. The tumor was staged as FIGO stage IB, and the patient was addressed to strict follow-up.

However, just one month later (September 2017), the patient developed a local recurrence with a 3 cm nodule in the right vulvar area and a 0.8 cm lesion in the clitoris. A wide local excision was performed and histopathology examination revealed a poorly differentiated vulvar SCC in both lesions.

A restaging CT scan of the chest, abdomen, and pelvis showed multiple bilateral pulmonary metastases and multiple inguinal and pelvic lymph node involvement.

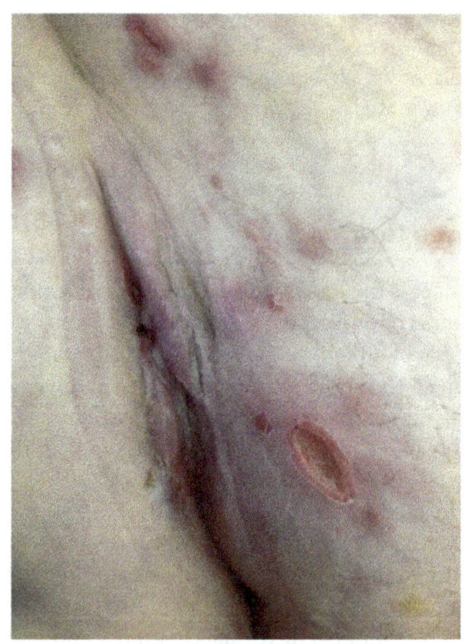

Figure 2: Further cutaneous progression during the second-line chemotherapy. Ulceration and fistulization of the right groin nodule.

Because of recurrence, systemic chemotherapy was started with carboplatin (AUC5 day 1 every 3 weeks) and paclitaxel (80 mg/m^2 days 1 and 8 every 3 weeks). After 3 cycles, a total body CT scan showed progression of metastatic disease in the lungs, lymph nodes, and liver. Moreover, a painful erythematosus nodule appeared on the skin of the right groin (Figure 1(a)) and right thigh (Figure 1(b)).

Because of disease progression, a second-line chemotherapy with capecitabine (1000 mg/m^2 bid, days 1-14 every

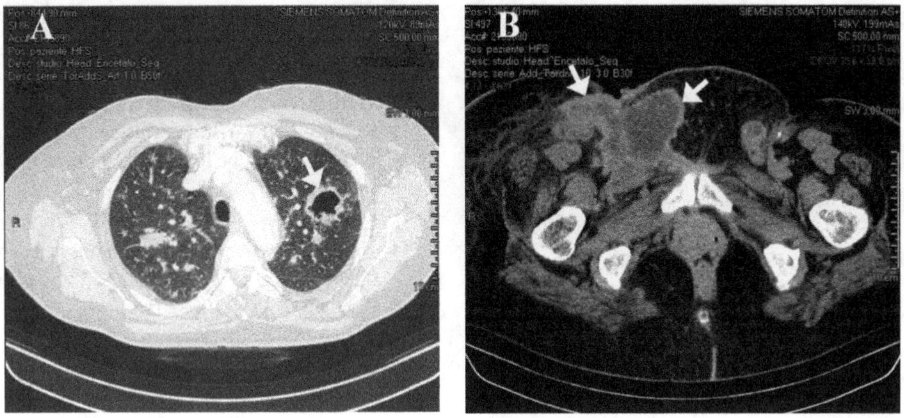

(a) (b)

FIGURE 3: Further systemic tumor progression during the second-line chemotherapy. CT scan showing multiple lesions in the lungs (a), some excavated (arrow), and matted metastatic lymph nodes in the iliac/inguinal region (b) (arrows).

21 days) was started (December 2017). After 3 cycles of treatment, the patient presented ulceration and fistulization of the groin lesion (Figure 2) and new skin nodules in the right thigh associated with extremities lymphedema. She complained of perineal pain and analgesic therapy was prescribed. Moreover, palliative radiotherapy to inguinal metastases (30 Gy in 10 fractions) was performed.

A reevaluation CT scan (February 2018) revealed further progression of the disease with multiple liver metastases, multiple excavated lesions in the lungs (Figure 3(a)), and matted metastatic iliac/inguinal lymph nodes (Figure 3(b)).

The patient died one month later, in March 2018, because of respiratory failure.

3. Discussion

We described a case of vulvar SCC that, despite an early-stage presentation at diagnosis, rapidly evolved into metastatic chemoresistant disease, leading the patient to death in a few months.

Vulvar SCC is a rare disease mainly occurring in postmenopausal women. The prognosis for patients with early-stage disease is generally good, but cancer can spread from its original site to locoregional nodes and/or distant organs by lymphatic embolization or hematogenous diffusion, respectively. Lymphatic spread represents an early event in the course of the disease and involves ipsilateral inguinal, femoral, and pelvic lymph nodes, usually in a sequential manner. Lymph node status remains the single most important prognostic factor. The 5-year overall survival is more than 90% for patients without nodal involvement, which reduces to less than 60% in the case of nodal involvement [9].

Our patient presented with a negative pathological nodal status at diagnosis, but unfortunately, her disease-free survival was very short, with local relapse occurring just one month after surgery. It is evident that other prognostic factors other than stage may influence the natural history of the disease. For example, tumor characteristics such as high-grade or lichen sclerosus-related etiopathogenesis, as in the case herein described, could play a pivotal role in determining a poor prognosis [4, 10].

Hematogenous spread to distant sites, including the lung, liver, and bone, usually occurs late in the natural history of the disease. Cutaneous metastases from vulvar carcinoma have been rarely described, but when documented, they are associated with short survival [11–15]. The median time to death from the diagnosis of skin metastasis has been estimated to be around 6 months [4, 15].

In our case, distant metastases developed shortly after diagnosis, in an early infiltrating phase of the disease (only 2.7 mm). Skin metastases also manifested early during the metastatic phase, in the course of the first-line systemic treatment. Consistent with literature data, the appearance of cutaneous metastases was a predictor of short survival for our patient. She died after only 4 months.

The rapid tumor progression was accompanied by a chemoresistant phenotype with a dismal prognosis. In fact, disease progressed during the first-line platinum-based chemotherapy in all the secondary sites and further progressed during the subsequent second-line treatment with capecitabine.

To date, the therapeutic management of metastatic vulvar SCC is heterogeneous and data are insufficient to recommend a preferred chemotherapeutic regimen in the palliative setting. Usually, regimens with proved efficacy in advanced cervical or anal cancers are chosen for the treatment of metastatic vulvar SCC [6].

Advances in the molecular biology of vulvar SCC may provide insight into the future management of this tumor [16]. At the moment, despite the two distinct etiologies, there is no specific recommended chemotherapeutic regimen for HPV-associated or HPV-independent tumors.

4. Conclusion

Vulvar SCC can unexpectedly evolve with a dismal prognosis even if diagnosed at an early stage. The disease can be rapidly progressive and refractory to chemotherapy. Novel therapeutic approaches are required.

Acknowledgments

This work was supported by the Consorzio Interuniversitario Nazionale per la Bio-Oncologia (CINBO).

References

[1] American Cancer Society, *Cancer facts & figures 2018*, American Cancer Society, Atlanta, GA, USA, 2018, November 2018, https://www.cancer.org/research/cancer-facts-statistics/all-cancer-facts-figures/cancer-facts-figures-2018.html.

[2] Y. Ueda, T. Enomoto, T. Kimura, K. Yoshino, M. Fujita, and T. Kimura, "Two distinct pathways to development of squamous cell carcinoma of the vulva," *Journal of Skin Cancer*, vol. 2011, Article ID 951250, 7 pages, 2011.

[3] C. Crum, C. Herrington, W. McCluccage, S. Regauer, and E. Wilkinson, "Tumours of the vulva; epithelial tumors," in *WHO Classification of Tumours of Female Reproductive Organs*, R. J. Kurman, M. L. Carcangiu, R. H. Young, and C. S. Herrington, Eds., pp. 232–236, International Agency for Research on Cancer, 2014.

[4] K. Prieske, N. Haeringer, D. Grimm et al., "Patterns of distant metastases in vulvar cancer," *Gynecologic Oncology*, vol. 142, no. 3, pp. 427–434, 2016.

[5] F. Hinten, A. Molijn, L. Eckhardt et al., "Vulvar cancer: two pathways with different localization and prognosis," *Gynecologic Oncology*, vol. 149, no. 2, pp. 310–317, 2018.

[6] M. H. M. Oonk, F. Planchamp, P. Baldwin et al., "European Society of Gynaecological Oncology guidelines for the management of patients with vulvar Cancer," *International Journal of Gynecological Cancer*, vol. 27, no. 4, pp. 832–837, 2017.

[7] M. Y. Kataoka, E. Sala, P. Baldwin et al., "The accuracy of magnetic resonance imaging in staging of vulvar cancer: a retrospective multi-centre study," *Gynecologic Oncology*, vol. 117, no. 1, pp. 82–87, 2010.

[8] J. M. Woolderink, G. H. de Bock, J. A. de Hullu, M. J. Davy, A. G. J. van der Zee, and M. J. E. Mourits, "Patterns and frequency of recurrences of squamous cell carcinoma of the vulva," *Gynecologic Oncology*, vol. 103, no. 1, pp. 293–299, 2006.

[9] S. Edge, D. Byrd, C. Compton, A. Fritz, F. Greene, and A. Trotti, Eds., *AJCC Cancer Staging Manual*, Springer, New York, NY, USA, 7th edition, 2010.

[10] N. C. te Grootenhuis, A. F. W. Pouwer, G. H. de Bock et al., "Prognostic factors for local recurrence of squamous cell carcinoma of the vulva: a systematic review," *Gynecologic Oncology*, vol. 148, no. 3, pp. 622–631, 2018.

[11] D. H. Tobias, H. O. Smith, J. G. Jones, P. Anderson, C. D. Runowicz, and G. L. Goldberg, "Cutaneous metastases from squamous cell carcinoma of the vulva. A case report and review of the literature," *European Journal of Gynaecological Oncology*, vol. 16, no. 5, pp. 382–386, 1995.

[12] W. A. A. Tjalma and K. Watty, "Skin metastases from vulvar cancer: a fatal event," *Gynecologic Oncology*, vol. 89, no. 1, pp. 185–188, 2003.

[13] F. Ghaemmaghami, M. Modares, N. Behtash, and A. Z. Moosavi, "Multiple, disseminated cutaneous metastases of vulvar squamous cell carcinoma," *International Journal of Gynecological Cancer*, vol. 14, no. 2, pp. 384–387, 2004.

[14] A. R. Wang, M. O'Brien, R. Ross, T. Long, and L. Robinson-Bostom, "Epidermotropic metastasis from vulvar squamous cell carcinoma: a rare cutaneous manifestation," *Journal of the American Academy of Dermatology*, vol. 63, no. 6, pp. 1088–1091, 2010.

[15] N. Bizzarri, V. G. Vellone, L. Parodi et al., "Cutaneous metastasis from vulvar squamous cell carcinoma: a rare occurrence that should not be forgotten," *Journal of Obstetrics and Gynaecology*, vol. 37, no. 8, pp. 975–981, 2017.

[16] A. A. Clancy, J. N. Spaans, and J. I. Weberpals, "The forgotten woman's cancer: vulvar squamous cell carcinoma (VSCC) and a targeted approach to therapy," *Annals of Oncology*, vol. 27, no. 9, pp. 1696–1705, 2016.

2

Regionally Metastatic Merkel Cell Carcinoma Associated with Paraneoplastic Anti-*N*-methyl-D-aspartate Receptor Encephalitis

Sophia Z. Shalhout,[1] Kevin S. Emerick,[2] Peter M. Sadow,[3] Jenny J. Linnoila,[4] and David M. Miller[1]

[1]Division of Hematology/Oncology, Department of Medicine, and Department of Dermatology, Massachusetts General Hospital, Harvard Medical School, Boston, MA 02114, USA
[2]Department of Otolaryngology, Massachusetts Eye and Ear Infirmary, Harvard Medical School, Boston, MA 02114, USA
[3]Department of Pathology, Massachusetts General Hospital, Harvard Medical School, Boston, MA 02114, USA
[4]Department of Neurology, Massachusetts General Hospital, Harvard Medical School, Boston, MA 02114, USA

Correspondence should be addressed to David M. Miller; dmiller4@mgh.harvard.edu

Academic Editor: Mauro Cives

Merkel cell carcinoma (MCC) is a rare and aggressive cutaneous neuroendocrine cancer with a high risk of recurrence and metastasis. MCC is generally associated with advanced age, fair skin, sun exposure, immunosuppression, and in the majority of cases, the Merkel cell polyomavirus. Neuroendocrine malignancies are associated with a variety of paraneoplastic neurological syndromes (PNS), characterized as autoimmune responses to malignancy-associated expression of neural antigens. Our literature review underscores previous case reports of MCC-associated PNS with voltage-gated calcium channel (VGCC) and anti-Hu (or ANNA-1) autoantibodies. We present the case of a 59-year-old male with regionally metastatic Merkel cell carcinoma complicated by the paraneoplastic manifestation of anti-*N*-methyl-D-aspartate receptor (NMDAR) encephalitis. His primary lower neck subcutaneous MCC and metastasis were initially treated with surgery. Additional recurrent lymph node metastases were successfully treated with definitive intensity-modulated radiation therapy. His PNS improved with rituximab therapy. Although rare, this case highlights that in the setting of seizures and prominent psychiatric symptoms accompanying an MCC diagnosis, evaluation for autoimmune paraneoplastic encephalitis is warranted. Awareness and detection of preexisting PNS are crucial in the era of immune checkpoint inhibitors (ICI) for advanced MCC, where treatment with ICI has the potential to exacerbate preexisting autoimmune PNS and lead to worsened or even lethal neurologic immune-related adverse events (nirAEs).

1. Introduction

Paraneoplastic neurological syndromes (PNS) are a heterogenous group of immune-mediated disorders associated with neural autoantibodies directed against antigens expressed by both the tumor and the nervous system. These syndromes may affect any part of the nervous system and are exceptionally rare [1], with a higher incidence in small-cell lung cancer and gynecological tumors [2].

Anti-*N*-methyl-D-aspartate receptor (NMDAR) encephalitis is a recently described PNS. When associated with cancer, NMDAR encephalitis is found to predominantly affect young women with ovarian teratomas [3]. Autoantibody production against the NMDAR leads to internalization of the receptors and profound dysregulation of neurotransmission, with prominent neuropsychiatric manifestations. The onset may begin with a viral-like prodrome, followed by a wide spectrum of clinical features including seizures, memory loss, psychosis, aphasia, and hallucinations [3, 4]. With rare incidence, in case reports, anti-NMDAR encephalitis has been described in association with neuroendocrine differentiated neoplasms of the uterus, pancreas, and liver, as well as small-cell lung carcinomas, typically in older individuals (Table 1).

Table 1: Reports of neuroendocrine neoplasms associated with anti-NMDA receptor encephalitis.

Reference(s)	Sex/age	Neuroendocrine neoplasm
Lim and Yip [14]	M/65	Hepatic neuroendocrine carcinoma
Bost et al. [9]	F/50	Pancreatic neuroendocrine tumor (NMDAR+ tumor)
Afanasiev et al. [15]	F/51	Pancreatic neuroendocrine tumor (NMDAR+ tumor)
Hara et al. [16]	F/65	Carcinosarcoma with neuroendocrine differentiation of the uterus (NMDAR+ tumor)
Kobayashi et al. [17]	F/44	Large-cell neuroendocrine carcinoma of the uterus (NMDAR+ tumor)
Boangher et al. [18]	F/66	Small-cell lung cancer
Jeraiby et al. [19]	F/62	Small-cell lung cancer (NMDAR+ tumor)
Titulaer et al. [20]	NA	Small-cell lung cancer

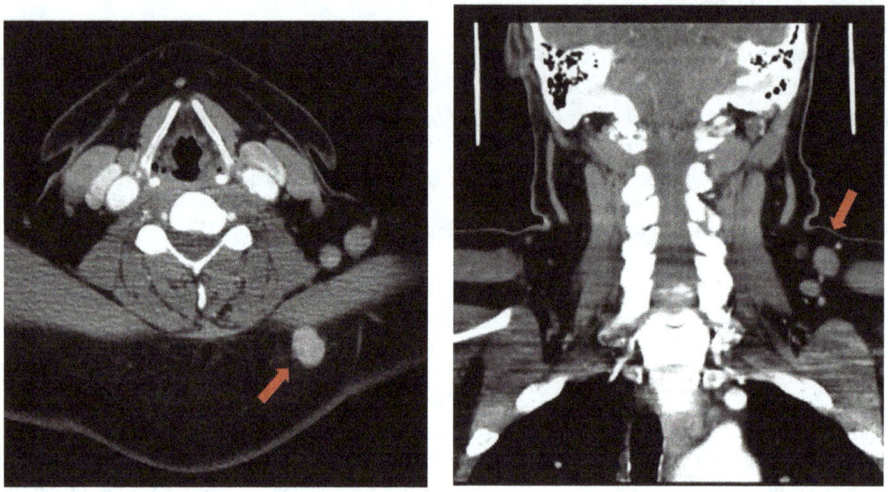

(a) (b)

Figure 1: (a, axial view) CT scan with contrast demonstrated a hyperdense rounded mass in the subcutaneous tissue of the left side of the neck, posterior to the trapezius muscle, corresponding to the patient's palpable primary mass (red arrow). (b, coronal view) Several lymph nodes (red arrow) in the posterior triangle anterior to the trapezius muscle ranging in size up to 1.5 cm in diameter were demonstrated on CT scan.

We report the case of a 59-year-old male who developed anti-NMDAR encephalitis as a paraneoplastic manifestation of Merkel cell carcinoma (MCC). This rare and aggressive cutaneous neuroendocrine cancer has a high risk of recurrence and metastasis, often occurring within the first two years after initial diagnosis [5]. His regionally metastatic MCC was Merkel cell polyomavirus (MCPyV) positive. He underwent surgical-wide local excision with neck lymph node dissection and was successfully treated with definitive intensity-modulated radiation. His anti-NMDAR encephalitis showed slow but steady improvement upon treatment with rituximab. In this report, we highlight the potential complications associated with the evaluation and management of MCC when treatment is initiated for anti-NMDAR encephalitis, since the interpretation of contemporaneous MCPyV oncoprotein antibody serum titers [6] may be affected. Furthermore, the timely identification of an underlying autoimmune PNS is critical when considering immune checkpoint inhibitors (ICI) for the treatment of advanced MCC. Treatment and close monitoring of PNS, including anti-NMDAR encephalitis, before ICI therapy may reduce the possibility of worsened or even lethal neurologic immune-related adverse events [7].

2. Case Report

A 59-year-old male with a history of posttraumatic stress disorder and depression presented for evaluation of a palpable mass on the left posterior aspect of his neck that grew over the course of a few months. A computed tomography (CT) scan of the neck with omnipaque contrast demonstrated a hyperdense rounded mass that corresponded to the patient's palpable neck abnormality in the subcutaneous tissue, posterior to the trapezius muscle. Several lymph nodes in the posterior triangle anterior to the trapezius muscle ranging in size up to 1.5 cm in diameter were also appreciated on CT scans (Figure 1).

A fine needle aspiration biopsy (FNA) was performed, and a poorly differentiated carcinoma with neuroendocrine features was identified on cytology. An MRI of the brain was unremarkable, and a PET-CT revealed that the nodule in the subcutaneous fat of the left posterior neck was FDG-avid. The left trapezius muscle had six FDG avid nodules in the posterior aspect of the left side of the neck. The patient was taken to the operating room one week later for a wide local excision and a comprehensive level 5 posterior neck lymph node dissection. The immunohistochemical profile

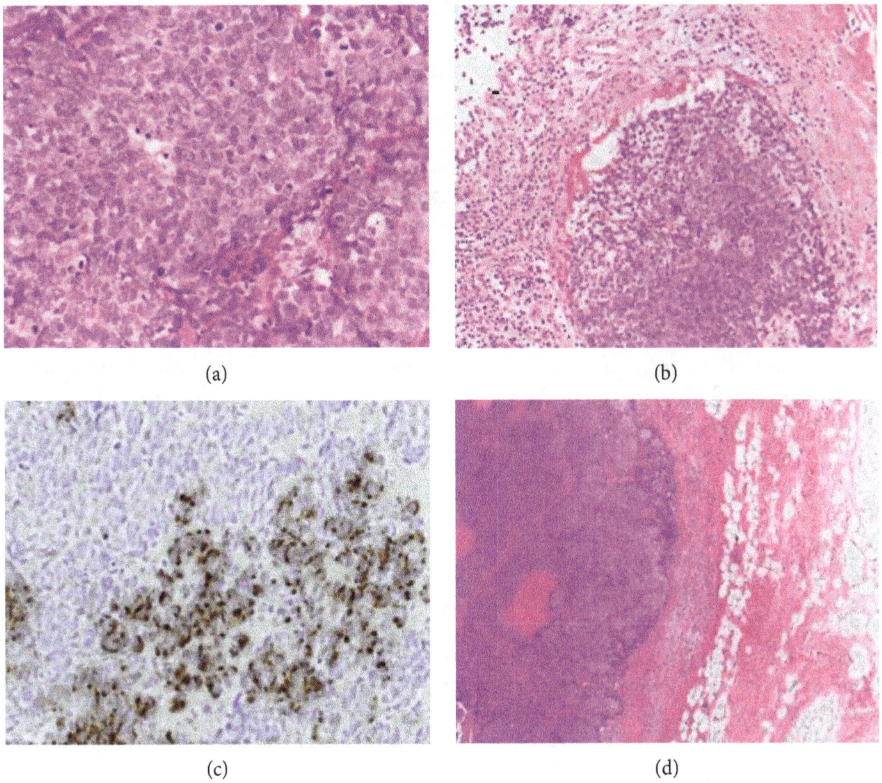

FIGURE 2: (a) Magnification 400x, hematoxylin and eosin stain of the left neck; Merkel cell carcinoma primary tumor demonstrates numerous mitoses and neuroendocrine nuclei. (b) Magnification 200x, MCC left neck primary highlighting lymphovascular invasion. (c) Magnification 400x, immunohistochemistry demonstrates perinuclear dot like immunostaining positive for cytokeratin 20. (d) Magnification 40x, MCC primary tumor of the left neck in subcutaneous tissue.

of the primary left neck mass demonstrated features consistent with MCC. The tissue was positive for synaptophysin, chromogranin, and cytokeratin 20 in a perinuclear dot-like distribution (Figure 2) as well as CAM5.2 and p16. The cells were negative for keratin 7, p40, TTF-1, PAX 8, and calcitonin. The upper level left neck dissection demonstrated 3 of 8 lymph nodes positive for metastatic MCC, and the lower left neck dissection demonstrated metastatic MCC to 6 of 36 lymph nodes. No extranodal extension was detected. A baseline anti-Merkel cell panel serology test (AMERK, University of Washington Medical Center) was positive for MCPyV oncoprotein antibodies at 7440 standard titer units (STU). The primary tumor was ≤2 cm in diameter, and he presented with clinically and radiologically detected regional lymph node metastasis and therefore was pathologically staged as Stage IIIB (T1pN1b) according to AJCC 8th edition.

Following his excision and lymph node dissection, adjuvant radiotherapy was recommended and planned to manage his MCC. However, prior to the initiation of his adjuvant radiation, the patient presented to the emergency department (ED) of an outside hospital due to seizure activity, with two witnessed seizures in the ED. He was afebrile with the absence of infectious symptoms and displayed expressive aphasia, dyskinesias, altered mental status, and auditory hallucinations. Levetiracetam (750 mg) was initially administered twice daily, and upon discharge, he had another generalized tonic-clonic seizure in the waiting room with a right-sided tongue bite and stool incontinence. He returned to the ED and was administered 1 g of levetiracetam. His aphasia and memory impairment continued, and he was started on empiric acyclovir for herpes simplex virus (HSV) encephalitis coverage, but therapy was discontinued due to acute renal injury. A head CT and brain MRI were unremarkable. A lumbar puncture showed normal chemistries, and his CSF meningoencephalitis panels were negative for any infectious process. He continued to be agitated and confused, with minimal improvement of his aphasia. A repeat brain MRI was unremarkable for abnormalities. The patient's CSF autoimmune encephalopathy panel returned positive for NMDA receptor GluN1 antibodies (1 : 80 titer) and negative for other neural antibodies. His symptoms were attributed to NMDAR encephalitis, likely an autoimmune paraneoplastic syndrome due to his MCC. He received a 5-day course of intravenous immunoglobulin and was started on 60 mg of prednisone per day. His expressive aphasia and neurological exams improved, and he was discharged to a rehab facility on levetiracetam (500 mg twice a day) and divalproex (750 mg twice a day). On the neurologic follow-up at this hospital, the patient still had significant cognitive deficits, particularly in his short-term memory. It was decided to slowly reduce his prednisone dose and to initiate rituximab instead.

A PET-CT three months after his surgical excision demonstrated two FDG-avid nodules along the left levator scapulae muscle. Moderate FDG uptake to his left axillary lymph

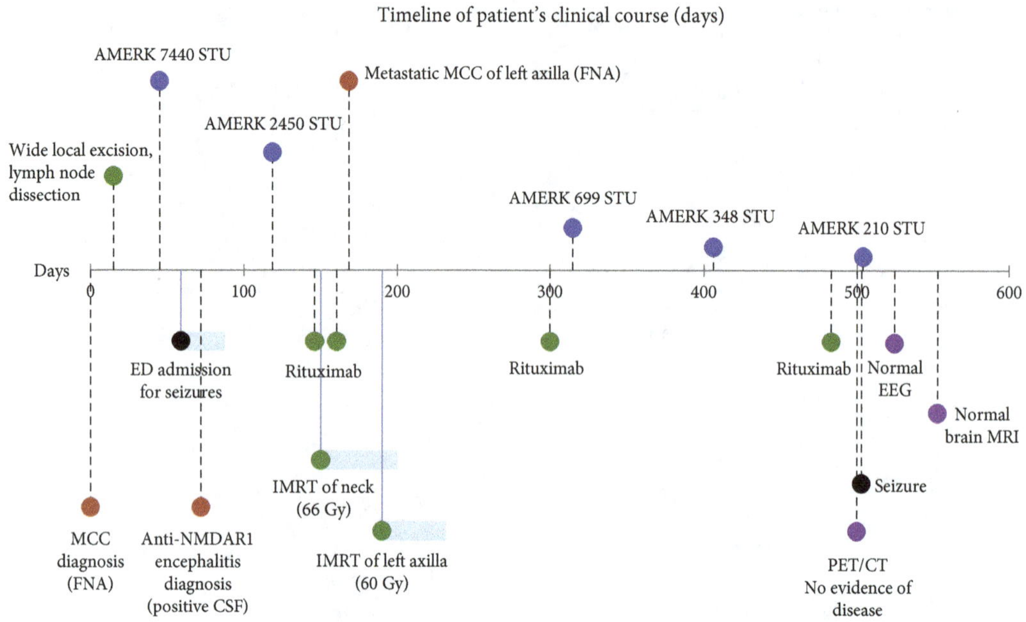

FIGURE 3: Timeline of patient's clinical course highlighting surgical excision, radiation, and MCPyV antibody panel AMERK results for the treatment and management of his MCC, as well as rituximab infusions for his paraneoplastic autoimmune encephalitis. Day 0 is set to his initial MCC diagnosis. Red: diagnoses; blue: AMERK titers; green: treatment interventions for MCC and encephalitis, including wide local excision, IMRT, and rituximab infusions (1 g); black: seizures; purple: latest follow-up scans and EEG.

nodes, consistent with recurrence of his MCC, was also observed. His AMERK test revealed a ~67% decrease in MCPyV oncoprotein serum titers (2450 STU). During this time, he completed two doses of rituximab for his anti-NMDAR encephalitis (Figure 3). He was slowly tapered off of levetiracetam and divalproex. An FNA of his left axillary mass confirmed metastatic MCC, with no evidence of metastatic brain disease demonstrated on MRI. He began intensity-modulated radiation therapy (IMRT) to his neck and left axillae. At this stage, he continued to need assistance with activities of daily living to improve his memory. He successfully completed IMRT and was continued on rituximab, dosed every six months. A few weeks after his latest dose, he experienced a single seizure. He was restarted on levetiracetam. A follow-up routine EEG was normal. His AMERK tests continued to trend downward to 210 STU but remained positive for oncoprotein antibody in serum (AMERK of <74 STU is considered negative) (Figure 3). He continues to be followed every three months for close monitoring, with full body skin exams and surveillance PET-CT scans, which continue to be reassuring for no evidence of recurrence or metastatic MCC disease. His cognitive status has continued to improve on rituximab, with a recent brain MRI revealing no abnormalities and no evidence of intracranial metastatic disease.

3. Discussion

Merkel cell carcinoma is an aggressive and rare neuroendocrine skin cancer. This report highlights a patient who was treated with surgical therapy and IMRT for regionally metastatic MCC and achieved complete regional control both clinically and radiologically, one year post definitive radiotherapy. The clinical psychiatric and neurological manifestations in our patient were typical of anti-NMDAR encephalitis, generally characterized by altered mental status, hallucinations, orofacial dyskinesias, seizures, and autonomic instability. The detection of anti-NMDAR antibodies in his CSF makes a paraneoplastic manifestation, with MCC as the inciting malignancy, probable [8]. Large cohort studies have demonstrated that the underlying tumor associated with paraneoplastic anti-NMDAR encephalitis in the majority of cases is an ovarian teratoma, either mature or immature [8, 9]. Nervous tissue components of ovarian teratomas from patients with anti-NMDAR encephalitis were shown to express NMDAR subunits [10]. A few previous cases have described anti-NMDAR encephalitis associated with neuroendocrine neoplasms of the uterus, liver, lung, and pancreas, with 5 reports demonstrating tumors positive for NMDAR subunits (Table 1).

A review of the literature of PNS associated with a diagnosis of MCC highlights case reports of neurologic and prominent psychiatric symptoms associated with VGCC and anti-Hu (or ANNA-1) autoantibodies. Cases describing novel antibodies against nerve fibers or filamentous nervous system structures have also been reported in patients with PNS secondary to MCC (Table 2). We report a rare case of anti-NMDAR encephalitis as a paraneoplastic manifestation due to MCPyV-positive MCC. The treatment of his encephalitis with rituximab complicates the interpretation of the AMERK MCPyV serology tests used to manage virus-positive patients who produce oncoprotein antibodies. An oncoprotein antibody test is typically obtained within 2-3 months of initial evident disease, to establish a baseline in virus-positive MCC patients. After successful treatment, oncoprotein antibodies usually decrease rapidly, falling

Table 2: Autoimmune paraneoplastic syndromes associated with Merkel cell carcinoma.

Reference(s)	Symptoms/syndrome	Autoimmune antibodies
Lopez et al. [21]	Painless proximal muscle weakness	Anti-Hu/ANNA-1 antibodies
Balegno et al. [22]	Paraneoplastic cerebellar ataxia	Antibodies against cerebellar nerve fibers
Greenlee et al. [23]	Sensorimotor and autonomic neuropathy, encephalopathy	Anti-Hu/ANNA-1 antibodies
Cher et al. [24]	Paraneoplastic brainstem encephalitis	Antibodies against brain and cerebellum filamentous structures
Eggers et al. [25], Nguyen et al. [26], and Iyer et al. [27]	Lambert-Eaton myasthenic syndrome	Antibodies against VGCCs
Sharobeam et al. [28]	Subacute cerebellar degeneration	Anti-Hu/ANNA-1 antibodies
Zhang et al. [29]	Paraneoplastic cerebellar degeneration	Antibodies against VGCCs
Hocar et al. [30]	Severe necrotizing myopathy	Anti-Hu/ANNA-1 antibodies
Current case	Expressive aphasia, altered mental status, memory loss, seizures/NMDAR encephalitis	Anti-NMDAR antibodies

~90% one year after successful treatment. However, upon recurrence, metastases, or increased tumor burden, titers increase rapidly [11]. Treating PNS with rituximab in our patient complicates the interpretation of the titer results, and we highlight the need for further studies and exploration of the effects on antibody levels used to track MCC burden in patients treated with anti-CD-20-directed therapies for PNS.

The timely identification and treatment of an underlying autoimmune PNS is critical when considering approved ICI therapies, such as avelumab and pembrolizumab, for the treatment of advanced MCC. Treatment and close monitoring of PNS, including anti-NMDAR encephalitis, before and during ICI therapy, may reduce the potential for worsening or lethal immunotherapy-related neurologic adverse events. PNS are typically associated with poor prognosis, and upon treatment with ICIs, these patients may have worsening of their PNS. Cases of severe and long-term disability as well as death have been reported in patients on anti-PD-1 inhibitors for lung cancer due to exacerbation of preexisting autoimmune PNS, with increased titers of anti-Hu/ANNA-1 and anti-voltage gated potassium channel (VGKC) antibodies [7, 12]. There were also 2 reports of cases of severe disability and death in patients on nivolumab and pembrolizumab for metastatic MCC due to exacerbation of preexisting anti-Hu/ANNA-1 and anti-VGKC autoimmune PNS and nirAEs [13]. Given the rarity of these conditions, awareness of PNS in the setting of prominent neurologic symptoms in association with MCC is of critical importance.

Abbreviations

AMERK: Anti-Merkel cell panel antibody titer serology test, University of Washington Medical Center
CSF: Cerebrospinal fluid
ICI: Immune checkpoint inhibitors
FDG: ^{18}F-fluorodeoxyglucose
ED: Emergency department
FNA: Fine needle aspiration biopsy
HSV: Herpes simplex virus
IMRT: Intensity modulated radiation therapy
MCC: Merkel cell carcinoma
MCPyV: Merkel cell polyomavirus
MRI: Magnetic resonance imaging
NA: Not available
nirAE: Neurologic immune-related adverse events
NMDAR: *N*-Methyl-D-aspartate receptor
PET-CT: Positron emission tomography-computed tomography
PNS: Paraneoplastic neurological syndrome
STU: Standard titer units
VGCCs: Voltage gated calcium channels
VGKCs: Voltage gated potassium channels.

Consent

Written informed consent was obtained from the patient for publication of this case report and any accompanying images. The patient involved in the case report gave the approval to treatments.

Acknowledgments

The Harvard Cancer Center Merkel Cell Carcinoma Patient Registry is funded by Project Data Sphere (DMM, SZS). SZS was supported by the Mass General Cancer Center Cutaneous Oncology Research Fellowship. JJL is a Phyllis & Jerome Lyle Rappaport Foundation Fellow and McCance Transformative Scholar from the MGH Department of Neurology with a K08 grant through NIH/NINDS: K08NS101084-01.

References

[1] R. B. Darnell and J. B. Posner, "Paraneoplastic syndromes involving the nervous system," *The New England Journal of Medicine*, vol. 349, no. 16, pp. 1543–1554, 2003.

[2] J. Dalmau and M. R. Rosenfeld, "Paraneoplastic syndromes of the CNS," *The Lancet Neurology*, vol. 7, no. 4, pp. 327–340, 2008.

[3] J. Dalmau, E. Lancaster, E. Martinez-Hernandez, M. R. Rosenfeld, and R. Balice-Gordon, "Clinical experience and laboratory investigations in patients with anti-NMDAR encephalitis," *The Lancet Neurology*, vol. 10, no. 1, pp. 63–74, 2011.

[4] J. Dalmau and F. Graus, "Antibody-mediated encephalitis,"

The New England Journal of Medicine, vol. 378, no. 9, pp. 840–851, 2018.

[5] K. L. Harms, M. A. Healy, P. Nghiem et al., "Analysis of prognostic factors from 9387 Merkel cell carcinoma cases forms the basis for the new 8th edition AJCC staging system," *Annals of Surgical Oncology*, vol. 23, no. 11, pp. 3564–3571, 2016.

[6] K. G. Paulson, C. W. Lewis, M. W. Redman et al., "Viral oncoprotein antibodies as a marker for recurrence of Merkel cell carcinoma: a prospective validation study," *Cancer*, vol. 123, no. 8, pp. 1464–1474, 2017.

[7] P. Raibagkar, D. Ho, K. S. Gunturu, and J. Srinivasan, "Worsening of anti-Hu paraneoplastic neurological syndrome related to anti-PD-1 treatment: case report and review of literature," *Journal of Neuroimmunology*, vol. 341, article 577184, 2020.

[8] J. Dalmau, A. J. Gleichman, E. G. Hughes et al., "Anti-NMDA-receptor encephalitis: case series and analysis of the effects of antibodies," *The Lancet Neurology*, vol. 7, no. 12, pp. 1091–1098, 2008.

[9] C. Bost, E. Chanson, G. Picard et al., "Malignant tumors in autoimmune encephalitis with anti-NMDA receptor antibodies," *Journal of Neurology*, vol. 265, no. 10, pp. 2190–2200, 2018.

[10] J. Dalmau, E. Tüzün, H. Y. Wu et al., "Paraneoplastic anti-N-methyl-D-aspartate receptor encephalitis associated with ovarian teratoma," *Annals of Neurology*, vol. 61, no. 1, pp. 25–36, 2007.

[11] K. G. Paulson, J. J. Carter, L. G. Johnson et al., "Antibodies to Merkel cell polyomavirus T antigen oncoproteins reflect tumor burden in Merkel cell carcinoma patients," *Cancer Research*, vol. 70, no. 21, pp. 8388–8397, 2010.

[12] H. Matsuoka, H. Kimura, H. Koba et al., "Nivolumab-induced limbic encephalitis with anti-Hu antibody in a patient with advanced pleomorphic carcinoma of the lung," *Clinical Lung Cancer*, vol. 19, no. 5, pp. e597–e599, 2018.

[13] A. Gill, M. A. Perez, C. M. Perrone, C. J. Bae, A. A. Pruitt, and E. Lancaster, "A case series of PD-1 inhibitor-associated paraneoplastic neurologic syndromes," *Journal of Neuroimmunology*, vol. 334, article 576980, 2019.

[14] E. W. Lim and C. W. Yip, "Anti-N-methyl-D-aspartate receptor encephalitis associated with hepatic neuroendocrine carcinoma: a case report," *Journal of Clinical Neuroscience*, vol. 41, pp. 70–72, 2017.

[15] V. Afanasiev, M. L. Brechemier, W. Boisseau et al., "Anti-NMDA receptor antibody encephalitis and neuroendocrine pancreatic tumor: causal link?," *Neurology*, vol. 87, no. 1, pp. 112-113, 2016.

[16] M. Hara, A. Morita, S. Kamei et al., "Anti-*N*-methyl-D-aspartate receptor encephalitis associated with carcinosarcoma with neuroendocrine differentiation of the uterus," *Journal of Neurology*, vol. 258, no. 7, pp. 1351–1353, 2011.

[17] M. Kobayashi, K. Nishioka, M. Takanashi et al., "Anti-NMDA receptor encephalitis due to large-cell neuroendocrine carcinoma of the uterus," *Journal of the Neurological Sciences*, vol. 383, pp. 72–74, 2017.

[18] S. Boangher, P. Mespouille, C. M. Filip, and S. Goffette, "Small-cell lung cancer with positive anti-NMDAR and anti-AMPAR antibodies paraneoplastic limbic encephalitis," *Case Reports in Neurological Medicine*, vol. 2016, Article ID 3263718, 3 pages, 2016.

[19] M. Jeraiby, A. Depince-Berger, V. Bossy, J. C. Antoine, and S. Paul, "A case of anti-NMDA receptor encephalitis in a woman with a NMDA-R$^+$ small cell lung carcinoma (SCLC)," *Clinical Immunology*, vol. 166-167, pp. 96–99, 2016.

[20] M. J. Titulaer, L. McCracken, I. Gabilondo et al., "Treatment and prognostic factors for long-term outcome in patients with anti-NMDA receptor encephalitis: an observational cohort study," *The Lancet Neurology*, vol. 12, no. 2, pp. 157–165, 2013.

[21] M. C. Lopez, C. Pericay, M. Agusti, M. Martinez-Gallo, R. Bordes, and C. Gelpi, "Merkel cell carcinoma associated with a paraneoplastic neurological syndrome," *Histopathology*, vol. 44, no. 6, pp. 628-629, 2004.

[22] S. Balegno, M. Ceroni, M. Corato et al., "Antibodies to cerebellar nerve fibres in two patients with paraneoplastic cerebellar ataxia," *Anticancer Research*, vol. 25, no. 5, pp. 3211–3214, 2005.

[23] J. E. Greenlee, J. D. Steffens, S. A. Clawson, K. Hill, and J. Dalmau, "Anti-Hu antibodies in Merkel cell carcinoma," *Annals of Neurology*, vol. 52, no. 1, pp. 111–115, 2002.

[24] L. M. Cher, F. H. Hochberg, M. Nitschke et al., "Therapy for paraneoplastic neurologic syndromes in six patients with protein a column immunoadsorption," *Cancer*, vol. 75, no. 7, pp. 1678–1683, 1995.

[25] S. D. Eggers, D. R. Salomao, R. P. Dinapoli, and S. Vernino, "Paraneoplastic and metastatic neurologic complications of Merkel cell carcinoma," *Mayo Clinic Proceedings*, vol. 76, no. 3, pp. 327–330, 2001.

[26] N. D. Nguyen, D. B. Simmons, A. R. Bersabe et al., "Lambert-Eaton myasthenic syndrome and Merkel cell carcinoma," *Cutis*, vol. 103, no. 5, pp. E19–E23, 2019.

[27] J. G. Iyer, K. Parvathaneni, S. Bhatia et al., "Paraneoplastic syndromes (PNS) associated with Merkel cell carcinoma (MCC): a case series of 8 patients highlighting different clinical manifestations," *Journal of the American Academy of Dermatology*, vol. 75, no. 3, pp. 541–547, 2016.

[28] A. Sharobeam, J. Ray, J. Dong, and V. Chong, "Subacute cerebellar degeneration due to a paraneoplastic phenomenon associated with metastatic Merkel cell carcinoma: a case report," *Case Reports in Oncology*, vol. 10, no. 2, pp. 764–768, 2017.

[29] C. Zhang, L. Emery, and E. Lancaster, "Paraneoplastic cerebellar degeneration associated with noncutaneous Merkel cell carcinoma," *Neurology - Neuroimmunology Neuroinflammation*, vol. 1, no. 2, article e17, 2014.

[30] O. Hocar, E. Poszepczynska-Guigne, O. Faye, J. Wechsler, M. Bagot, and V. Buffard, "Severe necrotizing myopathy subsequent to Merkel cell carcinoma," *Annales de Dermatologie et de Vénéréologie*, vol. 138, pp. 130–134, 2011.

3

A Case of Advanced Gastric Cancer with Folfiri as a Preoperative Chemotherapy

Hieu Van Nguyen,[1,2] Hung Van Nguyen,[1] Long Thanh Nguyen,[1] Nga Quynh Pham,[1,2] Hau Xuan Nguyen,[1,2] Hien Xuan Nguyen,[1] and Vuong Thi Nguyen[1,2]

[1]*Department of Oncology, Hanoi Medical University, Hanoi, Vietnam*
[2]*Department of Oncology and Palliative Care, Hanoi Medical University Hospital, Hanoi, Vietnam*

Correspondence should be addressed to Hung Van Nguyen; dr.hungnguyen.hmu@gmail.com

Academic Editor: Peter F. Lenehan

Introduction. In advanced gastric cancer, preoperative chemotherapy is associated with survival benefit. FOLFIRI has demonstrated promising results in terms of survival and tolerance, especially in patients with poor performance status. *Case Presentation.* A 59-year-old male, diagnosed with pT4bN2M0 gastric cancer, underwent gastrointestinal anastomosis and three cycles of EOX chemotherapy. Due to disease progression, he was switched to FOLFIRI regimen. After 12 cycles, the patient received a subtotal gastrectomy and D2 lymphadenectomy. Microscopic examination achieved pCR, and the patient has been surviving 34 months without recurrence. No severe toxicities of chemotherapy were recorded. *Conclusions.* FOLFIRI might be a safe and effective option in neoadjuvant treatment for advanced gastric cancer among patients with poor performance status or progression after first-line chemotherapy.

1. Introduction

Gastric cancer currently is the third most frequent cause of cancer-related deaths worldwide [1]. In Vietnam, there were approximately 17,527 new cases and 15,065 deaths due to gastric cancer in 2018 [1].

Gastric cancer treatment is a multidisciplinary strategy, in which surgery plays an essential role. As a means of down-staging prior to an attempt of curative resection, recent guidelines has recommended preoperative chemotherapy, especially for patients with locally advanced gastric cancer [2]. Various clinical trials have been conducted to investigate the efficacy of preoperative regimens, such as ECF/ECX (epirubicin, cisplatin, and 5-FU/capecitabine) in MAGIC and REAL 2 trials and FLOT (5-FU, leucovorin, oxaliplatin, and docetaxel) in FLOT4-AIO trial [3–5]. These regimens, however, have significant toxicity and cannot be administered to patients with poor performance status. Moreover, in cases that are unresponsive to the above regimens, the second-line treatment options are currently controversial and have remarkably lower response rates than the first-line regimen [6].

FOLFIRI (5-FU, leucovorin, and irinotecan) regimen in advanced gastric cancer treatment has been evaluated in some phase III trials, revealing promising results in terms of response rate, overall survival, and tolerance [7, 8]. To our knowledge, there are limited evidences on using FOLFIRI as a preoperative chemotherapy in patients with locally advanced gastric cancer. In this article, we reported a case diagnosed as advanced gastric cancer treated with second-line preoperative FOLFIRI regimen and following gastrectomy, resulting in a pathological complete response (pCR).

2. Case Presentation

A 59-year-old male, with a history of hypertension and type 2 diabetes, came to a national hospital complaining of epigastric pain, early satiety, nausea, and vomiting. On esophagogastroduodenoscopy, a pyloric ulcer was found which caused gastric outlet obstruction. A biopsy was done, revealing a poorly differentiated adenocarcinoma with signet ring cell features. The patient was diagnosed as gastric carcinoma with pyloric stenosis and then underwent exploratory surgery. During operation, the tumor was found at the antrum and pylorus region invading the duodenum, the head of the pancreas and the mesentery of transverse colon and small intestine, along with multiple enlarged and hard regional lymph nodes. A gastrointestinal anastomosis and a peritoneal lesion biopsy were performed. The pathology result of peritoneal lesion was signet ring cell carcinoma (SRCC), confirming the postoperative diagnosis of advanced gastric cancer (pT4bN2M0).

Afterwards, the patient was transferred to our institution for chemotherapy. After three cycles of EOX regimen (epirubicin, oxaliplatin, and capecitabine) [2], the disease was found to have progression. An abdominal CT scan at this time showed a broadly invasive gastric tumor, multiple enlarged lymph nodes, and secondary mesenteric lesions. Laboratory data indicated an increase in the level of tumor markers compared to pretreatment values, including CEA 12.47 ng/mL (from 3.91 ng/mL) and CA19-9 9.82 U/mL (from 5.99 U/mL).

We accordingly changed the chemotherapy regimen to FOLFIRI (5-fluorouracil, calcium folinate, and irinotecan) [2]. After two months (4 cycles), the tumor markers reduced below a normal range and CT scan also showed less-invasive lesions. Another CT scan done after six months (12 cycles) only showed a wall thickening of the gastric antrum (41 mm in length) with no surrounding fatty infiltration, no enlarged lymph nodes, and a well confined cyst posterior to the head of the pancreas (Figure 1). Endoscopic examination revealed no gross lesion of gastric mucosa. FOLFIRI chemotherapy has down-staged the patient from T4bN2M0 to ycT3N0M0. During chemotherapy treatment, the only significant toxicity was anemia which did not require blood transfusion and no grade 3-4 toxicities were recorded.

Then, we decided to perform a subtotal gastrectomy and a D2 lymphadenectomy on this patient. During surgery, the surgeons recorded a thickening of the antrum, without any enlarged lymph nodes or peritoneal metastases. The postoperative pathology result was gastric chronic inflammation, fibrosis, and intestinal metaplasia, with negative lymph nodes (7/7 nodes of stations 1, 3, 7, and 9 and 2/2 nodes of small intestinal mesentery) as well as negatively greater omentum lesions, giving a postop stage of ypT0N0M0. The patient was closely followed up afterwards. No adverse events were recorded during the follow-up, and a CT scan was performed 34 months after the second operation showed no recurrence.

3. Discussion

In this paper, we reported a patient with locally advanced gastric cancer, unresponsive to first-line chemotherapy (EOX regimen), then being treated with FOLFIRI regimen. Normally, patients who are switched to second-line regimen have poor prognosis, in which treatment is mostly palliative. However, in our case, the patient who was initially inoperable and subjected to palliative chemotherapy only became a candidate for curative resection after receiving 12 cycles of FOLFIRI. Postoperative microscopic examination demonstrated a pCR, and no recurrence has been detected 34 months after surgery.

The main purposes of neoadjuvant therapy are to downstage the tumor and increase the opportunity of curative resection. In some large-scaled clinical trials including MAGIC and REAL-2, EOX/ECF/ECX regimen has been shown to increase the rate of curative resection, improve overall survival (OS) and progression-free survival (PFS), and minimize local recurrence and distant metastases [3, 4]. With this evidence, EOX/ECF/ECX regimen had become the standard treatment at the time our patient was diagnosed. However, after three cycles of EOX, his imaging and laboratory tests indicated a disease progression. Although many second-line regimens have been evaluated, such as docetaxel-cisplatin and irinotecan-cisplatin, there has been still no consensus on which regimen is superior to others [2]. In 2014, a phase III clinical trial in France, comparing the efficacy of FOLRIFI and ECX regimen in patients with advanced gastric cancer, demonstrated no significant difference in response rate, OS, and PFS between the two regimens, but better tolerance in the FOLFIRI arm [7]. Especially, in cases that were unresponsive to first-line ECX, second-line FOLFIRI still achieved a response rate of 13.7% [7]. Until now, there have been some additional studies on chemotherapy options for advanced gastric cancer. A docetaxel-based regimen (FLOT) has been shown to have higher pathological response rate compared to EOX/ECF (16% vs. 6%), as well as better OS and PFS [9]. As a result, this regimen has been recommended to be the new standard treatment. However, its toxicity rate was considerably high, including 52% with grade 3-4 neutropenia and 12% with infection [9]. FOLFIRI regimen, meanwhile, is well-tolerated with a hematological toxicity rate of 38% [7]. Therefore, FOLFIRI could be an effective regimen for patients with poor performance status or those who are unresponsive to first-line treatment.

In this case, the patient with a SRCC, a pathological type commonly considered to have poor prognosis, achieved a pCR. pCR is an important factor in the prognosis of gastric cancer. Patients with pCR have a significantly lower relative risk (RR) of death from any cause (RR for one-year, three-year, and five-year mortalities of 0.5, 0.334, and 0.44, respectively) [10]. Many factors could be related to the pCR rate, including chemotherapy regimen, neutrophil-lymphocyte ratio, depth of tumor invasion, and histopathological type [9, 11]. Previous studies have shown that there might be a difference in molecular features, carcinogenesis, and chemosensitivity profile of SRCC compared to non-SRCC [12]. In two phase 3 clinical trials, adding irinotecan to chemotherapy regimen was associated with a longer survival time in patients with Lauren's diffuse type gastric cancer [13, 14]. Further studies are needed to clarify the reason behind this heterogeneity in the response to chemotherapy between different pathological types.

4. Conclusion

Selecting chemotherapy regimen depends on various factors, including patient's performance status and pathological type.

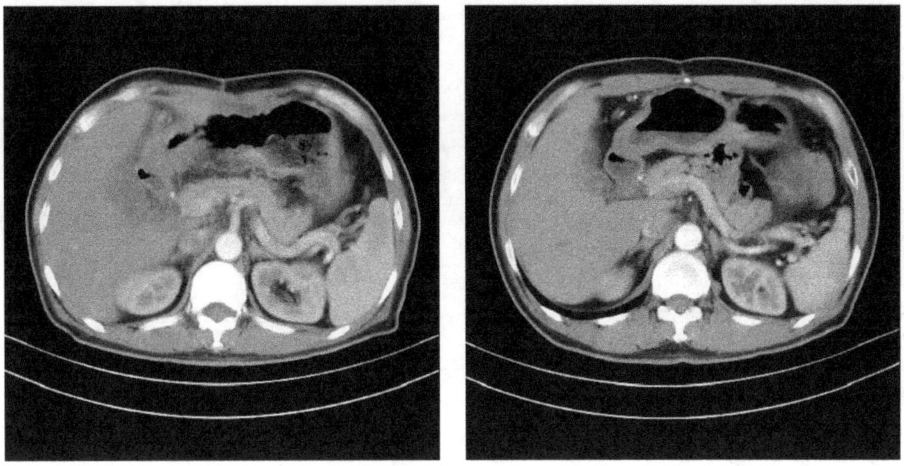

(a) (b)

FIGURE 1: CT scan images of the patient: (a) after 3 cycles of EOX regimen and (b) after 12 cycles of FOLFIRI regimen.

In cases with poor performance status, progression after first-line chemotherapy, or signet ring cell carcinoma, FOLFIRI might be a safe and effective option.

Additional Points

Highlights. In some cases, patients with advanced gastric cancer have good response to FOLFIRI regimen, even with pCR. pCR is an important prognostic factor, which is associated with a significantly longer survival time and decreased recurrence rate.

Ethical Approval

This study was approved by our research committee.

Consent

The publication of this study has been consented by the patient.

Disclosure

Hieu Van Nguyen and Vuong Thi Nguyen are coprimary authors.

Authors' Contributions

Vuong Thi Nguyen and Nga Quynh Pham are the medical oncologists who treated the patient. Hung Van Nguyen and Long Thanh Nguyen are the assistant doctors who wrote the manuscript. Hieu Van Nguyen is a professor and the main surgeon who revised the manuscript. Hau Xuan Nguyen and Hien Xuan Nguyen are the assistant surgeons, who also revised the manuscript. Hieu Van Nguyen, Prof., MD, Ph.D., is the guarantor. Hieu Van Nguyen and Vuong Thi Nguyen are equal contributors.

References

[1] F. Bray, J. Ferlay, I. Soerjomataram, R. L. Siegel, L. A. Torre, and A. Jemal, "Global cancer statistics 2018: GLOBOCAN estimates of incidence and mortality worldwide for 36 cancers in 185 countries," *CA: a Cancer Journal for Clinicians*, vol. 68, no. 6, pp. 394–424, 2018.

[2] J. A. Ajani, T. A. D'Amico, K. Almhanna et al., "Gastric cancer, version 3.2016, NCCN clinical practice guidelines in oncology," *Journal of the National Comprehensive Cancer Network*, vol. 14, no. 10, pp. 1286–1312, 2016.

[3] D. Cunningham, W. H. Allum, S. P. Stenning et al., "Perioperative chemotherapy versus surgery alone for resectable gastroesophageal cancer," *The New England Journal of Medicine*, vol. 355, no. 1, pp. 11–20, 2006.

[4] D. Cunningham, N. Starling, S. Rao et al., "Capecitabine and oxaliplatin for advanced esophagogastric cancer," *The New England Journal of Medicine*, vol. 358, no. 1, pp. 36–46, 2008.

[5] S.-E. Al-Batran, N. Homann, H. Schmalenberg et al., "Perioperative chemotherapy with docetaxel, oxaliplatin, and fluorouracil/leucovorin (FLOT) versus epirubicin, cisplatin, and fluorouracil or capecitabine (ECF/ECX) for resectable gastric or gastroesophageal junction (GEJ) adenocarcinoma (FLOT4-AIO): A multicenter, randomized phase 3 trial," *Journal of Clinical Oncology*, vol. 35, 15_supplement, pp. 4004–4004, 2017.

[6] R. Wesolowski, C. Lee, and R. Kim, "Is there a role for second-line chemotherapy in advanced gastric cancer?," *The Lancet Oncology*, vol. 10, no. 9, pp. 903–912, 2009.

[7] R. Guimbaud, C. Louvet, P. Ries et al., "Prospective, randomized, multicenter, phase III study of fluorouracil, leucovorin, and irinotecan versus epirubicin, cisplatin, and capecitabine in advanced gastric adenocarcinoma: a French intergroup (Fédération Francophone de Cancérologie Digestive, Fédération Nationale des Centres de Lutte Contre le Cancer, and Groupe Coopérateur Multidisciplinaire en Oncologie) study," *Journal of Clinical Oncology*, vol. 32, no. 31, pp. 3520–3526, 2014.

[8] M. Dank, J. Zaluski, C. Barone et al., "Randomized phase III study comparing irinotecan combined with 5-fluorouracil and folinic acid to cisplatin combined with 5-fluorouracil in chemotherapy naive patients with advanced adenocarcinoma of the stomach or esophagogastric junction," *Annals of Oncology*, vol. 19, no. 8, pp. 1450–1457, 2008.

[9] S.-E. Al-Batran, R. D. Hofheinz, C. Pauligk et al., "Histopatho-

logical regression after neoadjuvant docetaxel, oxaliplatin, fluorouracil, and leucovorin versus epirubicin, cisplatin, and fluorouracil or capecitabine in patients with resectable gastric or gastro-oesophageal junction adenocarcinoma (FLOT4-AIO): results from the phase 2 part of a multicentre, open-label, randomised phase 2/3 trial," *The Lancet Oncology*, vol. 17, no. 12, pp. 1697–1708, 2016.

[10] Z. Li, F. Shan, Y. Wang et al., "Correlation of pathological complete response with survival after neoadjuvant chemotherapy in gastric or gastroesophageal junction cancer treated with radical surgery: a meta-analysis," *PLoS One*, vol. 13, no. 1, p. e0189294, 2018.

[11] U. Ribeiro, M. F. K. P. Ramos, M. A. Pereira et al., "Predictors of pathological response and tumor regression following neoadjuvant therapy in advanced gastric cancer patients," *J Clin Oncol*, vol. 35, 4_supplement, p. 206, 2017.

[12] S. Pernot, T. Voron, G. Perkins, C. Lagorce-Pages, A. Berger, and J. Taieb, "Signet-ring cell carcinoma of the stomach: impact on prognosis and specific therapeutic challenge," *World Journal of Gastroenterology*, vol. 21, no. 40, pp. 11428–11438, 2015.

[13] N. Boku, S. Yamamoto, H. Fukuda et al., "Fluorouracil versus combination of irinotecan plus cisplatin versus S-1 in metastatic gastric cancer: a randomised phase 3 study," *The Lancet Oncology*, vol. 10, no. 11, pp. 1063–1069, 2009.

[14] H. Narahara, H. Iishi, H. Imamura et al., "Randomized phase III study comparing the efficacy and safety of irinotecan plus S-1 with S-1 alone as first-line treatment for advanced gastric cancer (study GC0301/TOP-002)," *Gastric Cancer*, vol. 14, no. 1, pp. 72–80, 2011.

4

Leiomyosarcoma of the Rectum as a Radiation-Induced Second Malignancy after Cervical Cancer Treatment: Case Report with Review of the Literature

Dmytro E. Makhmudov[1] **Olena O. Kolesnik,**[1] **Natalia N. Lagoda,**[2] **and Maryna O. Volk**[1]

[1]*Oncocoloproctology Department, National Cancer Institute, Lomonosova str. 33/43, Kyiv 03022, Ukraine*
[2]*Department of Pathomorphology, National Cancer Institute, Lomonosova str. 33/43, Kyiv 03022, Ukraine*

Correspondence should be addressed to Dmytro E. Makhmudov; dmahmudoff@gmail.com

Academic Editor: Peter F. Lenehan

Background. Incidence of cervical cancer among women of reproductive age still remains significantly high. In regard to prognostic features and risk factors, the standard treatment for most types of cervical cancer represents a combination of surgical treatment and radiation therapy, such as external beam radiation therapy and brachytherapy. Despite significant advances of long-term oncological outcomes, radiation-induced secondary malignancies among cervical cancer survivors are still an issue. Current case report describes an incredibly rare case of radiation-induced leiomyosarcoma of the rectum, which occurred 32 years after cervical cancer treatment. *Case Presentation.* A 62-year-old female had a past medical history of FIGO stage IIB cervical cancer (squamous cell carcinoma pT2bN0M0). In 1987, she underwent radical hysterectomy with bilateral iliac lymph node dissection, followed by adjuvant radiation therapy—70 Gy external beam pelvic irradiation followed by 30.5 Gy of brachytherapy. Thirty-two years later, she presented with signs of rectal bleeding. Regarding past medical history, radiologic, endoscopic, and pathologic data, the patient was initially diagnosed with a malignant nonepithelial lower rectal tumor of the unknown origin and staged as mrT3a mrN0 cM0. Total mesorectal excision with complete mesocolic excision and central vascular ligation (CME/CVL) carried by an open approach was carried out. In an attempt to identify the tissue of origin, an immunohistochemistry assay had been performed. Tumor cells showed a high rate of mitotic activity with a 45% rate of Ki-67 expression, positive reaction for desmin, and SMA in all samples. Negative reaction for CD117 and S100 was observed. As a conclusion, the immunophenotype was identified as a grade 3 leiomyosarcoma (ISD-code 8890/3). *Conclusions.* We suggest that up to date, radical surgery with curative intent, as it was performed in our study, is the most evidence-based treatment option for patients with radiation-induced sarcomas of the rectum.

1. Background

Primary colorectal sarcomas are an extremely rare group of malignant mesenchymal tumors. They represent up to 0.1% of all primary diagnosed colorectal malignancies [1]. Leiomyosarcomas appear to be the most common histological subtype of primary colorectal sarcomas with incidence up to 90%. More rare of their subtypes are liposarcomas, fibrous histiocytomas, and desmoplastic small cell tumors [2]. Regarding the small number of documented cases and their scattered features, prognostic factors and optimal treatment strategy for primary colorectal sarcomas remain indeterminate. However, pooled data from a majority of recently published case series suggest that primary colorectal sarcomas are characterized by both rapid progression and very poor oncological outcomes with a median of survival ranging from 30 to 53 months and a local recurrence rate of up to 85% [3–6]. Overall five-year survival rate of patients with primary colorectal sarcomas is significantly lower comparing to those with colorectal cancer—43%

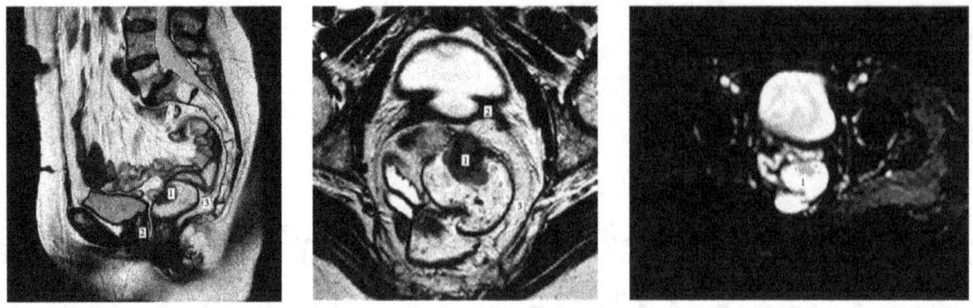

(a) (b) (c)

Figure 1: Radiologic data from a high-resolution pelvic MRI. Tumor of the lower rectum (1) situated on the anterior wall was observed on sagittal (a) and axial T2-weighted scans (b) with signs of mesorectal invasion (blue arrowheads) ranging up to 3 mm and no radiologic features of lymph node metastases (3). Vaginal stump and rectovaginal sept (2) had a significantly low intensity MR signal due to their fibrotic transformation. On a series of diffusion-weighted images (c), a significant delay of diffusion together with intense signaling on high b-factors was observed at the level of a tumor (blue arrowheads).

and 52%, respectively [7]. Tumor grade of primary colorectal sarcomas is the most important prognostic factor for overall five-year survival—38% for high grade and 61% for low grade [8]. Besides, inappropriate staging algorithm and wide use of local excision as a surgical option for primary treatment results in high rates of R1 and R2 resections with a local recurrence rate of 12.7%. Nevertheless, a number of authors suggest that curative surgery should be the main treatment option because data regarding chemotherapy and radiation therapy is either lacking or it is controversial [9, 10]. Colorectal sarcomas as a radiation-induced second malignancy after cervical cancer treatment, on contrary to primary ones, are an exceptionally rare entity. Up to date, only five cases had been described in the literature [11–15]. In our current paper, we provide data on the sixth case of similar malignancy.

2. Case Presentation

A 62-year-old female had a past medical history of FIGO stage IIB cervical cancer (squamous cell carcinoma pT2bN0M0). In 1987, she underwent radical hysterectomy with bilateral iliac lymph node dissection, followed by adjuvant radiation therapy—70 Gy external beam pelvic irradiation followed by 30.5 Gy of brachytherapy. Thirty-two years later, she presented with signs of rectal bleeding.

Digital rectal examination revealed a solid exophytic tumor on 5 cm above the anal verge. During rigid proctosigmoidoscopy, a 3 cm anterior wall rectal tumor with irregular margins and swollen mucosa was observed. Additional flexible colonoscopy showed no signs of synchronous colorectal neoplasms. Snare biopsy result showed an undifferentiated malignant nonepithelial tumor of unidentified histological origin. An attempt of immunohistochemistry assay was undertaken unsuccessfully due to an insufficient amount of tissue.

Consecutively, a pelvic MRI with a 1.5 Tl Philips Intera machine had been performed for local staging. MERCURY protocol for high resolution imaging was applied.

On a series of sagittal and axial MR scans, a lower rectal tumor was observed on 4 cm above the anorectal junction with maximal extent of 30 mm in the greatest dimension. Mesorectal infiltration with maximal depth of 3 mm (mrT_{3b}) was also identified. No radiological signs of either mesorectal fascia involvement or extramural vascular invasion ($mrCRM^-$ and $mrEMVI^-$) had been observed (see Figures 1(a) and 1(b)). Visible mesorectal lymph nodes had homogenous MR signal, smooth external margins, and a regular size, thus showing no radiologic signs of lymph node involvement (mrN_0). It was noticeable that the stump of the vagina and rectovaginal sept had prominent signs of fibrosis regarding a highly intensive MR signal on T2-weighted images. Malignant tumor features were also observed on a series of diffusion-weighted images (see Figure 1(c)).

A CT scan with intravenous enhancement showed no signs of neither distant metastases neither thoracic or intra-abdominal lymphadenopathy. Upper GI endoscopy and laboratory data of standard blood, serum, and urine counts revealed no signs of pathology.

3. Surgical Treatment

Regarding past medical history, radiologic, endoscopic, and pathologic data, the patient was initially diagnosed with a malignant nonepithelial lower rectal tumor of the unknown origin and staged as mrT3a mrN0 cM0. Being aware of primary colorectal sarcomas, their recurrence and progression patterns and a threatening rate of R1 and R2 resections, an institutional multidisciplinary board suggested curative surgery as a primary treatment option. Total mesorectal excision (TME) with complete mesocolic excision and central vascular ligation (CME/CVL) carried by an open approach was selected as proper extent of surgery. Standardized surgical technique in this case included complete left flexure mobilization, ligation of the inferior mesenteric artery at its origin near the aorta and inferior mesenteric vein just below the pancreatic tail with consecutive total mesorectal excision up to the level of the pelvic diaphragm (see Figure 2). Accurate TME procedure had been exacerbated by severe fibrotic changes of surrounding pelvic tissues due to postoperative changes after iliac lymphadenectomy for cervical cancer and radiation-induced fibrosis as well. Regarding the significant fibrotic transformation of the anterior rectal wall with adjacent tissues, an intraoperative decision was made to avoid reconstruction aware of an estimated high risk of

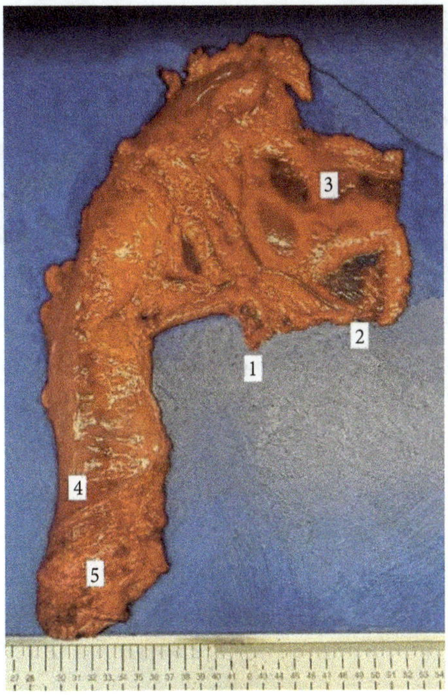

FIGURE 2: Resected gross specimen. 1: stump of the inferior mesenteric artery, 2: stump of the inferior mesenteric vein, 3: preserved peritoneal window, 4: level of the peritoneal reflection, and 5: mesorectum.

anastomotic leakage. Closure of the pelvic peritoneum was avoided as well.

On postoperative day 5, the patient developed such clinical signs as nausea, vomiting, and loss of flatus and stool. Computed tomography of the chest, abdomen, and pelvis revealed multiple "levels" of gas and liquid throughout the small intestine with a breakdown of peroral contrast at the level of distal ileal loop, which was situated at the cavity of minor pelvis, adherent to the stumps of both the rectum and the vagina (see Figure 3). At that level, a noticeable deformation of the intestinal loop with difference of luminal diameters was observed. On contrary, the lumen of a large intestine was collapsed.

By taking in regard both clinical and radiologic findings, the patient was diagnosed with postoperative ileus and an immediate reoperation had been carried out. During abdominal examination, dilated intestinal loops with block of passage at the level of the pelvic diaphragm were identified (see Figure 4). An adherent bowel wall was fixed between vaginal and rectal stumps as it was previously described on a series of CT scans. By the end of abdominal and pelvic exploration, no additional pathological findings were observed. After detachment of adhesions, the strangulated bowel was delivered back in the abdominal cavity. Closure of the pelvis was performed with mobilized body of the urinary bladder and remnant flaps of pelvic peritoneum. Postoperative period was uneventful within 30 days. The patient was safely discharged on postoperative day 14 after initial surgery. At one year of follow-up, the patient is alive and has no radiological signs of neither local nor distant recurrence.

4. Pathologic Findings

Macroscopically, the tumor was represented an exophytic homogenous lesion 45 × 25 mm with irregular margins and ulcerated surface covered with clots of fibrin. The tumor originated from the muscular layer of the rectum with concomitant mucosal invasion. Twelve regional lymph nodes were additionally examined. Initial histological appearance revealed a mixture of chaotic cellular and fibrotic vegetations. Among them, a subgroup of heterogeneous polykaryocytes with significant nuclear polymorphism (so called "monster cells") was identified (see Figure 5). Those and other morphological features corresponded to a malignant low-grade mesenchymal tumor. All examined lymph nodes had no signs of metastases.

In an attempt to identify the tissue of origin for a current tumor, an immunohistochemistry assay had been carried out. A panel of Ki-67, CD117, S100, smooth muscle actin (SMA), and desmin was used to conduct a differential diagnosis between leiomyosarcoma and gastrointestinal stromal tumor. Tumor cells showed a high rate of mitotic activity with a 45% rate of Ki-67 expression (see Figure 6). There was a positive reaction for desmin and SMA in all samples (see Figures 7 and 8). On contrary, all samples had negative reaction for CD117 and S100 (see Figures 9 and 10). As a conclusion, the observed immunophenotype was identified as a grade 3 leiomyosarcoma (ISD-code 8890/3).

5. Discussion

In the current paper, we present the sixth case of radiation-induced leiomyosarcoma of the rectum which developed 32 years after completion of cervical cancer treatment. Throughout the last decades, significant success was achieved in the treatment of patients with pelvic malignancies, especially those who require either adjuvant or neoadjuvant radiation therapy. As a consequence of overall survival improvement, the problem of metachronous secondary malignancies among those patients who were exposed to radiation had arisen. According to the data of the National Cancer Institute of USA, over 40% of all patients diagnosed with primary malignancy will have to undergo radiation therapy [16]. Most of primary malignancies which require radiation therapy as a treatment standard are breast, prostate, cervical, rectal, and urinary bladder cancer. Among long-term cancer survivors exposed to radiation, 16% are at risk of developing a secondary malignancy. Recent data from a SEER database suggests that 6–9.9% of all patients who underwent radiation therapy for prostate cancer are at a 34% risk of developing secondary lung, rectal, or urinary bladder cancer. Majority of those patients develop secondary malignancies mostly after 10 years from treatment discontinuation [17, 18].

Cervical cancer remains one of the leading cause of cancer-related morbidity and mortality among females [19]. It is known that only surgical treatment can be appropriate only in a relatively small subgroup of patients, particularly among those who were initially diagnosed with FIGO stage IA1 (T1a1 by TNM) or less, i.e., with a depth of stromal

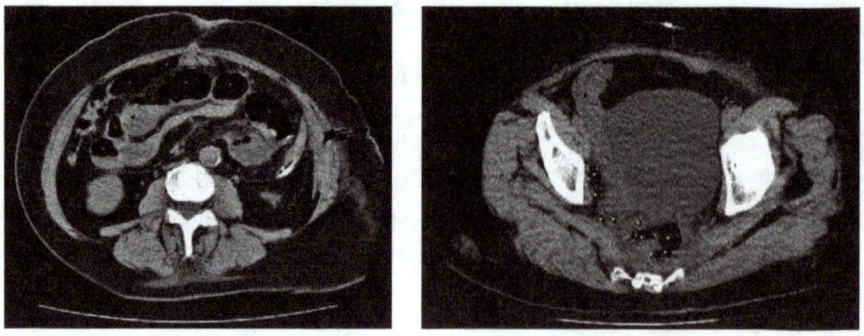

(a) (b)

Figure 3: Patient's CT scans on the 6th postoperative day. Multiple intestinal "levels" of gas and fluid throughout the abdominal cavity were observed ((a), red arrowheads). Part of the distal intestinal loop with difference in lumen diameters was situated at the level of the pelvic floor ((b), yellow arrowheads) and was adherent to both rectal and vaginal stumps.

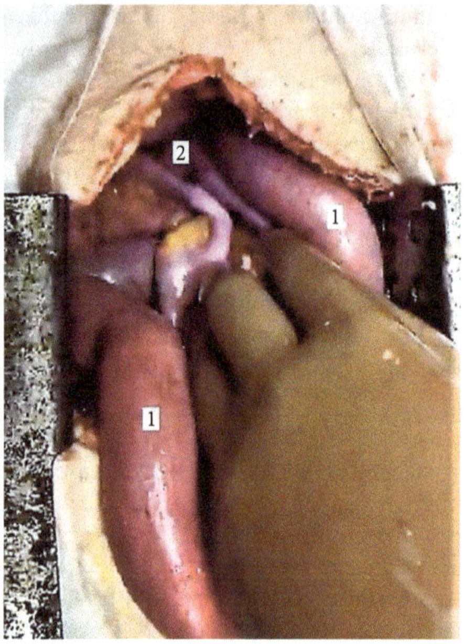

Figure 4: Intraoperative photo during reoperation. Dilated intestinal loops up to the level of distal ileum (1) are observed. The loop of a strangulated bowel (2) was adherent to the stump of the rectum and vagina deep inside the pelvic cavity.

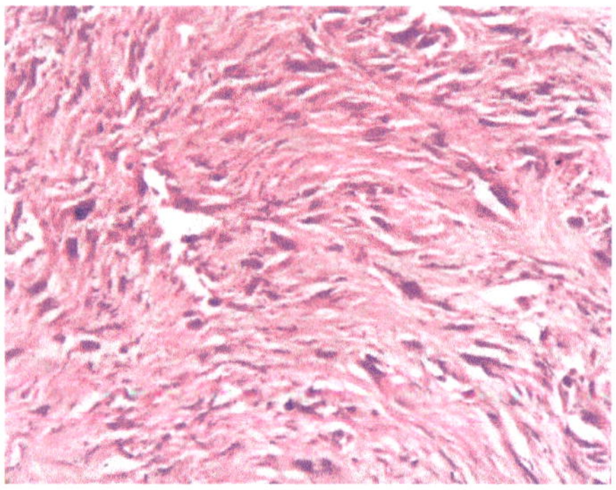

Figure 5: Poorly differentiated malignant mesenchymal tumor. Multiple sites of cellular and nuclear polymorphism are observed. Hematoxylin-eosin staining, ×100.

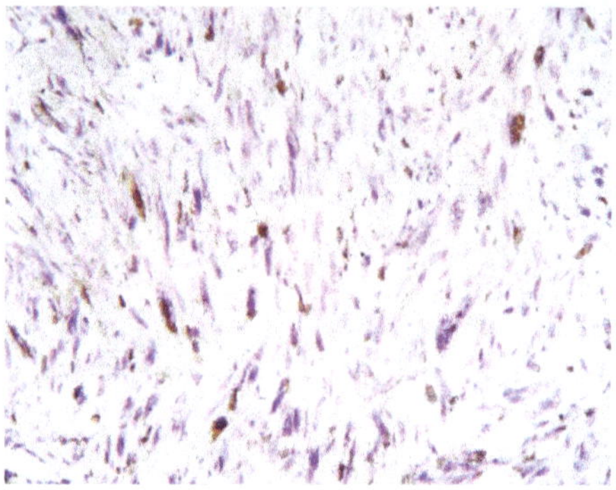

Figure 6: Poorly differentiated malignant mesenchymal tumor. Immunohistochemistry assay with Ki-67 antibodies.

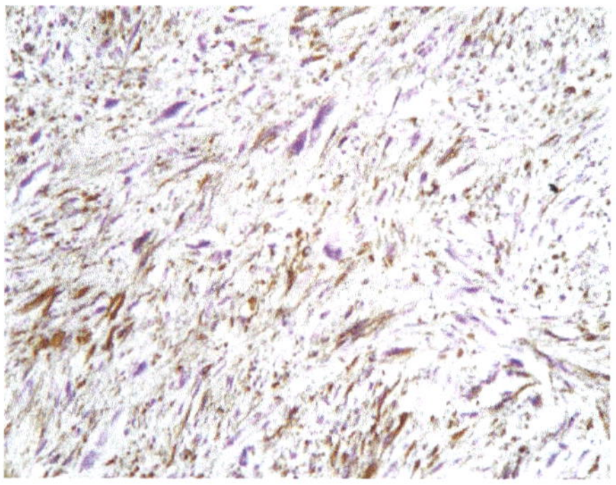

Figure 7: Poorly differentiated malignant mesenchymal tumor. Immunohistochemistry assay with desmin antibodies. Positive reaction in tumor cells observed.

invasion up to 3 mm and lateral spread up to 7 mm [20]. Recent NCCN guidelines suggest adjuvant radiation therapy for FIGO stage IA1 patients with a number of adverse risk features found at pathological examination, such as positive lymph nodes, parametrium invasion, or positive resection margins [21]. A standard approach for cervical cancer radiation therapy includes combination of external beam radiation therapy and brachytherapy. Overall radiation dosage depends on the range of primary tumor spread—in cases of tumors below 40 mm in maximum dimension, the overall dosage consists of 80 Gy and ≥85 Gy if above 40 mm.

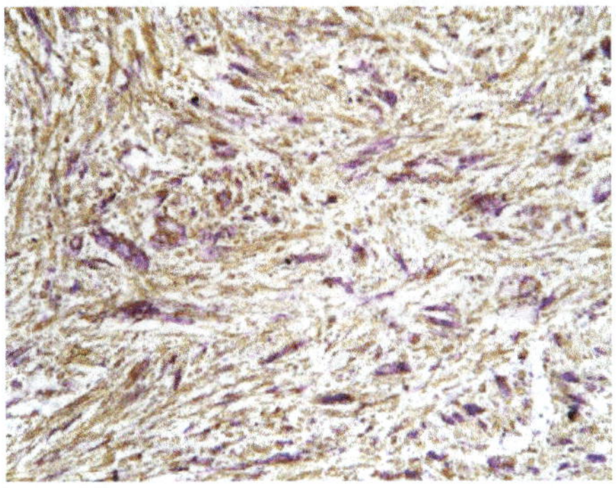

Figure 8: Poorly differentiated malignant mesenchymal tumor. Immunohistochemistry assay with SMA antibodies. Positive reaction in tumor cells observed.

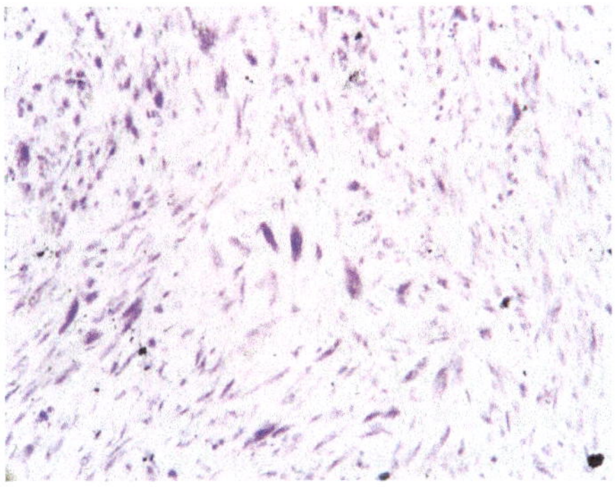

Figure 9: Poorly differentiated malignant mesenchymal tumor. Immunohistochemistry assay with CD117 antibodies. Negative reaction in tumor cells observed.

In cases of cervical cancer, the radiation field includes parametrium, sacrouterine ligaments, 3 cm of upper third of the vagina below the tumor, and presacral, obturator, external, and internal iliac lymph nodes. By taking in regard all the anatomical relations of the cervix, it becomes clear that the most critical radiation sites are represented by the vagina, the rectum, and the urinary bladder. In comparison, bony pelvis structures receive significantly lesser radiation dosages.

A successful combination of curative surgery and highly precise modalities of radiation therapy in either adjuvant or neoadjuvant regimens had given a unique opportunity to improve cervical cancer patient's overall and disease-free survival rates like never before. Hence, by dropping out of a cancer recurrence group, those patients consequently enter another one—a risk group of developing a secondary malignancy. The first population-based study which highlighted a relevance between previous exposure to pelvic irradiation and a risk of developing a second malignancy was presented by Boice et al., in 1984 [22]. The study included more than 95,000 patients after pelvic radiation therapy for cervical cancer within a 30-year study period. This population was compared with more than 99,000 patients who underwent only curative surgery. Throughout the study period, 3324 (3.5%) secondary radiation-induced malignancies had been observed, of which 1622 (1.7%) were located at the organs covered by the irradiation field. The main risk factor of

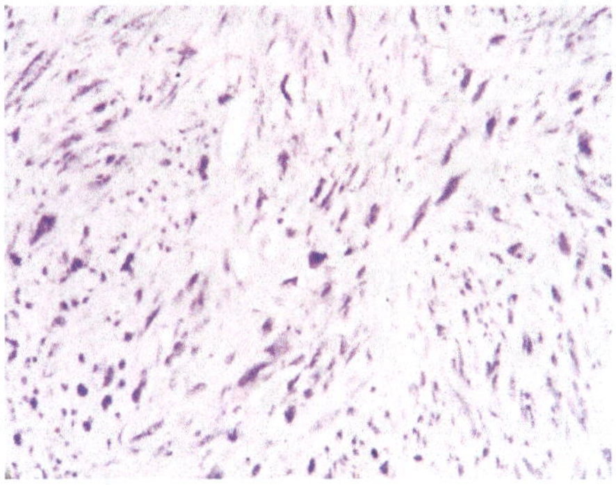

Figure 10: Poorly differentiated malignant mesenchymal tumor. Immunohistochemistry assay with S100 antibodies. Negative reaction in tumor cells observed.

secondary malignancy development was the age under 30 years at primary diagnosis of cervical cancer. Urinary bladder (4.5), vagina (2.7), stomach (2.1), and hematopoietic tissue (2.5) had the highest relative risk for secondary malignancy. It was noticeable that the rectum had the lowest relative risk among other pelvic organs (1.8). Other data from a study of Samerdokiene et al. suggest that secondary radiation-induced malignancies occur in 5.3% of cervical patients after a combination of external beam and brachytherapy. Among them, rectal malignancies consisted only 8.6% [23]. A population study of 37,757 patients based on a data from SEER database demonstrated a 2.6-fold increase in a number of secondary malignancies among those cervical cancer patients who underwent pelvic radiation therapy comparing to surgery alone [24]. Nevertheless, the authors acknowledged that metachronous bronchopulmonary, esophageal, and oropharyngeal cancer were mostly caused by continuous smoking and vaginal, vulval, and anal canal cancer—by HPV infection rather than by previous radiation exposure. Similar retrospective population-based data concerning a consistent pattern of an increased secondary malignancy rate among cervical cancer survivors was obtained from the Netherlands and Taiwan [25, 26]. Even though all secondary colon, rectal, and anal malignancies in those studies were united in one subgroup, their relative risk ratio still remained one of the lowest. A study by Ohno et al., based on a pooled data from 2167 patients after a combination of external beam and brachytherapy for cervical cancer, reports a 9.7% rate of secondary radiation-induced malignancies with 19% of them related to adjacent irradiated organs [27]. Soft tissue and bone sarcomas (22.0), leukemias (3.1), and urinary bladder cancer (2.2) had the greatest relative risk rates. On the other hand, rectal cancer, hepatocellular carcinoma, and gastric cancer (1.0, 1.2 and, respectively) possessed the lowest relative risk rates. Lim et al. came up with a data of 72,805 invasive cervical cancer patients after pelvic irradiation within a study period of 7.34 years [28]. A 3.68% rate (2678 cases) of secondary radiation-induced malignancies with similar relative risk patterns—vagina (9.36), soft tissues and bones (2.7), vulva (2.58), and anus and anal canal (2.42)—was observed. It is noticeable that among the 35 sites of secondary malignancy occurrence, rectal cancer had the lowest relative risk of 0.74. Correlation between previously treated cervical

Table 1: Pooled data of all identified case reports of radiation-induced leiomyosarcoma of the rectum after pelvic radiation therapy for cervical cancer.

Authors	Year of publication	Patient's age at diagnosis	Overall irradiation dosage (Gy)	Radiation modality	Time to diagnosis of a secondary malignancy (years)	Selected treatment strategy
Drumea et al. [11]	1993	62	70	40 Gy EBRT[1]+30 Gy BT[2]	17	Intra-abdominal resection of the rectum
Caporale et al. [12]	2003	N/A	N/A	N/A	N/A	N/A
Basu et al. [13]	2012	79	N/A	N/A	26	Intra-abdominal resection of the rectum
Garcia-Ortega et al. [14]	2018	58	85	50 Gy EBRT+35 Gy BT	8	Sigmostomy+ chemotherapy+pelvic exenteration+vulvectomy
Jayakumar et al. [15]	2015	58	N/A	N/A	15	Local excision
Current case report	2019	62	100.5	70 Gy EBRT+ 30.5 Gy BT	32	TME+CME/CVL

[1]EBRT: external beam radiation therapy. [2]BT: brachytherapy.

cancer secondary colorectal cancer had been recently highlighted in a paper of Rodriguez et al. [29]. After 35 years of follow-up, an estimated risk of colon cancer was 2.5% in a surgery alone group and 6.5% in a radiation therapy group. For rectal cancer, the difference was more significant—0.8% and 3.7%, respectively. Regression analysis survival model demonstrated a significant increase of relative risk for colon cancer development after 8 years and rectal cancer—after 15 years of follow-up. The authors suggest that 8 years should be a cutoff edge for colorectal cancer screening among cervical cancer survivors.

First studies about the influence of ionizing radiation on the development of malignancies were provided after a nuclear attack in Japan at 1945. Three main issues had been discovered then: tissues with higher proliferative index (i.e., epithelial and hematopoietic) are mostly affected; very small number of radiation-induced sarcomas and a ratio of 8%/1 Gray, which is a distribution of those who shall develop a malignancy among one hundred people exposed to an irradiation dosage of 1 Gy [30]. Mechanisms and conditions for radiation sarcoma development were firstly described by Cahan et al. in 1948 [31]. It was noticed that the occurrence of pathologically confirmed secondary sarcomas is related to an irradiation field previously exposed to a dosage of at least 50 Gy. However, the only uncertainty was timing of occurrence which could range from months to decades. Despite meeting all of Cahan's criteria, radiation-induced sarcomas in cervical cancer patients after pelvic radiation therapy are a very rare entity. Among all primary diagnosed soft tissue sarcomas, a range of 0.03% to 5.5% could be considered as radiation induced [32, 33].

According to the largest published series of Cha et al., only 125 (2.5%) out of 4884 primary soft tissue sarcomas satisfied Cahan's criteria and were considered as radiation induced [32]. Vast majority of those patients previously underwent radiation therapy for breast cancer (29%), lymphomas (16%), and prostate cancer (14%) with thoracic cavity, thoracic wall, extremities, head and neck as a tumor site. Pathological features of leiomyosarcomas were identified only in 12% of radiation-induced sarcomas. However, there was absolutely no data regarding a radiation-induced leiomyosarcoma after previous pelvic radiation therapy with intra-abdominal or either intrapelvic localization.

Remarkably, but up to date, there were only 5 published case reports of a radiation-induced leiomyosarcoma of the rectum in a patient after previous radiation therapy for cervical cancer (see Table 1). On the contrary, one of the largest recent studies by Thiels et al. evaluates a series of 433 primary colorectal sarcomas discovered within a 14-year observation period [8]. Among the 29.3% of patients with the rectum as a primary tumor site, only 57.5% had leiomyosarcomas.

Although radiation-induced leiomyosarcomas of the rectum appear to be an extremely rare type of secondary malignancies, there is an emerging data suggesting an intrinsically different sequence of molecular events responsible for their development and occurrence comparing to primary sarcomas [14]. Gonin-Laurent et al. recognize a mutation of TP53 and RB1 genes as a key molecular event in the development of radiation-induced sarcomas. Consecutive mutation of a TP53 gene was identified in 58% of radiation-induced sarcomas and was related to deletion of other oncogenes in 52% [34, 35]. It was also mentioned that mutation of a TP53 gene led to inactivation of RB1, which showed no signs of genetic alterations [35]. Hyperexpression of p53 is recognized as a specific pathogenic route for radiation-induced sarcoma development as well. Taubert et al. identified a p53 mutation in 9 out of 11 radiation-induced sarcoma cases [36]. Finally, a study of Nakanishi et al. revealed a p53 mutation pattern in a series of 14 secondary radiation-induced soft tissue sarcomas in patients who previously underwent pelvic radiation therapy for cervical cancer [37]. Real-time polymerase chain reaction detected polymorphism of p53 gene with an 88% rate of mutations in exons 5, 7, 8, 12, and 18. However, concomitant changes in the primary structure of a p53 protein were observed only in 31%. The authors conclude that such a biological mislead might be a reason for a long latency period between radiation exposure and clinical manifestation of secondary soft tissue sarcomas.

6. Conclusions

Among all radiation-induced malignancies affecting long-term cervical cancer survivors, soft tissue sarcomas occur quite frequently. However, radiation-induced leiomyosarcoma of the rectum represents a remarkably rare case. Although primary colorectal sarcomas represent a very small subgroup of malignant mesenchymal tumors, the data regarding its proper treatment is lacking. On contrary to primary ones, radiation-induced sarcomas possess a number of unique molecular features which make them biologically different. We suggest that up to date, radical surgery with curative intent, as it was performed in our study, is the most evidence-based treatment option for patients with radiation-induced sarcomas of the rectum. Fibrotic changes in the pelvis as a consequence of previous external beam and brachytherapy may significantly jeopardise the completion of a TME procedure. That is why a two-step surgical strategy with delayed reconstruction should be taken in regard.

Consent

Before the publication of the present clinical case, the patient filled out a written informed consent approving the use of her personal data in scientific purposes.

References

[1] M. Cuffy, F. Abir, and W. E. Longo, "Management of less common tumors of the colon, rectum, and anus," *Clinical Colorectal Cancer*, vol. 5, no. 5, pp. 327–337, 2006.

[2] S. Meijer, T. Peretz, J. J. Gaynor, C. Tan, S. I. Hajdu, and M. F. Brennan, "Primary colorectal sarcoma. A retrospective review and prognostic factor study of 50 consecutive patients," *Archives of Surgery*, vol. 125, no. 9, pp. 1163–1168, 1990.

[3] K. C. Conlon, E. S. Casper, and M. F. Brennan, "Primary gastrointestinal sarcomas: analysis of prognostic variables," *Annals of Surgical Oncology*, vol. 2, no. 1, pp. 26–31, 1995.

[4] C. L. Chou, S. C. Chang, T. C. Lin et al., "Clinical analysis and surgical results of primary colorectal sarcoma," *The Journal of Society of Colon and Rectal Surgeons (Taiwan)*, vol. 21, pp. 161–168, 2010.

[5] P. Luna-Pérez, D. F. Rodríguez, L. Luján et al., "Colorectal sarcoma: analysis of failure patterns," *Journal of Surgical Oncology*, vol. 69, no. 1, pp. 36–40, 1998.

[6] J. Yang, "Primary leiomyosarcoma in the colon: A case report," *Medicine (Baltimore)*, vol. 97, no. 7, 2018.

[7] C. R. Cooper, B. F. Scully, and S. Lee-Kong, "Colorectal sarcoma: more than a gastrointestinal stromal tumor," *Translational Gastroenterology and Hepatology*, vol. 3, pp. 42–42, 2018.

[8] C. A. Thiels, J. R. Bergquist, A. C. Krajewski et al., "Outcomes of primary colorectal sarcoma: a National Cancer Data Base (NCDB) review," *Journal of Gastrointestinal Surgery*, vol. 21, no. 3, pp. 560–568, 2017.

[9] C. D. Randleman, B. G. Wolff, R. R. Dozois, R. J. Spencer, L. H. Weiland, and D. M. Ilstrup, "Leiomyosarcoma of the rectum and anus," *International Journal of Colorectal Disease*, vol. 4, no. 2, pp. 91–96, 1989.

[10] B. D. Minsky, A. M. Cohen, S. I. Hajdu, and D. Nori, "Sphincter preservation in rectal sarcoma," *Diseases of the Colon and Rectum*, vol. 33, no. 4, pp. 319–322, 1990.

[11] K. Drumea, E. Sabo, E. Zuckerman, and J. E. Naschitz, "Leiomyosarcoma of the colon in the aftermath of pelvic irradiation for endometrial carcinoma," *The American Journal of Gastroenterology*, vol. 88, article 1302, 1993.

[12] A. Caporale, F. Angelico, M. U. Cosenza et al., "A late complication of pelvic radiotherapy: leiomyosarcoma of the rectum. Report of a case and review of the literature," *Hepatogastroenterology*, vol. 50, no. 54, pp. 1933–1936, 2003.

[13] I. Basu and P. Lemonas, "Leiomyosarcoma of the rectum following pelvic irradiation: a difficult histological diagnosis," *Annals of the Royal College of Surgeons of England*, vol. 94, no. 1, pp. e44–e45, 2012.

[14] D. Y. Garcia-Ortega, N. Reyes-Garcia, H. Martinez-Said, C. H. S. Caro-Sanchez, and M. Cuellar-Hubbe, "Radiation-induced leiomyosarcoma of the rectum after cervical cancer treatment," *Revista de Gastroenterología de México*, vol. 83, no. 4, pp. 465–467, 2018.

[15] R. Jayakumar, P. P. Basu, T. Huang, and C. A. Axiotis, "Post-irradiation leiomyosarcoma of rectum presenting as a polyp: case report and review of the literature," *International Journal of Surgical Pathology*, vol. 24, no. 2, pp. 163–169, 2015.

[16] L. B. Travis, C. S. Rabkin, L. M. Brown et al., "Cancer survivorship—genetic susceptibility and second primary cancers: research strategies and recommendations," *JNCI: Journal of the National Cancer Institute*, vol. 98, no. 1, pp. 15–25, 2006.

[17] D. J. Brenner, R. E. Curtis, E. J. Hall, and E. Ron, "Second malignancies in prostate carcinoma patients after radiotherapy compared with surgery," *Cancer*, vol. 88, no. 2, pp. 398–406, 2000.

[18] K. Moon, G. J. Stukenborg, J. Keim, and D. Theodorescu, "Cancer incidence after localized therapy for prostate cancer," *Cancer*, vol. 107, no. 5, pp. 991–998, 2006.

[19] L. A. Torre, F. Bray, R. L. Siegel, J. Ferlay, J. Lortet-Tieulent, and A. Jemal, "Global cancer statistics, 2012," *CA: a Cancer Journal for Clinicians*, vol. 65, no. 2, pp. 87–108, 2015.

[20] C. Marth, F. Landoni, S. Mahner et al., "Cervical cancer: ESMO clinical practice guidelines for diagnosis, treatment and follow-up," *Annals of Oncology*, vol. 28, supplement 4, pp. iv72–iv83, 2017.

[21] National Comprehensive Cancer Network, "Cervical cancer," 2019, https://www.nccn.org/professionals/physician_gls/pdf/cervical.pdf.

[22] J. D. Boice Jr., N. E. Day, A. Andersen et al., "Second cancers following radiation treatment for cervical cancer: an international collaboration among cancer registries," *JNCI: Journal of the National Cancer Institute*, vol. 74, no. 5, pp. 955–975, 1985.

[23] V. Samerdokiene, K. P. Valuckas, E. Janulionis, V. Atkocius, and M. J. Rivard, "Second primary malignancies after radiotherapy including HDR ^{252}Cf brachytherapy for cervical cancer," *Brachytherapy*, vol. 14, no. 6, pp. 898–904, 2015.

[24] R. E. Curtis, D. Michal Freedman, E. Ron et al., "New malignancies among cancer survivors: SEER cancer registries, 1973–2000," *National Cancer Institute*, 2006.

[25] M. Arnold, L. Liu, G. G. Kenter, C. L. Creutzberg, J. W. Coebergh, and I. Soerjomataram, "Second primary cancers in survivors of cervical cancer in the Netherlands: implications for

prevention and surveillance," *Radiotherapy and Oncology*, vol. 111, no. 3, pp. 374–381, 2014.

[26] C. J. Teng, L. K. Huon, Y. W. Hu et al., "Secondary primary malignancy risk in patients with cervical cancer in Taiwan: a nationwide population-based study," *Medicine*, vol. 94, p. 43, 2015.

[27] T. Ohno, S. Kato, S. Sato et al., "Long-term survival and risk of second cancers after radiotherapy for cervical cancer," *International Journal of Radiation Oncology·Biology·Physics*, vol. 69, no. 3, pp. 740–745, 2007.

[28] M. C. Lim, Y. J. Won, J. Lim et al., "Second primary cancer after diagnosis and treatment of cervical cancer," *Cancer Research and Treatment*, vol. 48, no. 2, pp. 641–649, 2016.

[29] A. M. Rodriguez, Y.-F. Kuo, and J. S. Goodwin, "Risk of colorectal cancer among long-term cervical cancer survivors," *Medical Oncology*, vol. 31, no. 5, p. 943, 2014.

[30] E. J. Hall and C. S. Wuu, "Radiation-induced second cancers: the impact of 3D-CRT and IMRT," *International Journal of Radiation Oncology, Biology, Physics*, vol. 56, no. 1, pp. 83–88, 2003.

[31] W. Cahan, H. Woodward, N. Higinbotham, F. W. Stewart, and B. L. Coley, "Sarcoma in irradiated bone. report of eleven cases," *Cancer*, vol. 1, no. 1, pp. 3–29, 1948.

[32] C. Cha, C. R. Antonescu, M. L. Quan, S. Maru, and M. F. Brennan, "Long-term results with resection of radiation-induced soft tissue sarcomas," *Annals of Surgery*, vol. 239, no. 6, pp. 903–910, 2004.

[33] A. Italiano, S. Bringer, J. Y. Blay et al., "Patterns of care and outcome radiation-induced soft tissue sarcomas," *International Journal of Radiation Oncology·Biology·Physics*, vol. 103, no. 2, pp. 449–452, 2019.

[34] N. Gonin-Laurent, N. S. Hadj-Hamou, N. Vogt et al., "RB1 and TP53 pathways in radiation-induced sarcomas," *Oncogene*, vol. 26, no. 41, pp. 6106–6112, 2007.

[35] N. Gonin-Laurent, A. Gibaud, M. Huygue et al., "Specific TP53 mutation pattern in radiation-induced sarcomas," *Carcinogenesis*, vol. 27, no. 6, pp. 1266–1272, 2006.

[36] H. Taubert, A. Meye, M. Bache et al., "p 53 status in radiation-induced soft-tissue sarcomas," *Strahlentherapie und Onkologie*, vol. 174, no. 8, pp. 427–430, 1998.

[37] H. Nakanishi, Y. Tomita, A. Myoui et al., "Mutation of the p 53 gene in postradiation sarcoma," *Laboratory Investigation*, vol. 78, no. 6, pp. 727–733, 1998.

5

A Histologically Complete Response to Immunotherapy using Pembrolizumab in a Patient with Giant Cell Carcinoma of the Lung: An Additional Report and Literature Review

Tomoo Kakimoto,[1] Mamoru Sasaki,[1] Tatsuya Yamamoto,[2] Arifumi Iwamaru,[2] Kentaro Ogata,[3] Ko Lee,[1] Shingo Nakayama,[1] and Naoto Minematsu[1]

[1]*Department of Internal Medicine Hino Municipal Hospital, Hino-shi, Tokyo, Japan*
[2]*Department of Surgery, Federation of National Public Service Personnel Mutual Aid Associations, Tachikawa Hospital, Tachikawa-shi, Tokyo, Japan*
[3]*Department of Pathology, Federation of National Public Service Personnel Mutual Aid Associations, Tachikawa Hospital, Tachikawa-shi, Tokyo, Japan*

Correspondence should be addressed to Naoto Minematsu; n.minematsu@hinohosp.jp

Academic Editor: Katsuhiro Tanaka

We previously reported a case of giant cell carcinoma in the lung, in which the use of antiprogrammed death 1 (PD-1) immunotherapy resulted in substantial tumor reduction. In the present study, we describe an additional clinical course. A 69-year-old woman was diagnosed with giant cell carcinoma of the lung in clinical stage IVB (T2bN0M1c, BRA). The tumor expressed programmed death ligand 1 (PD-L1) in a high proportion. The patient received stereotactic radiotherapy for two sites of small brain metastases, followed by immunotherapy using anti-PD-1 antibodies (pembrolizumab). The treatment exerted a substantial tumor reduction through four cycles. However, treatment was withdrawn due to renal dysfunction. The primary lung tumor continued to regress for an additional four months without any further therapy, resulting in a clinical stage of T1aN0M0. Salvage thoracic surgery was then performed to remove the tumor residue in the lung. Microscopic examination of the sample revealed no residual cancer. The patient was free from recurrence at 16 months post surgery. We then comprehensively reviewed lung sarcomatoid carcinoma cases in the literature, in which anti-PD-1 antibodies were implemented. The current literature and our own findings suggest sarcomatoid carcinomas express high levels of tumoral PD-L1 and can be effectively treated with anti-PD-1 antibodies.

1. Introduction

The development of immune checkpoint inhibitors (ICIs) has helped improve the treatment of non-small-cell lung carcinomas (NSCLCs). However, immunotherapy utilizing ICIs only results in clinical benefits in a portion of treated patients and rarely results in complete clinical remission. The molecular and genetic background and histological type of the specific cancer can alter the disease immunogenicity and modify the therapeutic efficacy of ICIs. We previously reported on a case of giant cell carcinoma in the lung, which is a rare form of sarcomatoid carcinoma, in which a substantial tumor reduction was accomplished through the immunotherapy using pembrolizumab [1].

In this report, we describe the additional clinical course of the patient since we first reported on that case. The patient has shown a complete response to immunotherapy, which has been confirmed by surgical sampling. The patient has continued to experience an excellent clinical course and a long period of progression-free survival. We also comprehensively review

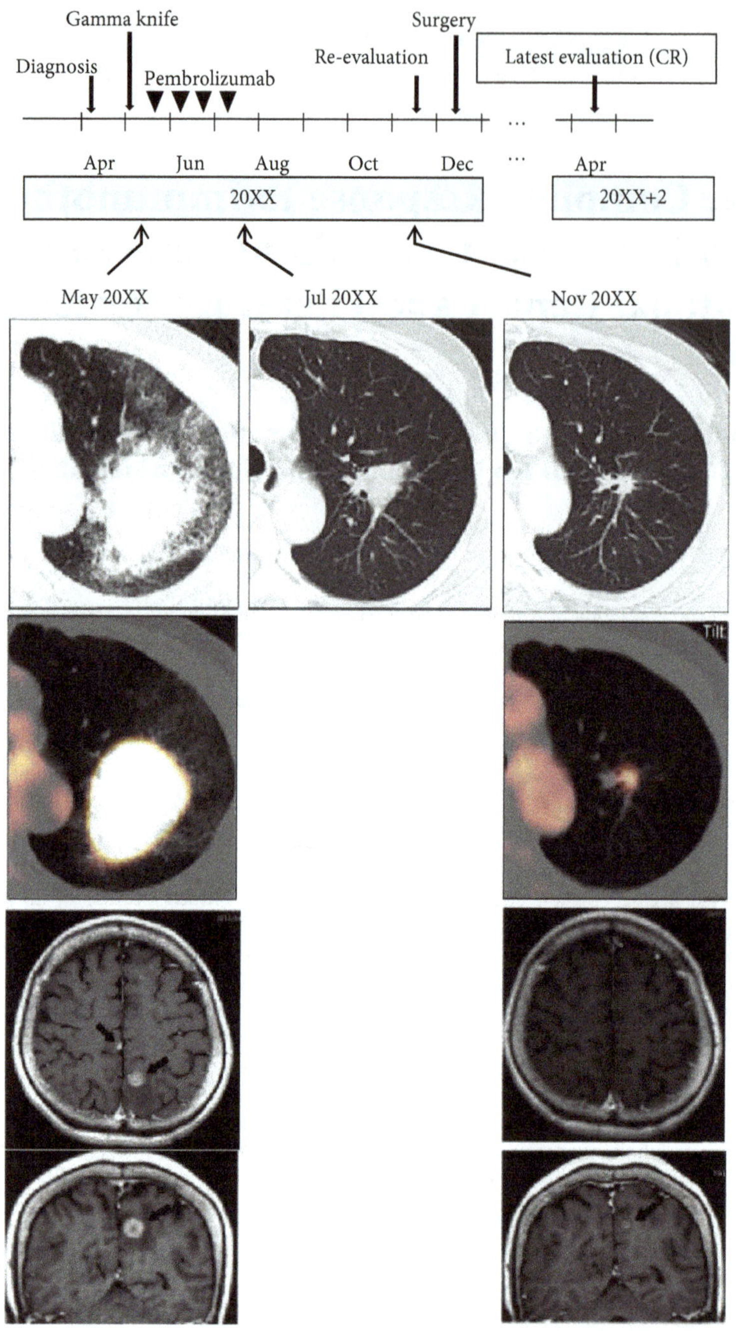

Figure 1: An outline of the clinical course is shown. CR: complete remission.

the literature and discuss the potential benefits of ICI immunotherapy as a treatment course for sarcomatoid carcinomas.

2. Case Presentation

A 69-year-old Japanese woman was diagnosed with giant cell carcinoma in the lung at the clinical stage of IVB (cT2bN0M1c, BRA). Briefly, the primary tumor was located in the upper lobe of the left lung (37 mm in diameter), on which a 2-[^{18}F]-fluoro-2-deoxy-D-glucose (FDG) positron emission tomography (PET) scan showed a high maximum standardized uptake value (SUV) of 28.4 (Figure 1). The PET scan also showed a marginal uptake of a maximum SUV of 3.49 in the mediastinum lymph nodes without any apparent enlargement. No other metastatic sites in the body were noted. A gadolinium-enhanced magnetic resonance imaging (MRI) scan detected two sites of small brain metastases (13 mm at the largest site) without any related neurological symptoms (Figure 1). A transbronchial biopsy aided in determining the pathological diagnosis of giant cell carcinoma. Stereotactic radiotherapy was indicated for the brain metastases in advance of implementing any anticancer medication. The primary tumor showed a high tumor proportion score (TPS) for programmed death ligand 1 (PD-L1) (75%). In response to this finding, the antiprogrammed death 1 (PD-1) antibody medication pembrolizumab (200 mg/body)

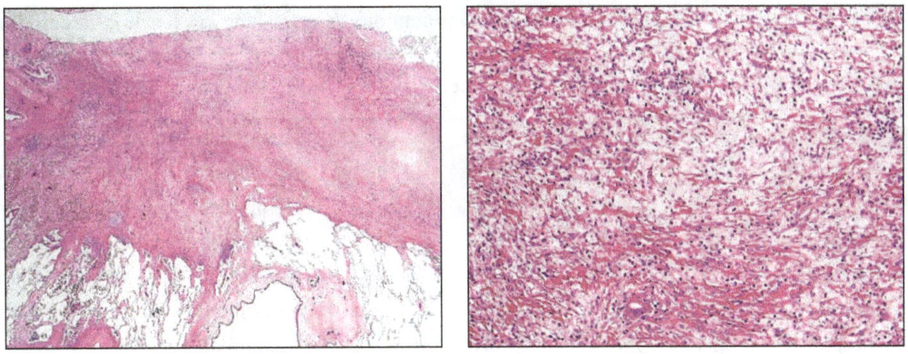

(a) (b)

FIGURE 2: Pathological images taken with a microscope are shown in low (a) and high (b) magnifications. No residual cancer cells existed in the primary resected lung site. Instead, scar formation and an infiltration of mononuclear cells and foamy macrophages were observed.

was administered every three weeks for four cycles. Pembrolizumab exerted an obvious antitumor effect, and the primary tumor size decreased from 48×41 to 24×16 mm (a tumor reduction rate of 80.0%) at the end of the four cycles of treatment (Figure 1). However, a diagnosis of grade 2 renal dysfunction (Common Terminology Criteria for Adverse Events (CTCAE) v4.0) was noted and the treatment was discontinued after four cycles (see Reference [1] for more details).

Within 12 weeks of withdrawing pembrolizumab administration, renal function was restored to the pretreatment baseline without any corticosteroid use. From this point, the patient did not need any readministration of pembrolizumab as the primary lung tumor continued to regress on CT scans (7×7 mm in size), even after a four-month treatment-free period (Figure 1). The brain metastases were well-controlled after the stereotactic radiotherapy as assessed using MRI scans. The ring enhancement of the brain metastases on an MRI scan suggested radiation necrosis (Figure 1). A FDG-PET scan scheduled four months after discontinuing pembrolizumab revealed a moderate uptake of FDG on a portion of the residual primary tumor (maximum SUV of 4.01) (Figure 1). However, there was no significant uptake in the lymph nodes or in the extrathoracic organs. The reduction rate of maximum SUV in the primary tumor was calculated at 85.9%. These data together with radiological assessments revealed the lung cancer was now in yT1aN0M0, stage IA1.

The patient and her family were intensely interested in a salvage surgery to remove the cancer residue in the left upper lobe of the lung to avoid a tumor regrowth and to diminish the risk of future dissemination. In general, a salvage surgery for a patient in clinical stage IVB is not efficacious and not recommended as part of a standard therapeutic strategy. This is true even when a patient is downgraded to stage I after chemotherapy. However, in this particular case, there were some medical reasons for the patient to consider a salvage surgery, including (i) an FDG uptake on the primary lung tumor suggesting a cancer residue *in situ*, (ii) the rapid tumor progression during the initial evaluation period, (iii) the fact that giant cell carcinomas are generally resistant to chemotherapy with cytotoxic antitumor agents resulting in a poor prognosis, and (iv) the brain being the only metastatic site, where stereotactic radiotherapy can be highly effective. After a substantial discussion on the risks of salvage surgery and informed consent, which included a conversation addressing the potential for no clinical benefit, the patient decided to move forward with the procedure. The patient received a left upper lobectomy and a lymphadenectomy at the Federation of National Public Service Personnel Mutual Aid Associations, Tachikawa Hospital, in the following month after a full radiological evaluation (Figure 1). Pathological examination of the resected surgical specimens resulted in surprising findings, with no evidence that any cancer residue existed in the primary site under vigorous microscopic examination (Figure 2). Instead, nonspecific inflammation and scar formation were observed with an infiltration of lymphocytes, plasmacytes, and foamy macrophages (Figure 2). Lymph node metastasis was pathologically absent.

The patient experienced a loss of appetite and body weight loss beginning two months after the surgery and six months after a discontinuation of pembrolizumab. This was diagnosed as isolated adrenocorticotrophic hormone deficiency, grade 3 (CTCAE v4.0). It was presumed that the deficiency was attributable to an immune-related adverse effect of pembrolizumab and an increased demand for steroid hormones elicited by surgical stress. Corticosteroid replacement therapy conferred a rapid and total recovery from this condition. As of 16 months post surgery, the patient was free from any recurrence of cancer, as assessed using body CT and brain MRI scans, and was in good health.

3. Discussion

In the present study, we report on a rare case of giant cell carcinoma in the lung demonstrating a histologically complete response to anti-PD-1 immunotherapy. Additionally, multidisciplinary treatment including brain radiotherapy, immunotherapy, and a salvage thoracic surgery successfully induced a clinically complete remission. Due to the progressive nature of giant cell carcinomas in the lung, a median survival time in advanced-stage cases is reportedly 5-6 months when treated with cytotoxic antitumor agents [2, 3]. Given these findings, the present case

Table 1: A summary of all case reports describing immunotherapy for lung sarcomatoid carcinomas.

	Age/sex	Pathology	PD-L1 TPS (%)	Tx line	Treatment	Response	Duration of ICI treatment	Ref
1	66/M	Pleomorphic	≧95	2nd	Nivolumab	PD	6 cycles/discontinue	[9]
2	59/F	Pleomorphic	80-90	3rd	Nivolumab	PR	19 cycles/ongoing	[9]
3	83/M	Pleomorphic	60-70	4th	Nivolumab	PR	10 cycles/ongoing	[9]
4	55/M	Pleomorphic	90	2nd	Nivolumab	PR	9 cycles/discontinue	[10]
5	62/M	Pleomorphic	70	2nd	Nivolumab	PR	12 cycles/ongoing	[11]
6	67/M	Pleomorphic	≧50	7th	Nivolumab	PR	8 cycles/ongoing	[12]
7	74/M	Pleomorphic	≧50	3rd	Nivolumab	PR	28 months/ongoing	[13]
8	75/M	Pleomorphic	90	3rd	Nivolumab	CR	3 cycles/ongoing	[14]
9	82/M	Pleomorphic	75	1st	Pembrolizumab	PR	3 cycles/discontinue	[15]
10	51/M	Pleomorphic	≧50	1st	Pembrolizumab	PR	3 cycles/ongoing	[16]
11	57/M	Sarcomatoid	80-90	1st (post operation recurrence)	Nivolumab	CR	3 months/ongoing	[17]
12	60/M	Sarcomatoid	100	1st (post operation recurrence)	Nivolumab	PR	8 months/ongoing	[17]
Present	69/F	Giant cell	75	1st	Pembrolizumab	CR	4 cycles/discontinue	—

represents an excellent clinical response and survival time as a result of the multidisciplinary treatments implemented in this study.

ICIs exert antitumor effects on cases with a wide variety of histological types in NSCLCs. Immunotherapy utilizing anti-PD-1/PD-L1 antibodies has been recommended as an option for the treatment of patients in advanced stages of cancer. However, it remains largely unknown whether lung carcinoma cases with minor histological types should be treated following the same strategy. It has become increasingly evident that lung sarcomatoid carcinomas present with a high tumoral PD-L1 expression (53-90% of all cases) [4–8]. This suggests a potential benefit of treating sarcomatoid carcinomas with PD-1/PD-L1 immunotherapy. We comprehensively searched the literature (written in English) for lung sarcomatoid carcinoma cases treated with anti-PD-1/PD-L1 inhibitors and summarized our findings in Table 1 [9–17]. Ten cases had pleomorphic carcinomas, and two cases had sarcomatoid carcinomas with unspecified subtypes. The present study was the only case of a giant cell carcinoma. PD-L1 expression was high (50-100% TPS), and anti-PD-1 antibodies (i.e., pembrolizumab or nivolumab) were used in all cases. The patients who were treated with nivolumab or pembrolizumab showed an objective response in 9 of 10 (90%) or in 3 of 3 (100%) cases, respectively. Two cases which received nivolumab treatment presented with a complete radiological response (Table 1). Further, treatment efficacy was not associated with any prior chemotherapy or thoracic surgery (recurrent cases). Given the findings of our literature review, we suggest the current case is unique in presenting a histologically complete response to anti-PD-1 immunotherapy in a case of giant cell carcinoma in the lung.

When investigating the efficacy of immunotherapy for the treatment of sarcomatoid carcinomas in other organs, we found the treatment of renal cell carcinomas (RCCs) particularly interesting. RCCs primarily manifest histologically as a type of clear cell carcinoma, while a sarcomatoid component only coexists in 5-8% of all cases [18]. It has been shown in histological examinations of resected tumors that PD-L1 expression is elevated in sarcomatoid RCCs when compared with nonsarcomatoid RCCs [19]. Interestingly, some cases have reported favorable clinical responses to nivolumab treatment in patients with sarcomatoid RCCs [20, 21]. However, to date, it has not been confirmed whether immunotherapy with ICIs is a superior therapy when compared to the standard treatment with cytotoxic antitumor agents in sarcomatoid RCCs.

In our review of basic research studies, we also noted that tumor mutation burden was recently proposed to be one of the predictors of ICI efficacy. For example, a study by Nakagomi et al. compared the genetic mutation burden between sarcomatoid and carcinomatous regions in four different lung sarcomatoid carcinoma cases. They showed that the sarcomatoid regions were more abundant in genetic mutations than in carcinomatous regions [22]. Given these findings and our current case report, we suggest ICIs targeting PD-1/PD-L1 could potentially play an important role in the antitumor treatment strategy of those patients with sarcomatoid carcinomas.

Another important observation we made was that a residual FDG uptake in a preoperative PET-CT scan was not associated with a pathological cancer residue in the present case. Recently, the immune PET Response Criteria in Solid Tumors (iPERCIST) was proposed to evaluate the metabolic response of solid tumors to immunotherapy [23]. In this assessment, a complete treatment response is defined as the disappearance of all metabolically active tumors. However, this approach could be difficult in evaluating cancer residues, since a restoration of antitumor immunity with ICIs can be associated with an upregulation of glucose metabolism. This could then lead to a misinterpretation on PET-CT scan images, as was shown in the present study.

In conclusion, we describe a giant cell carcinoma case in the lung which demonstrated a histologically complete response to PD-1/PD-L1 immunotherapy. A larger number of cases will be required to determine the potential role of immunotherapy in the treatment of sarcomatoid carcinomas in other patients and organs.

Consent

Written consent was obtained from the patient for the publication of this case report.

Acknowledgments

We would like to thank Editage (http://www.editage.jp) for English language editing.

References

[1] S. Nakayama, M. Sasaki, S. Morinaga, and N. Minematsu, "Nonsmall cell lung carcinoma with giant cell features expressing programmed death-ligand 1: a report of a patient successfully treated with pembrolizumab," *Case Reports in Oncological Medicine*, vol. 2018, Article ID 5863015, 4 pages, 2018.

[2] H. M. Bae, H. S. Min, S. H. Lee et al., "Palliative chemotherapy for pulmonary pleomorphic carcinoma," *Lung Cancer*, vol. 58, no. 1, pp. 112–115, 2007.

[3] T. Vieira, N. Girard, M. Ung et al., "Efficacy of first-line chemotherapy in patients with advanced lung sarcomatoid carcinoma," *Journal of Thoracic Oncology*, vol. 8, no. 12, pp. 1574–1577, 2013.

[4] V. Yvorel, A. Patoir, F. Casteillo et al., "PD-L1 expression in pleomorphic, spindle cell and giant cell carcinoma of the lung is related to TTF-1, p40 expression and might indicate a worse prognosis," *PLoS One*, vol. 12, no. 7, 2017.

[5] S. Kim, M. Y. Kim, J. Koh et al., "Programmed death-1 ligand 1 and 2 are highly expressed in pleomorphic carcinomas of the lung: comparison of sarcomatous and carcinomatous areas," *European Journal of Cancer*, vol. 51, no. 17, pp. 2698–2707, 2015.

[6] V. Velcheti, D. L. Rimm, and K. A. Schalper, "Sarcomatoid lung carcinomas show high levels of programmed death ligand-1 (PD-L1)," *Journal of Thoracic Oncology*, vol. 8, no. 6, pp. 803–805, 2013.

[7] T. Vieira, M. Antoine, C. Hamard et al., "Sarcomatoid lung carcinomas show high levels of programmed death ligand-1 (PD-L1) and strong immune-cell infiltration by TCD3 cells and macrophages," *Lung Cancer*, vol. 98, pp. 51–58, 2016.

[8] J. K. Sim, S. M. Chung, J. H. Choi et al., "Clinical and molecular characteristics of pulmonary sarcomatoid carcinoma," *Korean Journal of Internal Medicine*, vol. 33, no. 4, pp. 737–744, 2018.

[9] M. Kanazu, T. Uenami, Y. Yano et al., "Case series of pleomorphic carcinomas of the lung treated with nivolumab," *Thoracic Cancer*, vol. 8, no. 6, pp. 724–728, 2017.

[10] L. Marchand, V. Paulus, N. Fabien et al., "Nivolumab-induced acute diabetes mellitus and hypophysitis in a patient with advanced pulmonary pleomorphic carcinoma with a prolonged tumor response," *Journal of Thoracic Oncology*, vol. 12, no. 11, pp. e182–e184, 2017.

[11] S. Senoo, T. Ninomiya, G. Makimoto et al., "Rapid and long-term response of pulmonary pleomorphic carcinoma to nivolumab," *Internal Medicine*, vol. 58, no. 7, pp. 985–989, 2019.

[12] K. Ito, O. Hataji, K. Katsuta et al., ""Pseudoprogression" of pulmonary pleomorphic carcinoma during nivolumab therapy," *Journal of Thoracic Oncology*, vol. 11, no. 10, pp. e117–e119, 2016.

[13] M. Salati, C. Baldessari, F. Calabrese et al., "Nivolumab-induced impressive response of refractory pulmonary sarcomatoid carcinoma with brain metastasis," *Case Reports in Oncology*, vol. 11, no. 3, pp. 615–621, 2018.

[14] K. Okamura, Y. Fukuda, H. Soda et al., "Pulmonary pleomorphic carcinoma with few PD-1-positive immune cells and regulatory T cells that showed a complete response to nivolumab," *Thoracic Cancer*, vol. 9, no. 1, pp. 193–196, 2018.

[15] T. Tozuka, T. Sugano, R. Noro et al., "Pembrolizumab-induced agranulocytosis in a pulmonary pleomorphic carcinoma patient who developed interstitial lung disease and ocular myasthenia gravis," *Oxford Medical Case Reports.*, vol. 2018, no. 11, p. omy094, 2018.

[16] Y. Matsumoto, T. Miura, H. Horiuchi, and K. Usui, "The Successful Treatment of Pulmonary Pleomorphic Carcinoma with Pembrolizumab: A Case Report," *Case Reports in Oncology*, vol. 10, no. 2, pp. 752–757, 2017.

[17] C. Roesel, K. Kambartel, U. Kopeika, A. Berzins, T. Voshaar, and T. Krbek, "Lazarus-type tumour response to therapy with nivolumab for sarcomatoid carcinomas of the lung," *Current Oncology*, vol. 26, no. 2, pp. e270–e273, 2019.

[18] B. C. Leibovich, C. M. Lohse, P. L. Crispen et al., "Histological subtype is an independent predictor of outcome for patients with renal cell carcinoma," *Journal of Urology*, vol. 183, no. 4, pp. 1309–1316, 2010.

[19] R. W. Joseph, S. Z. Millis, E. M. Carballido et al., "PD-1 and PD-L1 expression in renal cell carcinoma with sarcomatoid differentiation," *Cancer Immunology Research*, vol. 3, no. 12, pp. 1303–1307, 2015.

[20] G. Noguchi, S. Tsutsumi, M. Yasui et al., "Significant response to nivolumab for metastatic chromophobe renal cell carcinoma with sarcomatoid differentiation: a case report," *BMC Urology*, vol. 18, no. 1, p. 26, 2018.

[21] D. M. Geynisman, "Anti-programmed cell death protein 1 (PD-1) antibody nivolumab leads to a dramatic and rapid response in papillary renal cell carcinoma with sarcomatoid and rhabdoid features," *European Urology*, vol. 68, no. 5, pp. 912–914, 2015.

[22] T. Nakagomi, T. Goto, Y. Hirotsu et al., "New therapeutic targets for pulmonary sarcomatoid carcinomas based on their genomic and phylogenetic profiles," *Oncotarget*, vol. 9, no. 12, pp. 10635–10649, 2018.

[23] N. Aide, R. J. Hicks, C. le Tourneau, S. Lheureux, S. Fanti, and E. Lopci, "FDG PET/CT for assessing tumour response to immunotherapy: report on the EANM symposium on immune modulation and recent review of the literature," *European Journal of Nuclear Medicine and Molecular Imaging*, vol. 46, no. 1, pp. 238–250, 2019.

6

Ductal Adenocarcinoma Ex Pleomorphic Adenoma of the Lacrimal Gland: A Rare and Morbid Malignancy

Prashanth Ashok Kumar[1] **Shweta Paulraj,**[1] **Kanish Mirchia**[2] **Seung Shin Hahn,**[3] **and Abirami Sivapiragasam**[4]

[1]*Department of Internal Medicine, SUNY Upstate Medical University, Syracuse, NY 13210, USA*
[2]*Department of Pathology, SUNY Upstate Medical University, Syracuse, NY 13210, USA*
[3]*Department of Radiation Oncology, SUNY Upstate Medical University, Syracuse, NY 13210, USA*
[4]*Department of Hematology-Oncology, SUNY Upstate Medical University, Syracuse, NY 13210, USA*

Correspondence should be addressed to Prashanth Ashok Kumar; ashokkup@upstate.edu

Academic Editor: Raffaele Palmirotta

Carcinoma ex pleomorphic adenoma (Ca ex PA) is a rare malignant transformation of a benign primary pleomorphic adenoma (PA). We report the case of a 62-year-old male who presented with a swelling over his left temple. Imaging revealed a lytic lesion over the left orbital wall with soft tissue extension suggestive of malignancy. He underwent an en bloc resection of the mass with orbital exenteration, craniotomy, and reconstruction. Pathology demonstrated a lacrimal gland ductal adenocarcinoma arising from a PA which led to the diagnosis of ductal adenoCa ex PA. Postoperatively, he received chemotherapy with 6 cycles of cisplatin and concurrent radiation therapy (RT), but his course was complicated by recurrent bacterial meningitis and abscesses and he ultimately opted for comfort measures. Patients with PA of the lacrimal gland experience an insidiously enlarging painless swelling of the orbit with transformation to Ca ex PA highlighted by a rapid onset of bulbar enlargement, displacement, and often proptosis. Ductal adenoCa ex PA is aggressive with a poor prognosis and has no established standard of care. This case highlights the rarity of this condition and the need for more literature to help direct treatment.

1. Introduction

The lacrimal gland is an almond-shaped, bilobed, eccrine gland embedded in the superolateral aspect of the orbital wall and is composed of small lobules separated by connective tissue [1–4]. Lacrimal gland tumors occur in about 1 in 1,000,000 individuals per year and constitute 5-25% of all orbital malignancies [2, 3, 5]. Epithelial neoplasms are the most common followed by lymphoid and metastatic lesions. Epithelial lesions comprise around 50-60% of all benign and 40-50% of all malignant lesions [2]. Pleomorphic adenoma (PA) is the most common benign neoplasm of the lacrimal gland and has excellent prognosis after surgical excision like its salivary counterpart [3, 4]. It represents around 20% of all lacrimal gland tumors and 48% of all epithelial lacrimal gland lesions [2, 5]. Carcinoma ex pleomorphic adenoma (Ca ex PA) is a rare transformation of a benign primary PA to a malignant neoplasm [5, 6]. These rare tumors themselves show morphologic variations and one of them is ductal adenoCa ex PA [7, 8]. There are about 26 cases of ductal carcinomas of the lacrimal gland and very few cases of Ca ex PA, which makes our case a very uncommon presentation [5, 8]. The tumor is aggressive and carries a very poor prognosis. Most of the data on these tumors are extrapolated from its salivary gland counterpart. Even among salivary gland malignancies, Ca ex PA has a 5-year disease-specific survival rate of 37-44% which is lower than most other salivary gland tumors [6]. We present the clinical course of ductal adenoCa ex PA in a 62-year-old male and highlight the morbid nature of this malignancy.

2. Case Report

Our patient was a 62-year-old Caucasian male with a history significant for obstructive sleep apnea and osteoarthritis. He visited his primary care provider with a swelling over his left temple that was present for a long time but had gradually increased in size for the past several months. The swelling was around 3.5 × 3 cm in size on presentation with newly developing tenderness in the left temple. There was an initial suspicion for giant cell arteritis and hence a temporal artery biopsy was done which was negative. The swelling continued to progress causing proptosis, tearing, discharge from the left eye, and redness over the left temple and orbit. Initial laboratory investigations including SPEP, liver function testing, prostate-specific antigen, ESR, and CRP were within normal limits. CT maxillofacial with contrast showed a 3.8 × 2.7 cm lytic lesion on the left orbital wall with associated heterogeneous soft tissue that was suspicious for malignancy. CT head with and without contrast did not show any significant findings.

The interventional radiology (IR) team performed a CT-guided biopsy of the left periorbital soft tissue mass which showed soft tissue diffusely infiltrated by a moderately differentiated adenocarcinoma with a prominent cribriform pattern. Tumor cells had moderate cytologic atypia, numerous mitotic figures, and evidence of individual cell necrosis. Immunohistochemistry was positive for GATA-3 and negative for PSA and TTF-1. The consideration then was a primary adenocarcinoma of either lacrimal or sinonasal origin or a metastatic adenocarcinoma likely from the breast. MRI of the brain with and without contrast showed a fairly well demarcated, lobulated mass with mixed cystic and solid components along with heterogenous enhancement involving the left lacrimal gland and the lateral wall of the left orbit. The mass extended into the left suprazygomatic space and orbit. The left lateral rectus muscle was displaced. The overlying muscle in the left supra zygomatic masticator space demonstrated edema and enhancement. Nasal endoscopy did not reveal any evidence of malignancy in the upper aerodigestive tract. PET CT imaging from the skull to the thigh showed increased metabolic activity of the left orbital soft tissue mass with adjacent lytic changes involving the left orbit. There was no evidence of metabolically active lymphadenopathy in the head and neck nor any evidence of distant metastatic disease. ENT, neurosurgery, ophthalmology, medical oncology, and radiation oncology teams were involved in the care of the patient.

The patient underwent an en bloc resection of his lacrimal gland tumor which required orbital exenteration. Biopsies were sent. Since his tumor extended to the skull base, a craniotomy was performed and a small dural leak repaired with a pericranial graft. Figure 1 shows the relationship of the tumor to the eyelid. Microscopic examination demonstrated the adenocarcinoma to be arising from a PA of the lacrimal gland (Figure 2), with the PA component demonstrating p63 positivity (Figure 3). The tumor showed an invasive cystic growth pattern with papillary and cribriform arch formations, invading the fibroadipose tissue and adjacent bone. The cystic structures were lined by neoplastic

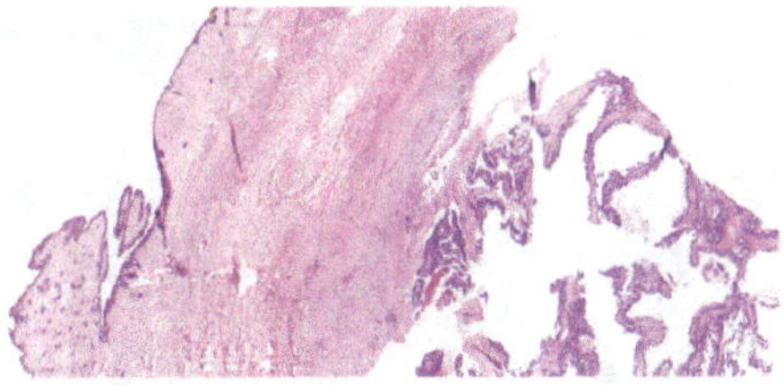

FIGURE 1: H&E sections (0.5x) showing relationship of the tumor with the overlying eyelid.

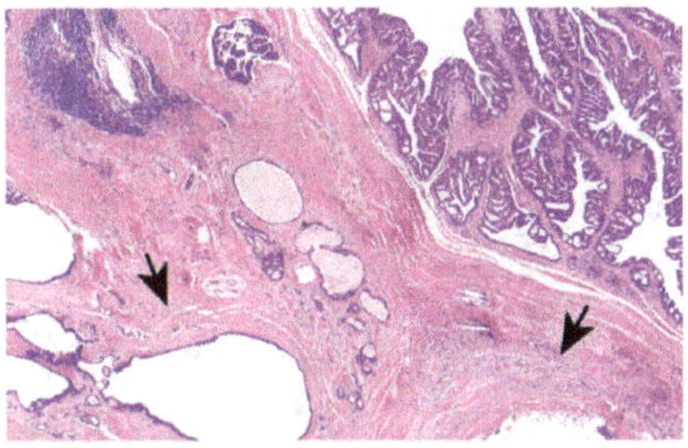

FIGURE 2: Hyalinized stroma of pleomorphic adenoma overtaken by the adenocarcinoma (H&E, 5x magnification).

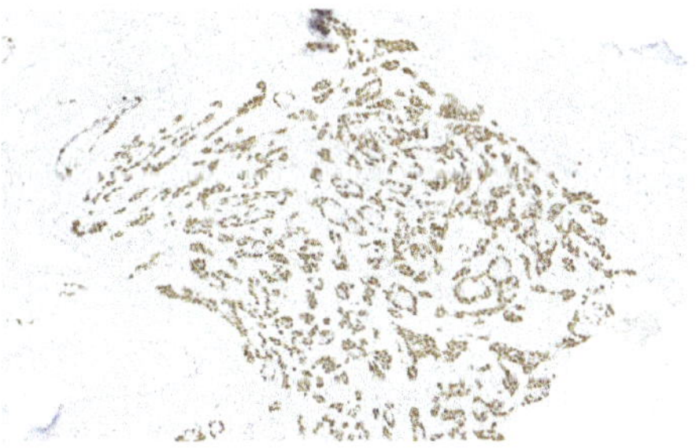

FIGURE 3: 20x magnification of pleomorphic adenoma with positive p63 staining.

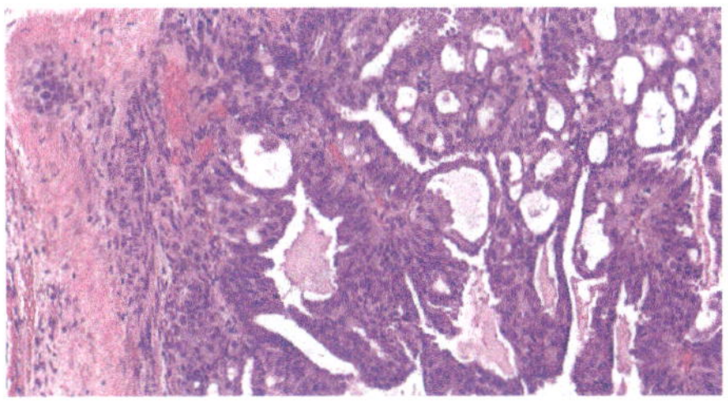

FIGURE 4: H&E sections (20x) showing neoplastic cells lining cystic structures with low- to high-grade pleomorphic nuclei.

cells with apocrine features and nuclear pleomorphism ranging from low to high grade. Up to 8 mitotic figures/10 high-power fields were seen within the areas of high-grade features. Foci of invasive solid component were identified with cribriform architecture and high nuclear atypia (Figure 4). There was no evidence of perineural or lymphovascular invasion. Foci of hemorrhage, granulation tissue,

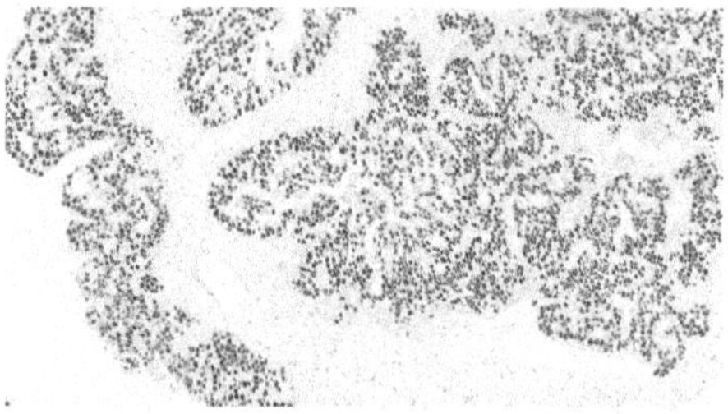

FIGURE 5: Carcinoma component showing positive androgen receptor (AR) staining (20x).

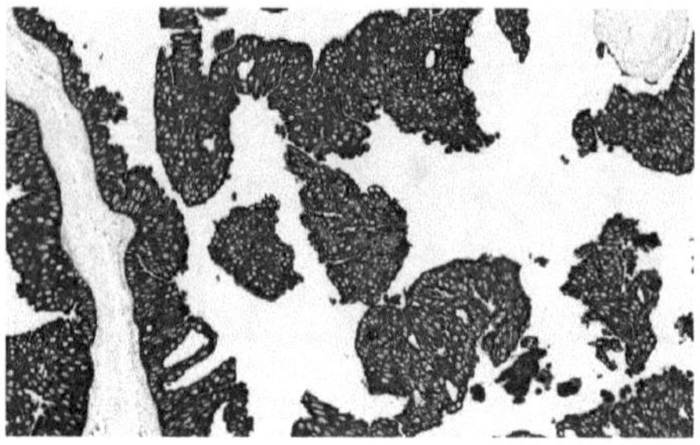

FIGURE 6: Carcinoma component showing positive staining for CAM 5.2 (20x).

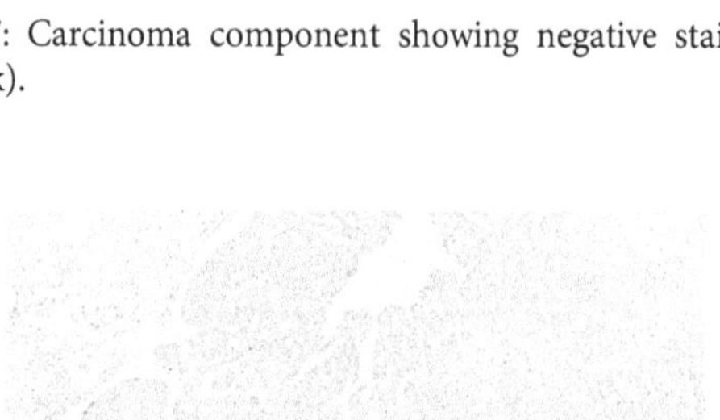

FIGURE 7: Carcinoma component showing negative staining for S100 (20x).

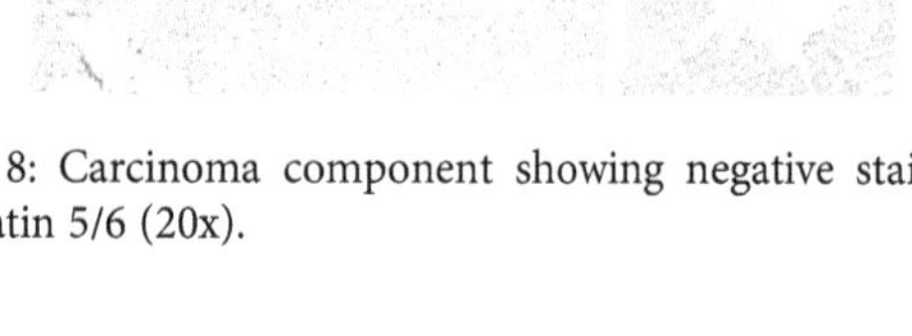

FIGURE 8: Carcinoma component showing negative staining for cytokeratin 5/6 (20x).

and dystrophic calcification were also identified within the cystic component of the tumor. Immunohistochemistry showed the carcinoma cells to be positive for androgen receptor (AR), GCDFP15, HMWK903, and CAM5.2, while staining negative for S100, cytokeratin 5/6, p53, HER2/neu, progesterone (PR), and estrogen receptor (ER) (Figures 5–8).

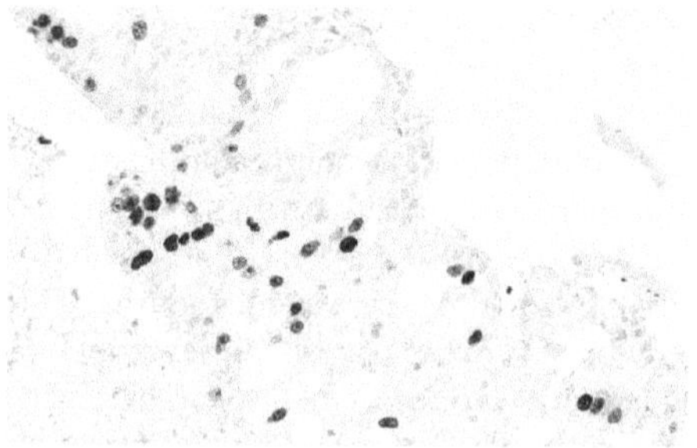

FIGURE 9: Areas of adenocarcinoma component showing focal areas of Ki 67 elevation (40x).

The Ki 67 index was focally elevated at 22% as shown in Figure 9. The overall findings supported the diagnosis of invasive ductal adenoCa ex PA of the lacrimal gland with the carcinoma component showing features ranging from low-grade papillary cystadenocarcinoma to intermediate-/high-grade ductal carcinoma.

Postoperatively, he received chemotherapy with 6 cycles of cisplatin with concurrent radiation therapy (RT). Six months after diagnosis and 2 months after completing chemoradiation, there was a suspicion for recurrence of the tumor and the patient had to undergo reexcision of the surgical site. Biopsies however did not show any definitive evidence of recurrence. Throughout his clinical course, he had multiple episodes of temporal abscesses and bacterial meningitis and had to undergo several craniotomies. Due to the complicated course and poor prognosis, the family decided to adopt comfort measures alone and the patient eventually succumbed to severe sepsis and cardiorespiratory arrest 1 year after his diagnosis.

3. Discussion

Lacrimal glands are sometimes considered a type of minor salivary gland and share histologic features with the main salivary glands [9]. Epithelial lacrimal gland tumors are grouped according to the classification of salivary gland tumors due to the common histopathologic features and lack of available data with regard to the former [10]. With PA, there always remains a risk of transformation into Ca ex PA and the risk increases with time [11]. There have been instances of malignant transformation noted 60 years after a diagnosis of PA [12]. Lacrimal and salivary PA and Ca ex PA have shown similar clinical and genomic profiles [13, 14]. Besides pure adenocarcinomas, there are other types of Ca ex PA such as myoepithelial carcinoma, adenoid cystic carcinoma, epithelial-myoepithelial carcinoma, squamous cell carcinoma, clear cell carcinoma, adenosquamous carcinoma, mucoepidermoid carcinoma, and acinic cell carcinoma. While adenocarcinoma is the most common type of Ca ex PA in salivary glands, there is insufficient information to comment on lacrimal Ca ex PA [15–18].

Patients with PA experience an insidiously enlarging painless swelling of the orbits over the years. Those with transformation to Ca ex PA experience a rapid onset of bulbar enlargement and displacement. Proptosis is often seen as in our patient [17, 19]. Lacrimal gland tumors

Table 1: Comparison of the present case and Ca ex PA reported by Nambu et al. in 2017 [8].

S. no		Present case	Nambu et al.
1	Age in years	62	72
2	Sex	Male	Male
3	Race	Caucasian	Japanese
4	Laterality	Left	Left
5	Presenting symptoms	Exophthalmos, redness, and swelling over the temple	Exophthalmos
6	Staging	T4cN0M0	T4cNxM0
7	AR	Positive	Positive
8	P53	Negative	Positive
9	HER2	Negative	Positive
10	GCDFP15, HMWK903, CAM5.2	Positive	Unknown
11	S100, cytokeratin 5/6	Negative	Unknown
12	ER, PR	Negative	Negative
13	Ki 67	Focally high-22%	Unknown
14	Treatment	Orbital exenteration and repair+chemotherapy+RT	Orbital exenteration and repair+RT
15	Outcome	Patient passed away	Unknown

are staged based on the TNM staging system and are assigned a grade based on the same [20]. Our patient would thus be T4cN0M0, G3.

The benign PA component is generally seen under the microscope as a pseudocapsule enclosed compilation of cuboidal ductal cells and polygonal or spindle-shaped myoepithelial cells in a chondromyxoid stroma [21]. The malignant component is characterized by nuclear pleomorphisms, atypical mitotic figures, hemorrhage, and necrosis. Various morphologies as mentioned above can be noticed [20]. Ca ex PA is noninvasive, minimally invasive, or invasive depending on its extension into the adjacent tissue. Noninvasive Ca ex PA remains within the fibrous capsule of the original PA. A minimally invasive tumor invades less than 1.5 mm in the extracapsular structures whereas an invasive Ca ex PA is characterized by greater than 1.5 mm invasion of the malignant component into the surrounding tissues [6, 22, 23]. Our case was thus invasive.

Hashimoto et al. showed that in salivary gland Ca ex PA, HER2 amplification played a significant role in the progression of the tumor and was associated with worse prognosis [24]. In Nambu and Tsukamoto et al.'s case of ductal adenoCa ex PA, HER2 gene amplification and protein overexpression was seen in the high-grade components, which was not the case in our patient. There is no available data on the use of anti-HER2-targeted therapies in ductal adenoCa ex PA of the lacrimal gland. AR positivity has been noted in some Ca ex PA, but no data on targeted therapies are available [8]. Ki-67 is a marker of DNA proliferation and malignant tumors usually have a high Ki-67 expression. The PA component being benign has a low expression, and the Ca ex PA is known to have a higher expression [6]. GCDFP-15 has been shown to be a biomarker for adenocarcinoma of the lacrimal gland, but its role in management is uncertain. Our patient was positive for the same [25]. p63 is a marker of myoepithelial elements and is positive in PA, whereas Ca ex PA is generally characterized by loss of p63 expression [26, 27]. Andreasen et al. in their report provide a summary of the demographics, stage, management, outcome, and certain receptor status of 25 cases of lacrimal gland ductal Ca from 1995 to 2016 [7]. Table 1 compares the present case to that of Nambu et al. who reported a high-grade invasive ductal Ca ex PA in 2017 [8].

Management of PA and Ca ex PA is surgical excision. If there is infiltration, the involved adjacent structures need to be removed followed by adjuvant RT and reconstructive procedures [18]. This is similar to our patient where orbital craniotomy was done. There is currently no standard protocol for chemotherapy or targeted therapy even for the more common salivary gland subtype. Sharon et al. reported a case of salivary HER2 positive Ca ex PA that was successfully treated with trastuzumab and capecitabine [22]. Similarly, in the salivary subtype, Chooback et al. showed a good response to a combination of cyclophosphamide, doxorubicin, and cisplatin. Paclitaxel-tamoxifen, cisplatin-5 fluorouracil, nedaplatin-docetaxel, and experimental wT1 peptide vaccine have demonstrated limited success in salivary Ca ex PA [22]. There is insufficient evidence of the successful use of chemotherapy or targeted therapies in lacrimal gland Ca ex PA in literature. When assessing the management of lacrimal Ca ex PA, it is to be noted that Ishida et al. and Daniel et al. used only surgical excision, whereas Nambu et al. used surgery with adjuvant RT [8, 18].

As seen with past experiences and in our patient, this rare tumor is aggressive and carries a very poor prognosis with a high predilection for recurrence and metastasis [20].

4. Conclusion

Ca ex PA is an extremely uncommon and aggressive tumor arising from a preexisting PA and carries a poor prognosis. Given the unpredictable nature of this tumor, we believe that it is important to make an early and correct pathologic diagnosis for which a high index of suspicion is needed. There are no guidelines to aid in management of this rare tumor. More case reports and, eventually, meta-analysis are needed to improve outcomes of this uncommon yet morbid malignancy.

Acknowledgments

Our sincere gratitude to the Department of Hematology Oncology and the Department of Pathology for all the support and guidance.

References

[1] C. D. Conrady, Z. P. Joos, and B. C. Patel, "Review: the lacrimal gland and its role in dry eye," *Journal of Ophthalmology*, vol. 2016, Article ID 7542929, 11 pages, 2016.

[2] S. Andreasen, B. Esmaeli, S. L. Holstein, L. H. Mikkelsen, P. K. Rasmussen, and S. Heegaard, "An update on tumors of the lacrimal gland," *Asia-Pacific Journal of Ophthalmology*, vol. 6, no. 2, pp. 159–172, 2017.

[3] W. Harrison, P. Pittman, and T. Cummings, "Pleomorphic adenoma of the lacrimal gland: a review with updates on malignant transformation and molecular genetics," *Saudi Journal of Ophthalmology*, vol. 32, no. 1, pp. 13–16, 2018.

[4] A. Skálová, P. Andrle, L. Hostička, and M. Michal, "Pleomorphic adenoma of salivary glands: diagnostic pitfalls and mimickers of malignancy," *Ceskoslovenská Patologie*, vol. 48, no. 4, pp. 179–183, 2012.

[5] E. Weis, J. Rootman, T. J. Joly et al., "Epithelial lacrimal gland tumors: pathologic classification and current understanding," *Archives of Ophthalmology*, vol. 127, no. 8, pp. 1016–1028, 2009.

[6] J. Antony, V. Gopalan, R. A. Smith, and A. K. Lam, "Carcinoma ex pleomorphic adenoma: a comprehensive review of clinical, pathological and molecular data," *Head and Neck Pathology*, vol. 6, no. 1, pp. 1–9, 2012.

[7] S. Andreasen, M. Grauslund, and S. Heegaard, "Lacrimal gland ductal carcinomas: clinical, morphological and genetic characterization and implications for targeted treatment," *Acta Ophthalmologica*, vol. 95, no. 3, pp. 299–306, 2017.

[8] N. Nambu, Y. Tsukamoto, H. Tsuji et al., "Invasive ductal carcinoma ex pleomorphic adenoma of the lacrimal gland - a long term follow-up case," *Human Pathology: Case Reports*, vol. 10, pp. 81–84, 2017.

[9] S. O. Baek, Y. J. Lee, S. H. Moon, Y. J. Kim, and Y. J. Jun, "Primary adenocarcinoma of the lacrimal gland," *Archives of Plastic Surgery*, vol. 39, no. 5, pp. 578–580, 2012.

[10] A. Touil, S. El Abbassi, Y. Echchikhi, M. Maher, T. Kebdani, and N. Benjaafar, "Adenocarcinoma of the lacrimal gland: a case report," *Journal of Medical Case Reports*, vol. 11, no. 1, p. 257, 2017.

[11] O. Binatli, O. Yaman, N. Ozdemir, and E. I. Gökçöl, "Pleomorphic adenoma of lacrimal gland," *Journal of Surgical Case Reports*, vol. 2013, no. 10, article rjt089, 2013.

[12] M. R. Vagefi, J. E. Hong, O. M. Zwick, E. H. Bedrossian Jr., S. R. Seiff, and K. P. Cockerham, "Atypical presentations of pleomorphic adenoma of the lacrimal gland," *Ophthalmic Plastic and Reconstructive Surgery*, vol. 23, no. 4, pp. 272–274, 2007.

[13] S. L. von Holstein, A. Fehr, M. Persson et al., "Lacrimal gland pleomorphic adenoma and carcinoma ex pleomorphic adenoma: genomic profiles, gene fusions, and clinical characteristics," *Ophthalmology*, vol. 121, no. 5, pp. 1125–1133, 2014.

[14] N. R. Rabade and N. A. Goel, "Clear cell myoepithelial carcinoma ex pleomorphic adenoma," *Indian Journal of Pathology & Microbiology*, vol. 57, no. 3, pp. 456–459, 2014.

[15] E. Avdagic, N. Farber, N. Katabi, and R. Shinder, "Carcinoma ex pleomorphic adenoma of the lacrimal gland with epithelial-myoepithelial carcinoma histologic type," *Ophthalmic Plastic and Reconstructive Surgery*, vol. 33, no. 3S, pp. S136–S138, 2017.

[16] B. P. Venkatesulu, S. Pathy, A. G. Vallonthaiel, and B. Chawla, "Epithelial–myoepithelial carcinoma of lacrimal gland from an ex pleomorphic adenoma," *BMJ Case Reports*, vol. 2015, article bcr2015210795, 2015.

[17] M. Covinsky, Z. Cai, M. Ambelil, J. Liu, and H. Zhu, "Low grade carcinoma ex-pleomorphic adenoma: diagnosis and diagnostic challenges caused by fine needle aspiration: report of three cases and review of literature," *Head and Neck Pathology*, vol. 12, no. 1, pp. 82–88, 2018.

[18] L. Daniel, S. Rao, R. Muthusamy, and D. Yerramsetti, "Mucoepidermoid carcinoma ex pleomorphic adenoma of the lacrimal gland: a rare presentation," *Indian Journal of Ophthalmology*, vol. 62, no. 6, pp. 743–746, 2014.

[19] S. L. von Holstein, S. E. Coupland, D. Briscoe, C. Le Tourneau, and S. Heegaard, "Epithelial tumours of the lacrimal gland: a clinical, histopathological, surgical and oncological survey," *Acta Ophthalmologica*, vol. 91, no. 3, pp. 195–206, 2013.

[20] J. Mallen-St Clair, A. Arshi, B. Tajudeen, E. Abemayor, and M. St John, "Epidemiology and treatment of lacrimal gland tumors: a population-based cohort analysis," *JAMA Otolaryngology Head & Neck Surgery*, vol. 140, no. 12, pp. 1110–1116, 2014.

[21] P. Zhang, L. J. Tang, H. H. Gao, W. X. Zhang, J. X. Lin, and H. S. Yang, "Immunohistochemical features of carcinoma ex pleomorphic adenoma and pleomorphic adenoma in the lacrimal gland," *International Journal of Ophthalmology*, vol. 12, no. 8, pp. 1238–1242, 2019.

[22] E. Sharon, R. J. Kelly, and E. Szabo, "Sustained response of carcinoma ex pleomorphic adenoma treated with trastuzumab and capecitabine," *Head & Neck Oncology*, vol. 2, no. 1, p. 12, 2010.

[23] A. Altemani, M. T. Martins, L. Freitas, F. Soares, N. S. Araújo, and V. C. Araújo, "Carcinoma ex pleomorphic adenoma (CXPA): immunoprofile of the cells involved in carcinomatous progression," *Histopathology*, vol. 46, no. 6, pp. 635–641, 2005.

[24] K. Hashimoto, H. Yamamoto, H. Shiratsuchi et al., "HER-2/neu gene amplification in carcinoma ex pleomorphic adenoma in relation to progression and prognosis: a chromogenic in-situ hybridization study," *Histopathology*, vol. 60, no. 6B, pp. E131–E142, 2012.

[25] M. M. Zhu, H. G. Cui, and X. D. Teng, "GCDFP-15, AR, and Her-2 as biomarkers for primary ductal adenocarcinoma of the lacrimal gland: a Chinese case and literature review," *OncoTargets and Therapy*, vol. 8, pp. 1017–1024, 2015.

[26] D. S. Rawat, D. Sonkhya, N. Sonkhya, and S. Gupta, "Myoepithelial cell-rich pleormorphic adenoma of minor salivary gland of parapharyngeal space," *Case Reports in Otolaryngology*, vol. 2012, Article ID 537381, 3 pages, 2012.

7

A Rare Case of Breast Implant-Associated Diffuse Large B-Cell Lymphoma

Christopher Larrimore and Annmarie Jaghab

Nova Southeastern University Dr. Kiran C. Patel College of Osteopathic Medicine, USA

Correspondence should be addressed to Christopher Larrimore; cl1398@mynsu.nova.edu

Academic Editor: Katsuhiro Tanaka

This is a case of an elderly female who presented for follow-up ultrasound of the right breast after routine mammogram revealed a small benign mass. A subsequent ultrasound detected a small nodular mass that was described as benign in appearance. Although the patient was asymptomatic, a fine-needle biopsy was performed to rule out malignancy. Results from immunohistochemistry and FISH studies of the biopsy were positive for diffuse large B-cell lymphoma (DLBCL). The patient underwent surgery for lumpectomy and removal of breast implants. Intraoperative tissue samples were analyzed by pathology using both flow cytometry and microscopy, and results confirmed DLBCL. With total tumor resection and implant removal completed, the patient did not require additional treatments as the prognosis of DLBCL status post implant removal is excellent. She returned for follow-up six months later and has since had no signs of reoccurrence.

1. Introduction

Primary breast lymphoma has a low rate of occurrence comprising an estimated 0.5% of breast malignancies [1, 2]. Even rarer are lymphomas associated with breast implants with the majority of the documented cases being T-cell lymphomas. Worldwide, over 500 cases of anaplastic large cell lymphoma associated with breast implants have been documented [3], including 4 cases of cutaneous T-cell lymphoma [1]. However, to date, only 5 cases of diffuse large B-cell lymphoma (DLBCL) associated with breast implants have been reported [1, 2, 4]. Because lymphomas associated with breast implants have been reported as well localized, implant removal and mass resection have proven to be satisfactory treatment. However, without many cases documented within the literature and without long-term outcome studies, it is difficult to know if additional treatments are required. In this case report, a patient with a newly diagnosed DLBCL is described. In the report, her clinical presentation, diagnostic studies, and outcome after surgery will be discussed.

2. Case Report

A 70-year-old female without significant past medical history presented to the clinic after the results of a routine mammogram revealed the continued presence of a small mass in her right breast. A mammogram dated 3 years prior detected this mass and reported it as small and benign, located inferior to an implant of her right breast. The more recent mammogram findings reported no change in size. The patient was asymptomatic and denied previous history of cancer and no family history of breast cancer, or other malignancies. She denied weight loss, fever, night sweats, or change in appetite. However, she did report mild discomfort with self-palpation to her lower right breast. Her breast implants were placed 28 years ago in Argentina for cosmetic reasons and have not since been revised. Additionally, she reported a long history of smoking tobacco daily.

To rule out malignancy, an ultrasound was performed and confirmed the presence of an elongated nodular density benign in appearance. The mass had multiple areas of

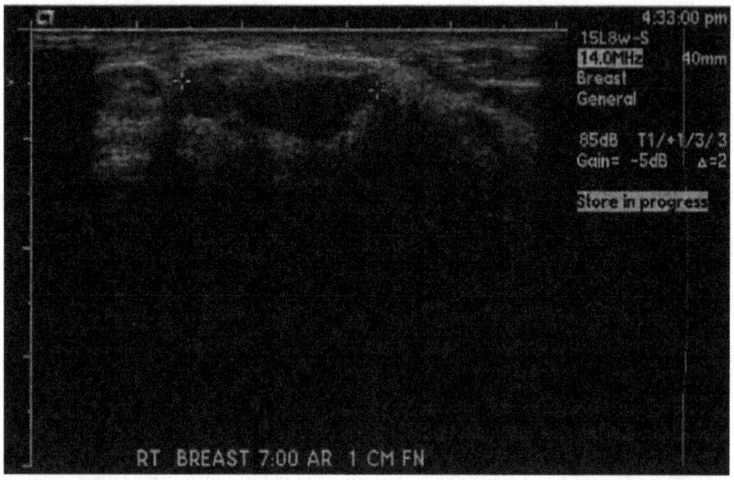

FIGURE 1: Ultrasound of the right breast before fine-needle biopsy shows a nodular density with multiple areas of hyperechoic densities within it.

hyperechoic densities within it and was located at the 8 o'clock position 10 cm from the right nipple. The size was measured to be 3.4 × 1.3 × 3.2 cm, with no evidence of shadowing or implant rupture reported (Figure 1). The impression of the ultrasound was the presence of a hamartoma, a benign lesion of the breast that corresponded with previous mammogram results. Despite recommendations for a follow-up mammogram at a later date, the patient was referred by her primary care provider for fine-needle biopsy and samples were sent for evaluation.

Biopsy samples were sent to pathology for analysis using histology, immunohistochemistry, and FISH studies. Histologic sections of the core biopsy fragments showed malignant lymphoma of diffuse pattern. The tumor cells were large in size with anaplastic and focally spindled morphology. Additionally, there were increased mitotic figures and cellular apoptosis. Immunohistochemistry revealed lymphoma cells positive for CD20, PAX5, BCL2, BCL6, and vimentin and negative for CD3, CD5, CD10, cyclin D1, smooth muscle myosin, S100, CD31, CD20, E-cadherin, and keratin. It was determined that the neoplasm had a nongerminal center phenotype with a proliferative index of 80-90%. FISH studies were completed to determine the presence of MYC, BCL2, or BCL6 gene rearrangements. All were negative; however, an abnormal signal pattern suggestive of gains of BCL2 was detected. Overall, testing of the fine-needle biopsy confirmed DLBCL.

The patient underwent surgery for lumpectomy of the right breast, as well as bilateral breast implant removal. During the operation, the presence of a calcified capsule surrounding each nontextured implant was noted. Found within the capsules was silicone. It was unclear if the nontextured implants had ruptured prior to surgery or if there was a rupture during the procedure. Both capsules were removed, and silicone was irrigated and aspirated from the sites. The tumor was found to be in direct contact with the calcified capsule but without evidence of capsule invasion into the tumor. The tumor was also widely excised with ample samples sent to pathology for further testing. The patient was given a one-time dose of cefazolin 1 gm IV and hydrocodone for pain management. She was discharged 2 days later with a complaint of moderate breast pain that was being managed well with hydrocodone.

Intraoperative tissue samples were sent to pathology. The breast lesion was noted to be well circumscribed and consisted of monomorphous cells with large lymphocytic features. No evidence of invasion from the calcified capsule was found. The cells had pleomorphic ovoid to round nuclei with occasional atypical mitotic figures. Atypical cells, as well as foamy macrophages, were present in the touch prep. Atypical lymphoid cells with anaplastic nuclear features were noted to infiltrate into collagenized-sclerotic stroma and at times adjacent fatty lobules. Immunohistochemistry was positive for CD45, BCL2, BCL6, CD43, CD79A, MUM1, and PAX5. Flow cytometry results, in addition to the histologic and immunohistochemistry staining, confirmed the diagnosis of DLBCL. The tumor was ultimately measured as 2.3 × 1.3 cm in maximal dimension, and the benign sclerotic capsule tissue provided evidence of the chronic rupture of implants.

The patient returned to the clinic 2 weeks after surgery and had well-healing scars without signs of infection. She returned again 6 months later and reported no pain at the surgical sites. Physical exam did not find any lymphadenopathy or mass with palpation. She continues to remain in good health.

3. Discussion

In this report, a rare case of DLBCL associated with breast implants is presented. The mass was first detected 3 years prior during routine mammogram. Findings reported the mass to be benign in appearance, which resulted in no additional work-up. Three years later, routine mammogram reported no change in size or appearance. While the patient continued to be asymptomatic, it was decided to order additional testing to rule out any potential malignancy.

Table 1: A listing of DLBCL diagnostic markers [4, 6].

Biomarker expression/genetic alterations	Percentage of cases
CD19, CD20, CD22, CD79A, CD45	Pan B-cell antigens, highly expressed
CD30	25% (anaplastic variant)
BCL2	25-80%
BCL6	70%
CD10	30-60%
MUM1/IRF4	35-65%
CD5	Uncommon, aggressive disease
(14;18) translocation	30%
MYC gene rearranged	5-15%

Fine-needle biopsy with ultrasound guidance was performed, and pathology results revealed the diagnosis of DLBCL.

DLBCL is a non-Hodgkin lymphoma (NHL). It is the most common type of lymphoid malignancy in adults and is B-cell in origin [1, 2]. In western countries, DLBCL accounts for 31% of NHLs [2]. While DLBCL does have a higher rate of occurrence in adults, its association with breast implants is extremely rare. With only 0.5% of breast malignancy being comprised of primary breast lymphomas [1], only 5 cases of DLBCL have been reported [1, 2, 4, 7]. The more frequent primary breast lymphoma is anaplastic large cell lymphoma (ALCL). This lymphoma is T-cell in origin, is associated most commonly with textured implants, and has been reported in over 500 cases worldwide [2, 3]. Regardless, both forms of primary breast lymphomas are rarely documented in the medical literature resulting in the pathogenesis being poorly understood.

NHLs are characterized by the abnormal growth of lymphocytes. In ALCL, the expression of T-cell markers CD4 and CD43 occurs in 82% and 77% of the cases, respectively [2]. Also present is a typical expression of CD30 and a characteristic horseshoe-shaped nucleus [2, 3]. While ALCL can be further divided into two groups based upon the presence of anaplastic lymphoma kinase (ALK), implant-associated ALCL is primarily ALK-negative [2, 3]. In contrast, DLBCL is heterogeneous in respect to morphology and biomarker expression. Based upon gene expression studies, DLBCL has been subdivided into separate molecular subtypes that arise at different stages of B-cell differentiation [5]. Although there is diversity in marker expression as outlined in Table 1, the more common diagnostic markers for DLBCL include BCL2, BCL6, c-MYC, and PAX5 [2, 5, 6]. With the detection of these cellular markers and the presence of specific morphologic changes, ALCL and DLBCL can be properly identified.

In this patient, the microscopy of the tissue samples from the fine-needle biopsy showed malignant lymphoma in a diffuse pattern. The tumor cells present were large in size and with an anaplastic morphology. DLBCL morphology can be diverse with variants that include centroblastic, immunoblastic, T-cell/histiocyte rich, or anaplastic [2]. To confirm the diagnosis, testing that included flow cytometry and immunohistochemistry of both the fine-needle biopsy and the intraoperative tissue samples was completed. Laboratory testing was consistently positive for CD45, BCL2, BCL6, CD43, CD79A, MUM1, and PAX5. All of these are markers that strongly correlate with DLBCL [2, 5, 7]. Further reinforcing the diagnosis was the lack of T-cell markers that would be present in ALCL. This included CD3 and CD5.

While DLBCL is an aggressive cancer and rapidly fatal if left untreated, DLBCL associated with breast implants has a far better prognosis and is often less aggressive. Nonbreast implant-associated DLBCL requires a treatment combination of cyclophosphamide, doxorubicin, vincristine, and prednisone (CHOP). Adding rituximab, a chimeric monoclonal antibody against CD20, has proven to increase survival rates [8]. Breast implant-associated DLBCL, if localized, requires no CHOP regimen. Instead, treatment is the complete resection of malignant tissue and removal of breast implants. If malignancy has invaded the lymph nodes, a treatment regimen should be considered.

In this case, a 70-year-old female with 28-year-old non-textured silicone breast implants developed a slow-growing mass in the right breast later identified as DLBCL. While symptomatology is dependent upon the severity of the disease, the common clinical presentation for DLBCL is breast swelling and tenderness. This patient was asymptomatic with benign mammogram findings. Because tumors associated with breast implants can be aggressive and are sometime associated with squamous cell tumors, additional testing was ordered that ultimately revealed the malignancy. Within 6 months from diagnosis, the patient underwent complete tumor resection and implant removal. There were no reported intraoperative or postoperative complications. Subsequent follow-up appointments at 2 weeks, 6 months, and 1 year were highly suggestive of a successful treatment as no new mass was noted and the patient remained asymptomatic.

References

[1] A. Messer, H. Jenkinson, W. Wang, and M. Duvic, "New B-cell lymphomas in the setting of a previous rare breast implant–associated B-cell lymphoma," *Plastic and Reconstruction Surgery*, vol. 4, no. 11, article e1148, 2016.

[2] A. Rupani, J. D. Frame, and D. Kamel, "Lymphomas associated with breast implants: a review of the literature," *Aesthetic Surgery Journal*, vol. 35, no. 5, pp. 533–544, 2015.

[3] F. Fitzal, S. Turner, and L. Kenner, "Is breast implant-associated anaplastic large cell lymphoma a hazard of breast implant surgery?," *Open Biology*, vol. 9, no. 4, article 190006, 2019.

[4] B. K. Smith and S. S. Gray, "Large B-cell lymphoma occurring in a breast implant capsule," *Plastic and Reconstructive Surgery*, vol. 134, no. 4, pp. 670e-671e, 2014.

[5] H. Nogai, B. Dorken, and G. Lenz, "Pathogenesis of non-Hodgkin's lymphoma," *Journal of Clinical Oncology*, vol. 29, no. 14, pp. 1803–1811, 2011.

[6] N. Johri, S. C. Patne, M. Tewari, and M. Kumar, "Diagnostic utility of PAX5 in Hodgkin and non-Hodgkin lymphoma: a study from northern India," *Journal of Clinical Diagnostic Research*, vol. 10, no. 8, pp. XC04–XC07, 2016.

[7] A. S. Freedman and J. C. Aster, *Epidemiology, clinical manifestations, pathologic features, and diagnosis of large B cell lymphoma*, UpToDate, 2018.

[8] B. Coiffier, E. Lepage, J. Brière et al., "CHOP chemotherapy plus rituximab compared with CHOP alone in elderly patients with diffuse large-B-cell lymphoma," *The New England Journal of Medicine*, vol. 346, no. 4, pp. 235–242, 2002.

8

An Exceptional Responder to Nivolumab in Metastatic Non-Small-Cell Lung Cancer: A Case Report and Literature Review of Long-Term Survivors

Babak Baseri,[1] **Bachar Samra**,[1] **Eric Tam**,[1] **Edwin Chiu**,[1] **and Andrea Leaf**[1,2]

[1]*Department of Hematology/Oncology, State University of New York Downstate Medical Center, Brooklyn, New York, USA*
[2]*Department of Hematology/Oncology, Veterans Affairs New York Harbor Healthcare System, Brooklyn Campus, New York, USA*

Correspondence should be addressed to Babak Baseri; bbaseri.82@gmail.com

Academic Editor: Constantine Gennatas

Background. Exceptional responders to immune checkpoint inhibitors in metastatic non-small-cell lung cancer (NSCLC) are rare. Furthermore, the optimal duration of immunotherapy in patients who achieve complete remission and the benefit of rechallenge after recurrence remain unknown. Studying the clinical course of exceptional responders can help identify potential predictors of response to immunotherapy and further fine-tune our management algorithms in the absence of standard of care in challenging scenarios. *Case Presentation.* We highlight the case of a 73 year old Vietnam War Veteran with active tobacco dependence who achieved complete response with nivolumab for metastatic NSCLC after four prior lines of chemotherapy. Nivolumab was discontinued after 10 cycles due to immune-mediated hepatitis that resolved with steroids. He remained in complete remission for 14 months while off therapy. Then, his tumor recurred twice locally in the mediastinum and he again achieved complete and durable responses after each recurrence with radiotherapy. Due to recurrence in both lungs one year later, he was rechallenged with nivolumab and achieved partial response after two months of therapy. He continues to do well five and a half years since his initial diagnosis of de novo metastatic NSCLC. *Conclusion.* Optimal management of exceptional responders to immune checkpoint inhibitors in metastatic NSCLC is largely unknown. Our case report adds to the limited data supporting the use of localized therapy for oligometastatic recurrences and rechallenge with immunotherapy for widespread disease in achieving disease control and long-term survival.

1. Introduction

The use of immune checkpoint inhibitors (ICI) in many malignancies including non-small-cell lung cancer (NSCLC) has revolutionized the field of oncology and has magnified the critical role of the immune system in fighting cancer [1, 2]. However, only a select group of patients derive clinically meaningful benefit from immunotherapy, ranging from improved quality of life to durable clinical responses, including rare complete remissions that may last many months even beyond immunotherapy discontinuation [3, 4]. The superior efficacy of immunotherapy in such exceptional responders has sparked an intense research interest in cancer immunobiology [1, 5]. Here, we describe the clinical course of a patient with heavily pretreated NSCLC who had an exceptional response to a short treatment course with nivolumab.

2. Case Presentation

A 73-year-old Vietnam War Veteran with active tobacco dependence ($1.5-2$ packs per day >50 years), prostate cancer in remission (status post definitive radiation in 2008), and alcoholic fatty liver disease was diagnosed in November 2013 with metastatic poorly differentiated lung adenocarcinoma of the left upper lobe (LUL) with biopsy-proven pleural and pericardial metastases after he presented with pneumonia and lung nodules. Molecular studies were negative for EGFR mutation and ALK rearrangement, and nondiagnostic for ROS-1.

He was started on chemotherapy in January 2014 and received five cycles of carboplatin, pemetrexed, and bevacizumab, followed by three cycles of maintenance pemetrexed and bevacizumab (see Figure 1 for therapy sequence). Due to progression of disease (PD) with new liver lesions, he was switched to second-line docetaxel and he completed six cycles. Although interim positron emission tomography/-computed tomography (PET/CT) showed stable disease, the patient developed a paraneoplastic syndrome of inappropriate antidiuretic hormone secretion (SIADH) during the sixth cycle, concerning for PD. Therapy was subsequently switched to erlotinib as third-line therapy. In the interim, the patient reported left shoulder pain that was attributed to a left apical lung tumor involving the pleura and was treated palliatively with RT (3000 cGy). Notably, hyponatremia resolved within one week of initiating RT, suggesting an abscopal effect given the high burden of disease outside of the radiation field. After three months of receiving erlotinib, PET/CT showed PD but the patient continued to have a good performance status. He was started on fourth-line therapy with vinorelbine and received a total of four cycles until he had recrudescence of SIADH. Imaging showed enlarging hepatic metastasis and left apical and hilar lung lesions, but no evidence of intracranial lesions. Thus, the decision was made to switch therapy to nivolumab (240 mg IV every two weeks) as fifth line. The patient received 10 cycles from August 2015 to January 2016 and his SIADH resolved after 2 months. Following four months of therapy, nivolumab was held due to grade II transaminitis, for which he was started on prednisone 100 mg daily and had a prolonged steroid taper (for six months). PET/CT following discontinuation of therapy showed no evidence of disease (NED). Nivolumab was not restarted as he was in complete remission, and it was deemed that the risks of nivolumab rechallenge outweighed its benefits. Repeat PET/CT scans (Figure 2) continued to show sustained complete remission, which lasted 14 months after discontinuation of nivolumab, until March 2017 when his tumor recurred in a 1.1 cm subcarinal node (biopsy proven, PDL-1 positive 80%; 22C3 pharmDX kit). Molecular studies showed RET rearrangement (10q11) in 84% of the cells (Leica BioSystems) and were negative for MET amplification and BRAF and HER2 mutations. Given local recurrence with very low disease burden, decision was made to treat the subcarinal node with RT (3000 cGy, 10 daily fractions of 300 cGy), with a resultant complete response. Nine months later, PET/CT showed a new hypermetabolic focus (SUV 8.7) in the right paratracheal lymph node (LN, 1.2 cm from 0.6 cm previously) and a new hypermetabolic focus (SUV 3.7) in the right middle paratracheal LN (0.7 cm). Given limited disease, RT was administered to the paratracheal LNs (3000 cGy), and complete response was again achieved until 12 months later, when his disease recurred in the lungs with new and growing bilateral subcentimeter nodules. He was rechallenged with nivolumab and has achieved a partial response after two months of therapy. He has no evidence of immune-mediated adverse events after 10 cycles. Of note, his SIADH has not recurred since the initial nivolumab therapy, and he continues to be asymptomatic with excellent performance status.

3. Discussion

Our case report highlights the oncologic management of a heavily pretreated patient with NSCLC who continues to be alive and well four years since his initial nivolumab treatment. The major benefit in the field of immunooncology in solid tumors, including lung cancer, has been the achievement of durable responses in a subset of patients receiving checkpoint inhibitors, with subsequent translation to longer survivals (Table 1). Most recently, the 5-year follow-up of nivolumab for pretreated advanced solid tumors (up to 5 prior lines of therapy) showed a 5-year overall survival (OS) rate of 16% across both squamous and nonsquamous NSCLC [6], compared with a historical 4% rate with traditional cytotoxic therapy [7]. Similarly, the 5-year OS rate for pembrolizumab was recently reported as 15.6% (previously treated) and 23.2% (frontline) in the Keynote 001 trial [8]. Furthermore, complete responses (CR) with ICIs are uncommon and have been reported in 1-6% of NSCLC (Table 1). A large meta-analysis of nine randomized clinical trials evaluating 4803 NSCLC patients treated with ICI reported the incidence of CR as 1.5% compared to 0.7% in chemotherapy groups [3], and found the use of ICIs as first line (relative risk (RR) 2.39, $P = 0.032$) or second line (RR 4.99, $P = 0.038$), and the use of nivolumab (RR 4.83, $P = 0.042$) and atezolizumab (RR 3.26, $P = 0.01$), but not pembrolizumab and ipilimumab, to be significantly associated with higher CR rates. However, no correlation was found between OS and CR ($r = 0.19$, $P = 0.75$). Limited data suggest that CRs may be more common in PDL-1-positive tumors and may be associated with the development of irAEs (Table 1) [9].

Predicting which patients will respond to checkpoint inhibitors is an evolving area of research. The current predictive markers of response to immunotherapy in NSCLC remain imperfect and can be divided into two main groups. The first group includes host and tumor/microenvironment factors that already exist prior to the initiation of immunotherapy. These factors include male gender [10], PDL-1 expression [11, 12], smoking status [13, 14], tumor mutation burden [15], microsatellite instability [16], presence or absence of CD8+ tumor-infiltrating lymphocytes (TILs) [11, 17], KRAS mutation or EGFR wild type [18], previous radiotherapy [19] or bevacizumab use [20], and baseline neutrophil-to-lymphocyte (NLR) ratio [21] and platelet-to-lymphocyte ratio [22]. The second group of predictors belongs to "evolving or developing" determinants that arise concurrently with immunotherapy treatment, which may be subject to exploitation by external factors. These predictive markers include but are not limited to change in gut microbiome [23], change in NLR [24] and lymphocyte-to-monocyte ratio [25], and immune-related adverse events (irAEs) [26, 27]. Based on current data, no new biomarkers have been identified in long-term survivors specifically. In the aforementioned nivolumab phase I CA209-003 trial [6], the majority of the long-term survivors were current smokers (14 out of 16 patients). In subgroup analysis, the 5-year OS rate was higher in patients with PDL-1 expression > 50% (43% vs. 20% in PDL-1 < 1, and 23% in PDL-1 ≥ 1%). Most

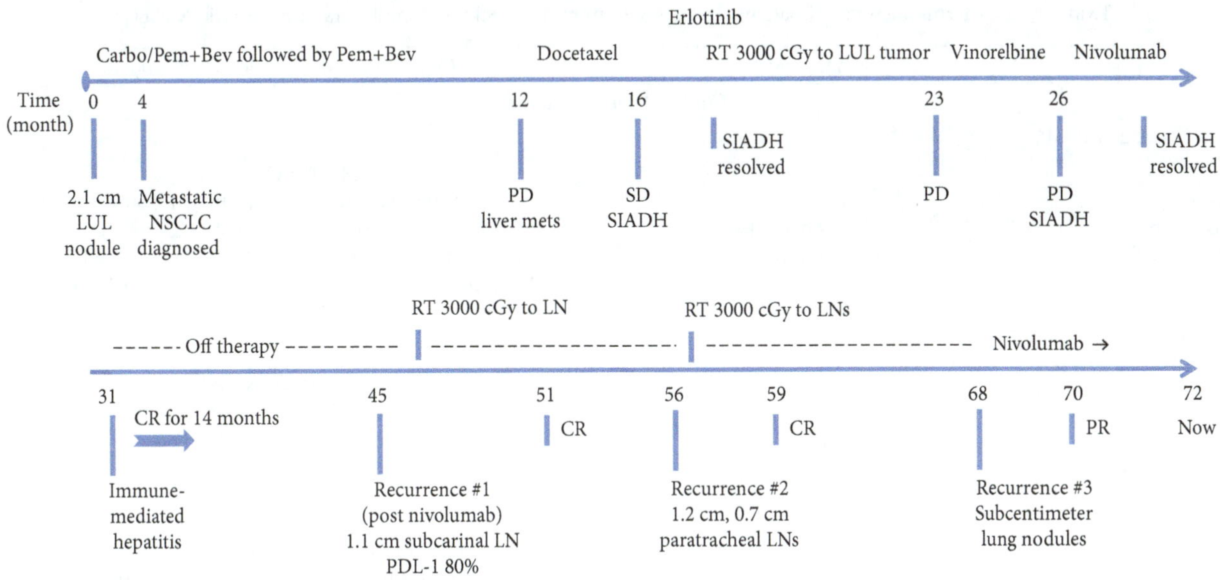

FIGURE 1: Treatment timeline. *The numbers below the axis represent the number of months since the initial presentation. Abbreviations: NSCLC—non-small-cell lung cancer; Carbo—carboplatin; Pem—pemetrexed; Bev—bevacizumab; LUL—left upper lobe of the lung; PD—progression of disease; SD—stable disease; CR—complete response; PR—partial response; LN—lymph node; PDL-1—programmed death ligand-1; SIADH—syndrome of inappropriate antidiuretic hormone secretion.

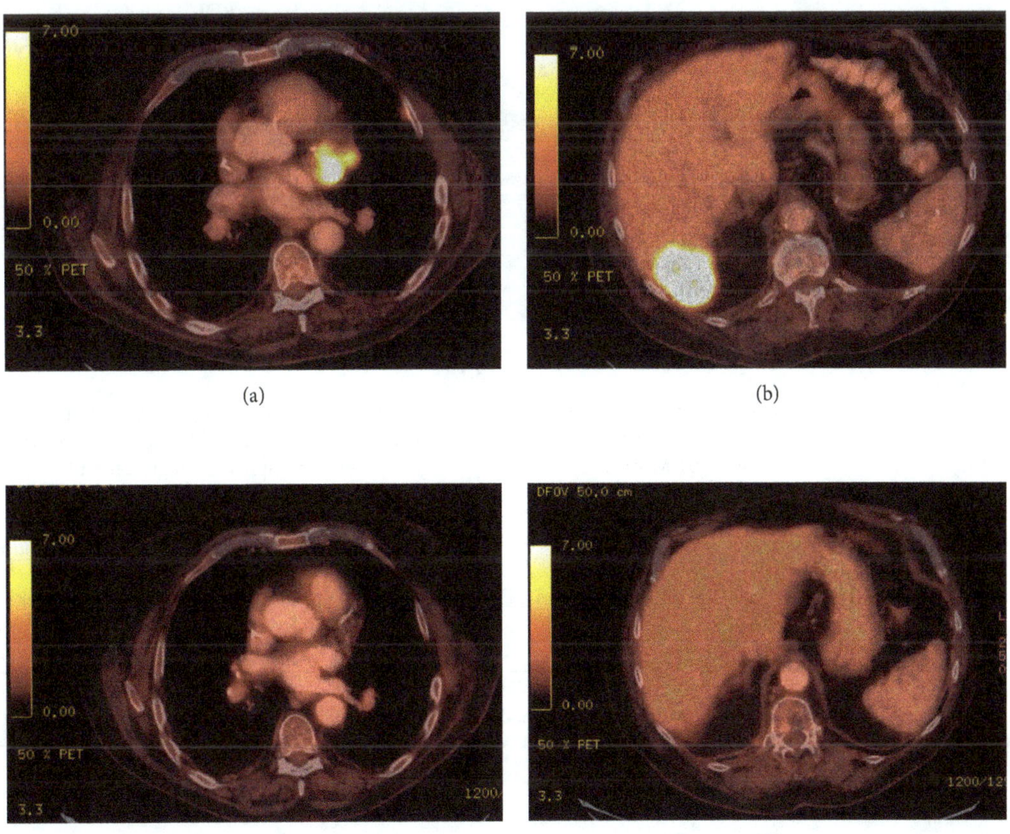

FIGURE 2: PET/CT images showing increased metabolic activity in the mediastinum (a) and in the liver (b) prior to initiating nivolumab. Resolution of FDG-avid lesions in the mediastinum (c) and in the liver (d) 10 months after discontinuation of nivolumab.

Table 1: Long-term outcomes of patients treated with immune checkpoint inhibitors in metastatic NSCLC.

	Characteristics	Outcomes and exceptional responders
	Clinical trials (5 yr data)	
Phase 1 (CA 209-003)		
Nivolumab 2nd line; Ref. [6]	129 patients Median follow-up: 58 m	Median OS 9.9 m 5-year OS 16% (43% for PDL-1 ≥ 50%) *For 5-year survivors:* 14/16 current or former smokers, 10/16 had received prior RT, 12/16 no further tx after stopping Nivo and without PD PDL-1 ≥ 1% in 7, ≥50% in 5, <1% in 3 pts
Phase Ib (Keynote 001)		
Pembrolizumab 1st line or later; Ref. [8]	101 tx naïve 449 previously treated Median follow-up: 60.6 m	*Treatment naïve:* Median DOR 16.8 m; CR 3% (3 patients) Median OS 22.3 m 5-year OS 23.2% (29.6% for PDL-1 ≥ 50%) *Previously treated:* Median DOR 38.9 m; CR 1.1% (5 patients) Median OS 10.5 m (15.5 m for PDL-1 ≥ 50%) 5-year OS 15.6% (25% for PDL-1 ≥ 50%)
	Clinical trials (3 yr data)	
Phase III (CheckMate 017, 057)		
Nivolumab vs. Doc 2nd line; Ref. [35]	854 patients Median follow-up: 40.3 m	Median DOR 23.8 m CR 6% for those alive at 3 years 3-year OS: 17% (vs. 8% Doc), 8% (vs. 2%) for patients with liver metastases
Phase III (Keynote 010)		
Pembrolizumab vs. Doc 2nd line or later; Ref. [49]	1033 patients Median follow-up: 42.6 m	PDL-1 ≥ 50%: Median OS 16.9 m (vs. 8.2 m Doc) 3-year OS: 35% (vs. 13% Doc) PDL-1 ≥ 1-49%: Median OS 11.8 m (vs. 8.4 m Doc) 3-year OS: 23% (vs. 11% Doc)
Phase II (POPLAR)		
Atezolizumab vs. Doc 2nd line; Ref. [50]	287 patients Minimum 3-year follow-up	Median DOR: 22.3 m (vs. 7.2 m docetaxel) 3-year OS: ITT 16.6% (vs. 10% docetaxel) IHC TC3 or IC3 37.5% (vs. 14.9%) IHC TC 2/3 or IC 2/3 21.2% (vs. 9.9%)
	Case reports	
Nivolumab 3rd line; Ref. [28]	67 male; squamous cell ca PDL-1 TPS > 50% TMB 87-91 Mut/Mb	Nivolumab-induced pneumonitis after 3 doses; following discontinuation of the drug, the patient continued to have complete remission for 14 months
Nivolumab 2nd line; Ref. [29]	80 male; squamous cell ca RT (3 months prior to Nivo) PDL-1 positive > 5%	Radiation-induced pneumonitis CR after 6 cycles, ongoing after 2 years of continuous nivolumab
Nivolumab 2nd line; Ref. [31]	47 male; adenocarcinoma Current smoker SBRT to LNs while on Nivo	PR after 6 cycles; CR after 13 cycles (10 weeks after RT) Nivo discontinued after cycle 17 due to pancreatitis; still in CR almost 2 years since discontinuation

Abbreviations: OS—overall survival; m—months; tx—treatment; DOR—duration of response; CR—complete response; PD—progressive disease; ITT—intention to treat; Nivo—nivolumab; doc—docetaxel; LN—lymph node; ca—carcinoma; NSCLC—non-small-cell lung cancer; RT—radiotherapy; SBRT—stereotactic body radiation therapy; IHC—immunohistochemistry; TC—tumor cells; IC—tumor-infiltrating immune cells; Mut/Mb—mutations per megabase; PDL-1—programmed death ligand-1.

interestingly, 75% of the long-term survivors received nivolumab for no more than two years, required no further cancer therapy afterwards, and remained without disease progression as of their last follow-up visit (median follow-up of 58 months). Majority of this cohort (75%) had partial response as their best response, and none had a CR.

Case reports of exceptional responders to ICI in NSCLC are rare and possibly underreported (Table 1) [28–33]. Our case is unique in several aspects. First, it is a real-world scenario of an exceptional responder to immunotherapy outside of a clinical trial. Second, our patient has been diagnosed with metastatic lung cancer more than 5.5 years and continues to do well with very limited disease burden following eight lines of therapy, including RT. Third, he exhibited many of the predictive markers mentioned above, including high PDL-1 expression (80%), smoking history, prior RT and bevacizumab use, and development of immune-mediated hepatitis requiring nivolumab to be held. Although he continues to smoke daily, it currently remains unclear if active smoking has any role in potentiating response to ICI. Interestingly, unlike what is reported in the literature on poor responses to ICI in liver metastasis [34], our patient had a CR to nivolumab and his disease never recurred in his liver despite having a relatively large liver metastasis (Figure 2), possibly due to the activation of the immune system that resulted in hepatitis. Notably, in phase III CheckMate 017 and 057 trials, nivolumab resulted in improved OS compared with docetaxel in patients with liver metastases, and their immune-mediated hepatic adverse events were higher than the overall pooled population (10% vs. 6%) [35]. Fourth, the clinical course following nivolumab discontinuation is interesting as he achieved CR lasting 14 months after a short course of nivolumab. Notably, the prolonged course of steroid taper for his hepatitis did not affect his duration of response nor did it affect his second response to nivolumab upon rechallenge. Ongoing responses following discontinuation of immunotherapy is a well-known phenomenon and has been documented in clinical trials, including the nivolumab trial above [6, 36]. Fifth, he was noted to have a RET rearrangement on repeat biopsy. In contrast to our case, a recent case series by Offin et al. [37] showed that majority of RET-rearranged lung cancers have low PDL-1 expression and low TMB, and exhibit poor responses to ICIs. However, only one patient in that series had PDL-1 expression > 50%, and hence no conclusions as to how to sequence targeted therapies in such patients can be drawn. In an ongoing global registry (IMMUNOTARGET), it was noted that ICI efficacy in oncogenic-driven lung cancers is inconsistent and depends on smoking history, PDL-1 expression, and the type of mutation (less benefit in RET/EGFR/ALK patients) [38]. In our case, we did not use a RET inhibitor as the patient's cancer recurrences were mostly localized, and it was thought that radiotherapy would provide the best local control with potential for greater disease-free and treatment-free intervals. Upon his last relapse, immunotherapy rechallenge was also more appealing given the patient's initial complete durable response and high PDL-1 expression. As expected, his local disease recurrences were successfully treated with radiation therapy, with responses lasting 9 and 12 months after each RT. Finally, rechallenge with nivolumab following his third tumor recurrence resulted in rapid partial response after four cycles. In the future, we plan to use a RET inhibitor as the next line of therapy once he progresses on nivolumab.

Optimal duration of immunotherapy in responders remains unclear and is an area of active investigation. A randomized trial of continuous (76 patients) vs. 1-year fixed duration (87 patients) nivolumab in advanced NSCLC (CheckMate 153, $n = 220$) showed significant improvement in progression-free survival (hazard ratio (HR) 0.42, 95% confidence interval (CI): 0.25, 0.71) and a trend towards better OS (HR 0.63, 95% CI: 0.33, 1.20) favoring the continuous nivolumab arm [39]. However, it should be noted that the continuous arm had a higher percentage of PDL-1 expression > 50% (28% vs. 23%) and higher rates of CR (10% vs. 2%) at baseline (1-year randomization mark) compared to the 1-year fixed duration arm. Notably, two patients who achieved CR in the 1-year treatment arm recurred 6 and 13 months after stopping treatment. Retreatment with nivolumab after disease progression while off therapy resulted in response in the majority of patients, although the duration of response to the rechallenge was short for those with early progression (<6 months) [39].

Immune-related adverse events are major causes of ICI interruption or discontinuation, complicating the subsequent management of patients, particularly those who have achieved durable clinical benefit. irAEs have been generally associated with better ICI efficacy as well as increased overall survival [26, 27, 40]. Although the optimal oncologic management of patients who discontinue therapy due to irAEs is unknown, current data [6, 28], including our case report, suggest that patients who achieve a CR are more likely to have prolonged duration of response off therapy. Whether resuming immunotherapy (if prior irAE grade ≤ 2) or adding chemotherapy in the absence of measurable metastatic disease further extends duration of response or even achieves the ultimate goal of cure is currently unknown. Limited data at this time suggest that it may be reasonable to rechallenge patients with immunotherapy upon recurrence [6, 33, 41–44], or treat oligometastatic recurrences with surgery or radiation therapy, with lower threshold to initiate systemic therapy following multiple recurrences or in those with higher burden of disease [6]. Furthermore, increased use of liquid biopsies (such as circulating tumor DNA) [45, 46], tumor markers (such as CEA, CA125) [47, 48], and blood parameters (such as NLR) [46] as biomarkers of response or relapse in ICI-treated patients will further identify early responders, discern CRs from occult disease, and guide therapy in patients with early progression.

4. Conclusion

Exceptional responders to immune checkpoint inhibitors are uncommon in metastatic NSCLC. Additionally, the optimal duration of immunotherapy in patients who achieve complete remission remains unknown. Our case report adds to the limited data in the management of exceptional responders following discontinuation of immunotherapy. Treatment of oligometastatic recurrences with localized therapy and rechallenge with immunotherapy may increase disease control and extend overall survival. Further understanding of tumor microenvironment and tumor/immune system interactions may help identify better predictors of response and further improve patients' outcomes.

References

[1] D. B. Doroshow, M. F. Sanmamed, K. Hastings et al., "Immunotherapy in non–small cell lung cancer: facts and hopes," *Clinical Cancer Research*, vol. 25, no. 15, pp. 4592–4602, 2019.

[2] J. Remon, M. J. Ahn, N. Girard et al., "Advanced-stage non-small cell lung cancer: advances in thoracic oncology 2018," *Journal of Thoracic Oncology*, vol. 14, no. 7, pp. 1134–1155, 2019.

[3] J. Li, Q. He, X. Yu, K. Khan, X. Weng, and M. Guan, "Complete response associated with immune checkpoint inhibitors in advanced non-small-cell lung cancer: a meta-analysis of nine randomized controlled trials," *Cancer Management and Research*, vol. 11, pp. 1623–1629, 2019.

[4] R. Chen, X. Hou, L. Yang, and D. Zhao, "Comparative efficacy and safety of first-line treatments for advanced non-small cell lung cancer with immune checkpoint inhibitors: a systematic review and meta-analysis," *Thoracic Cancer*, vol. 10, no. 4, pp. 607–623, 2019.

[5] A. Anichini, E. Tassi, G. Grazia, and R. Mortarini, "The non-small cell lung cancer immune landscape: emerging complexity, prognostic relevance and prospective significance in the context of immunotherapy," *Cancer Immunology, Immunotherapy*, vol. 67, no. 6, pp. 1011–1022, 2018.

[6] S. Gettinger, L. Horn, D. Jackman et al., "Five-year follow-up of nivolumab in previously treated advanced non-small-cell lung cancer: results from the CA209-003 study," *Journal of Clinical Oncology*, vol. 36, no. 17, pp. 1675–1684, 2018.

[7] K. Cetin, D. S. Ettinger, Y. J. Hei, and C. D. O'Malley, "Survival by histologic subtype in stage IV nonsmall cell lung cancer based on data from the surveillance, epidemiology and end results program," *Clinical Epidemiology*, vol. 3, pp. 139–148, 2011.

[8] E. B. Garon, M. D. Hellmann, N. A. Rizvi et al., "Five-year overall survival for patients with advanced non–small-cell lung cancer treated with pembrolizumab: results from the phase I KEYNOTE-001 study," *Journal of Clinical Oncology*, vol. 37, no. 28, pp. 2518–2527, 2019.

[9] E. Nadal, B. Massuti, M. Domine, R. Garcia-Campelo, M. Cobo, and E. Felip, "Immunotherapy with checkpoint inhibitors in non-small cell lung cancer: insights from long-term survivors," *Cancer Immunology, Immunotherapy*, vol. 68, no. 3, pp. 341–352, 2019.

[10] H. El-Osta and S. Jafri, "Predictors for clinical benefit of immune checkpoint inhibitors in advanced non-small-cell lung cancer: a meta-analysis," *Immunotherapy*, vol. 11, no. 3, pp. 189–199, 2019.

[11] R. S. Herbst, J. C. Soria, M. Kowanetz et al., "Predictive correlates of response to the anti-PD-L1 antibody MPDL3280A in cancer patients," *Nature*, vol. 515, no. 7528, pp. 563–567, 2014.

[12] J. Kim, J. Cho, M. H. Lee, and J. H. Lim, "Relative Efficacy of Checkpoint Inhibitors for Advanced NSCLC According to Programmed Death-Ligand-1 Expression: A Systematic Review and Network Meta- Analysis," *Scientific Reports*, vol. 8, no. 1, article 11738, 2018.

[13] E. B. Garon, N. A. Rizvi, R. Hui et al., "Pembrolizumab for the treatment of non-small-cell lung cancer," *The New England Journal of Medicine*, vol. 372, no. 21, pp. 2018–2028, 2015.

[14] H. Borghaei, L. Paz-Ares, L. Horn et al., "Nivolumab versus docetaxel in advanced nonsquamous non-small-cell lung cancer," *The New England Journal of Medicine*, vol. 373, no. 17, pp. 1627–1639, 2015.

[15] N. A. Rizvi, M. D. Hellmann, A. Snyder et al., "Cancer immunology. Mutational landscape determines sensitivity to PD-1 blockade in non-small cell lung cancer," *Science*, vol. 348, no. 6230, pp. 124–128, 2015.

[16] D. T. Le, J. N. Uram, H. Wang et al., "PD-1 blockade in tumors with mismatch-repair deficiency," *The New England Journal of Medicine*, vol. 372, no. 26, pp. 2509–2520, 2015.

[17] P. C. Tumeh, C. L. Harview, J. H. Yearley et al., "PD-1 blockade induces responses by inhibiting adaptive immune resistance," *Nature*, vol. 515, no. 7528, pp. 568–571, 2014.

[18] Q. Huang, H. Zhang, J. Hai et al., "Impact of PD-L1 expression, driver mutations and clinical characteristics on survival after anti-PD-1/PD-L1 immunotherapy versus chemotherapy in non-small-cell lung cancer: a meta-analysis of randomized trials," *Oncoimmunology*, vol. 7, no. 12, article e1396403, 2018.

[19] N. Shaverdian, A. E. Lisberg, K. Bornazyan et al., "Previous radiotherapy and the clinical activity and toxicity of pembrolizumab in the treatment of non-small-cell lung cancer: a secondary analysis of the KEYNOTE-001 phase 1 trial," *The Lancet Oncology*, vol. 18, no. 7, pp. 895–903, 2017.

[20] R. Giannicola, G. D'arrigo, P. Pastina et al., "Correlation of survival of NSCLC patients given nivolumab with treatment related-eosinophilia, autoimmunity and previous bevacizumab containing regimens," *Journal of Clinical Oncology*, vol. 36, article e21008, Supplement 15, 2018.

[21] S. J. Bagley, S. Kothari, C. Aggarwal et al., "Pretreatment neutrophil-to-lymphocyte ratio as a marker of outcomes in nivolumab-treated patients with advanced non-small-cell lung cancer," *Lung Cancer*, vol. 106, pp. 1–7, 2017.

[22] S. Diem, S. Schmid, M. Krapf et al., "Neutrophil-to-lymphocyte ratio (NLR) and platelet-to-lymphocyte ratio (PLR) as prognostic markers in patients with non-small cell lung cancer (NSCLC) treated with nivolumab," *Lung Cancer*, vol. 111, pp. 176–181, 2017.

[23] B. Routy, E. Le Chatelier, L. Derosa et al., "Gut microbiome influences efficacy of PD-1–based immunotherapy against epithelial tumors," *Science*, vol. 359, no. 6371, pp. 91–97, 2018.

[24] T. Kiriu, M. Yamamoto, T. Nagano et al., "The time-series behavior of neutrophil-to-lymphocyte ratio is useful as a predictive marker in non-small cell lung cancer," *PLoS One*, vol. 13, no. 2, article e0193018, 2018.

[25] K. Sekine, S. Kanda, Y. Goto et al., "Change in the lymphocyte-to-monocyte ratio is an early surrogate marker of the efficacy of nivolumab monotherapy in advanced non-small-cell lung cancer," *Lung Cancer*, vol. 124, pp. 179–188, 2018.

[26] A. Cortellini, R. Chiari, B. Ricciuti et al., "Correlations between the immune-related adverse events spectrum and efficacy of anti-PD1 immunotherapy in NSCLC patients," *Clinical Lung Cancer*, vol. 20, no. 4, pp. 237–247.e1, 2019.

[27] K. Haratani, H. Hayashi, Y. Chiba et al., "Association of immune-related adverse events with nivolumab efficacy in non-small-cell lung cancer," *JAMA Oncology*, vol. 4, no. 3, pp. 374–378, 2018.

[28] H. Li, W. Ma, K. Y. Yoneda et al., "Severe nivolumab-induced pneumonitis preceding durable clinical remission in a patient with refractory, metastatic lung squamous cell cancer: a case report," *Journal of Hematology & Oncology*, vol. 10, no. 1, p. 64, 2017.

[29] G. Lazzari, A. Terlizzi, G. Porrazzo et al., "Effective nivolumab sequential thoracic radiotherapy in elderly patients with

advanced squamous cell lung cancer: did radiation therapy play a role? A case report," *OncoTargets and Therapy*, vol. 11, pp. 4621–4629, 2018.

[30] D. Keohane and G. P. Fitzgerald, "The changing face of cancer treatments," *BMJ Case Reports*, 2018, bcr-2018-224784.

[31] C. Britschgi, O. Riesterer, I. A. Burger, M. Guckenberger, and A. Curioni-Fontecedro, "Report of an abscopal effect induced by stereotactic body radiotherapy and nivolumab in a patient with metastatic non-small cell lung cancer," *Radiation Oncology*, vol. 13, no. 1, p. 102, 2018.

[32] B. McCullar, T. Alloway, and M. Martin, "Durable complete response to nivolumab in a patient with HIV and metastatic non-small cell lung cancer," *Journal of Thoracic Disease*, vol. 9, no. 6, pp. E540–E542, 2017.

[33] R. Tay, A. Prelaj, and R. Califano, "Immune checkpoint blockade for advanced non-small cell lung cancer: challenging clinical scenarios," *Journal of Thoracic Disease*, vol. 10, Supplement 13, pp. S1494–S1502, 2018.

[34] P. C. Tumeh, M. D. Hellmann, O. Hamid et al., "Liver metastasis and treatment outcome with anti-PD-1 monoclonal antibody in patients with melanoma and NSCLC," *Cancer Immunology Research*, vol. 5, no. 5, pp. 417–424, 2017.

[35] E. E. Vokes, N. Ready, E. Felip et al., "Nivolumab versus docetaxel in previously treated advanced non-small-cell lung cancer (CheckMate 017 and CheckMate 057): 3-year update and outcomes in patients with liver metastases," *Annals of Oncology*, vol. 29, no. 4, pp. 959–965, 2018.

[36] L. Horn, D. R. Spigel, E. E. Vokes et al., "Nivolumab versus docetaxel in previously treated patients with advanced non-small-cell lung cancer: two-year outcomes from two random ized, open-label, phase III trials (CheckMate 017 and CheckMate 057)," *Journal of Clinical Oncology*, vol. 35, no. 35, pp. 3924–3933, 2017.

[37] M. Offin, R. Guo, S. L. Wu et al., "Immunophenotype and response to immunotherapy ofRET-Rearranged lung cancers," *JCO Precision Oncology*, vol. 3, no. 3, pp. 1–8, 2019.

[38] J. Mazieres, A. E. Drilon, L. Mhanna et al., "Efficacy of immune-checkpoint inhibitors (ICI) in non-small cell lung cancer (NSCLC) patients harboring activating molecular alterations (ImmunoTarget)," *Journal of Clinical Oncology*, vol. 36, Supplement 15, p. 9010, 2018.

[39] D. R. Spigel, M. Mcleod, M. A. Hussein et al., "1297ORandomized results of fixed-duration (1-yr) vs continuous nivolumab in patients (pts) with advanced non-small cell lung cancer (NSCLC)," *Annals of Oncology*, vol. 28, Supplement 5, 2017.

[40] A. Qin, L. Street, K. Cease et al., "Clinical determinants of durable clinical benefit of pembrolizumab in veterans with advanced non-small-cell lung cancer," *Clinical Lung Cancer*, vol. 18, no. 5, pp. 559–564, 2017.

[41] A. Bernard-Tessier, C. Baldini, P. Martin et al., "Outcomes of long-term responders to anti-programmed death 1 and anti-programmed death ligand 1 when being rechallenged with the same anti-programmed death 1 and anti-programmed death ligand 1 at progression," *European Journal of Cancer*, vol. 101, pp. 160–164, 2018.

[42] L. Horn, S. N. Gettinger, M. S. Gordon et al., "Safety and clinical activity of atezolizumab monotherapy in metastatic non- small-cell lung cancer: final results from a phase I study," *European Journal of Cancer*, vol. 101, pp. 201–209, 2018.

[43] K. Fujita, N. Uchida, O. Kanai, M. Okamura, K. Nakatani, and T. Mio, "Retreatment with pembrolizumab in advanced non-small cell lung cancer patients previously treated with nivolumab: emerging reports of 12 cases," *Cancer Chemotherapy and Pharmacology*, vol. 81, no. 6, pp. 1105–1109, 2018.

[44] K. Fujita, N. Uchida, Y. Yamamoto et al., "Retreatment with anti-PD-L1 antibody in advanced non-small cell lung cancer previously treated with anti-PD-1 antibodies," *Anticancer Research*, vol. 39, no. 7, pp. 3917-3921, 2019.

[45] P. Hofman, S. Heeke, C. Alix-Panabieres, and K. Pantel, "Liquid biopsy in the era of immuno-oncology: Is it ready for prime-time use for cancer patients?," *Annals of Oncology*, vol. 30, no. 9, pp. 1448–1459, 2019.

[46] F. Passiglia, A. Galvano, M. Castiglia et al., "Monitoring blood biomarkers to predict nivolumab effectiveness in NSCLC patients," *Therapeutic Advances in Medical Oncology*, vol. 11, 2019.

[47] M. G. Dal Bello, R. A. Filiberti, A. Alama et al., "The role of CEA, CYFRA21-1 and NSE in monitoring tumor response to Nivolumab in advanced non-small cell lung cancer (NSCLC) patients," *Journal of Translational Medicine*, vol. 17, no. 1, p. 74, 2019.

[48] M. Zhuo, H. Chen, T. Zhang et al., "The potential predictive value of circulating immune cell ratio and tumor marker in atezolizumab treated advanced non-small cell lung cancer patients," *Cancer Biomarkers*, vol. 22, no. 3, pp. 467–476, 2018.

[49] R. S. Herbst, E. B. Garon, D. W. Kim et al., "Long-term survival in patients (pts) with advanced NSCLC in the KEYNOTE-010 study overall and in pts who completed two years of pembrolizumab (pembro)," in *European Society for Medical Oncology*, Munich, Germany, October 2018.

[50] J. Mazières, K. Park, C. Lewanski et al., "136PD_PR 3-year survival and duration of response in randomized phase II study of atezolizumab (atezo) vs docetaxel (doc) in 2L+ NSCLC (POPLAR)," *Journal of Thoracic Oncology*, vol. 13, no. 4, p. S79, 2018.

9

Spontaneous Bilateral Hemothorax as a Case of Epithelioid Hemangioendothelioma (EHE)

Essa M. AlGhunaim,[1] **Hafsa AlNajem**,[2] **and Derar S. AlShehab**[1]

[1]*Thoracic and Foregut Surgery Unit, Chest Diseases Hospital, Kuwait*
[2]*General Surgery Department, Mubarak Al-Kabeer Hospital, Kuwait*

Correspondence should be addressed to Essa M. AlGhunaim; ealghunaim@thoracickuwait.org

Academic Editor: Constantine Gennatas

Epithelioid hemangioendothelioma (EHE) is a rare tumor that is vascular in origin, arising from the endothelial or preendothelial cells. It can occur at different sites of the body, commonly in the liver, lungs, and bone. Pulmonary EHE is usually symptomatic, sometimes presenting with a cough, dyspnea, or chest pain. Rarely, it presents with pleural effusion. Here, we are presenting a case of pleural epithelioid hemangioendothelioma presenting as a case of spontaneous bilateral hemothorax.

1. Introduction

Epithelioid hemangioendothelioma (EHE) is a rare vascular tumor of endothelial or preendothelial cell origin, and it represents less than 1% of all vascular tumors. EHE affects various sites of the body, but it typically affects the lungs and liver [1]. The presentations or manifestations of EHE are unspecific, and they vary according to the affected site. In this paper, we present a case of pleural EHE, which presented with bilateral spontaneous hemothorax. This case of EHE is reported due to its rare clinical presentation.

2. Case Report

A 49-year-old male, a smoker of 15 packs/year, previously healthy, presented with a ten-day history of a sudden cough, associated with shortness of breath and left-sided chest pain. The patient also gave a history of loss of appetite and weight loss of about 15 kilograms for the past three months. On admission, his blood test revealed a drop in hemoglobin from 14.3 g/dL to 8.6 g/dL. The chest X-ray on admission showed bilateral lung opacity (Figure 1), and pleural tapping was done, which revealed a bloody content. Thoracic surgery service was consulted to evaluate the hemothorax.

A CT scan of the chest with IV contrast was done, and it showed massive bilateral hemothorax, more on the left side causing lung collapse, but no evidence of contrast extravasations (Figures 2–5). Immediately, a chest tube (size: 28 Fr) was inserted in the left side, which yielded around 1000 mL of blood (Figure 6). The following day, the patient condition remained the same, and he was still complaining of shortness of breath and tachycardia. Thus, the patient was shifted under the care of thoracic surgery. A second chest tube (28 Fr) was inserted on the left side, and a pigtail was inserted on the right side. The right-sided pigtail yielded about 2700 mL of dark-colored blood. After the insertion of the previously mentioned tubes, the patient condition improved significantly, and the patient was stabilized. The following day, the patient underwent video-assisted thoracoscopy (VATS) pleural exploration and biopsy; it showed a nodular pleura and normal-looking lungs. Multiple biopsies were taken from the pleura and were sent for histopathology testing.

3. Pathological Findings

Histopathological examination of the pleural biopsies revealed extensive infiltration of the pleura by atypical epithelioid cells arranged in clusters, in strands, or lying

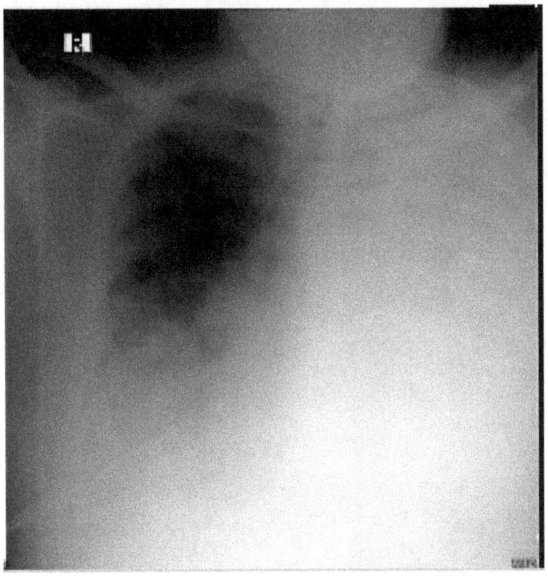

FIGURE 1: CXR of the case on admission showing the white out lung on the left side giving the impression of massive pleural effusion.

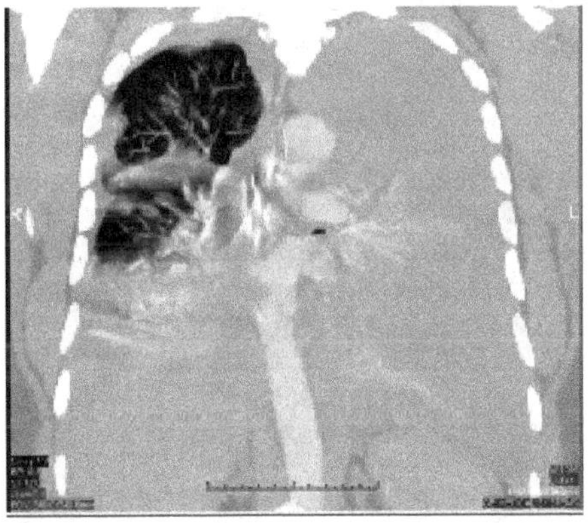

FIGURE 2: Initial CT chest of the patient (coronal view) with complete obliteration of the left hemithorax and some lung parenchyma seen in the right hemothorax. Hounsfield units were consistent with hemorrhagic effusion.

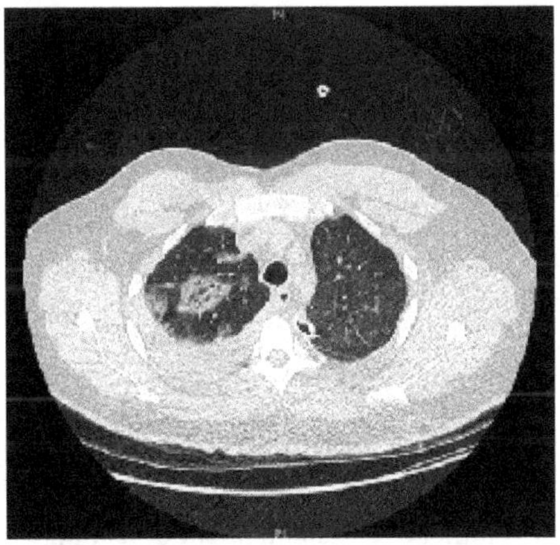

FIGURE 3: CT chest of the patient (axial view) showing the position of the chest tube and location of hemothorax.

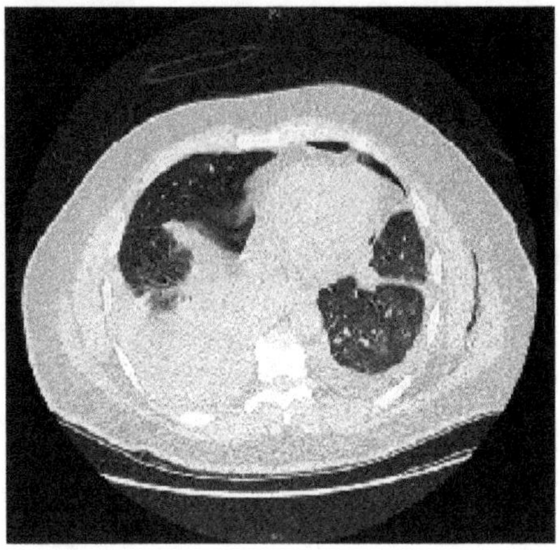

FIGURE 4: CT chest of the patient (axial view) showing the position of the chest tube and location of hemothorax.

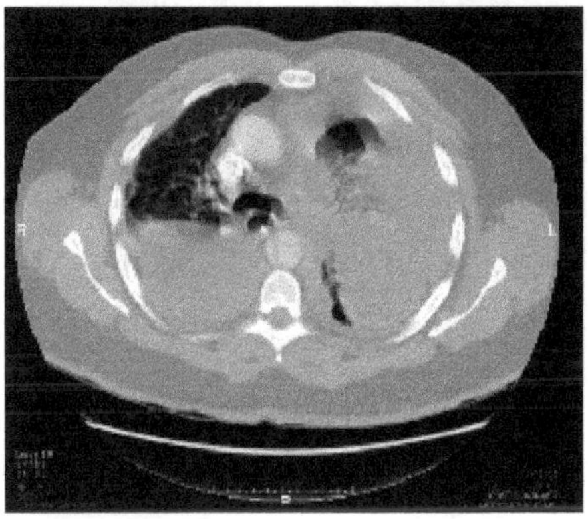

FIGURE 5: Another image of the CT chest (axial) in the lower chest showing cuts with massive hemothorax.

individually (Figures 7 and 8). The cells exhibit nuclear pleomorphism, mitosis, and intracytoplasmic vacuoles. There are irregular vascular channels lined by these atypical cells (Figure 9). The immunohistochemical stain showed positivity for CD34 and CD31 (Figure 10) but was negative for CK7, CK20, calretinin, TTF1, and napsin. It was consistent with epithelioid hemangioendothelioma.

The case was discussed in a multidisciplinary meeting, and the consensus is to start him on chemotherapy.

4. Discussion

Epithelioid hemangioendothelioma (EHE) is a rare vascular tumor of endothelial cell origin, with an estimated prevalence of less than one in 1 million [1, 2]. It was first described in 1975 by Dail and Liebow as an aggressive bronchoalveolar cell carcinoma [1]. EHE can involve a single organ or multiple organs simultaneously. The most commonly affected organs in EHE were the liver, lung, and bone. According to the observation and data analysis of Epithelioid Hemangioendothelioma and Related Vascular Disorders (HEARD) Support Group, the most common presentations for EHE were the liver alone

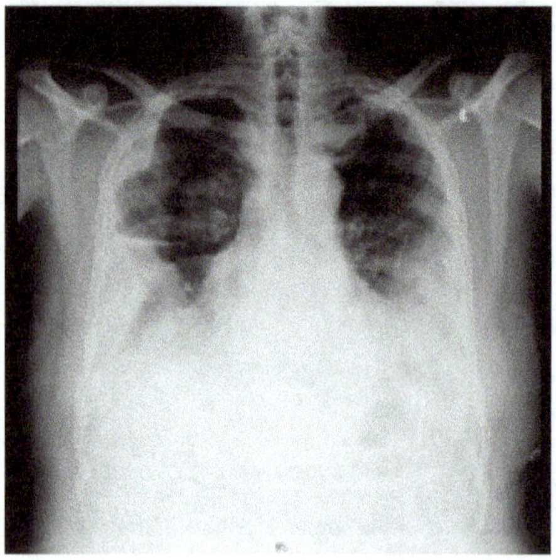

FIGURE 6: CXR postdrainage of hemothorax with abnormal pleura.

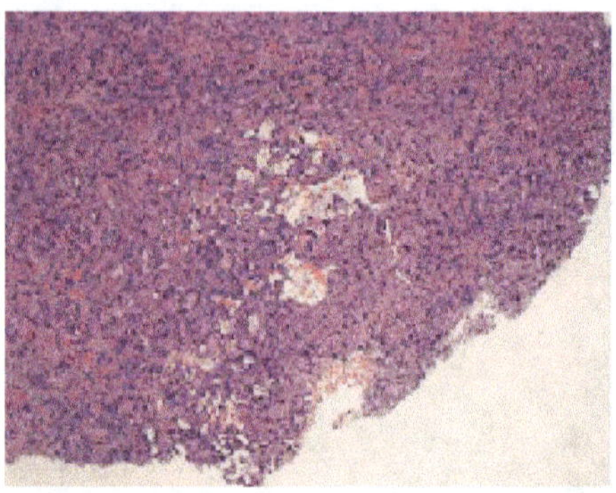

FIGURE 7: Histological photograph of the pleural specimen shows a pleural intraparenchymal tumor with focal irregular vascular spaces (H&E × 40x).

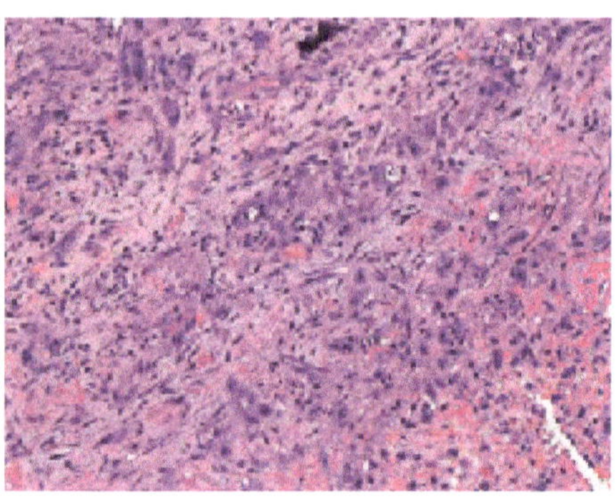

FIGURE 8: Cords and nests of epithelioid endothelial cells: some with intracytoplasmic vacuoles infiltrate the fibrous tissue (H&E × 100x).

(21%), liver plus lung (18%), lung alone (12%), and bone alone (14%) [3].

Histologically, the tumor is composed of small nests or short cords of rounded to slightly spindled endothelial cells that blend. A typical finding seen in immunohistochemistry is Weibel-Palade bodies seen in the cytoplasm of the endothelial cells [1]. In EHE, immunohistochemical stains for vascular endothelial markers are usually positive for CD31 and CD34 and negative for epithelial markers, like cytokines [4].

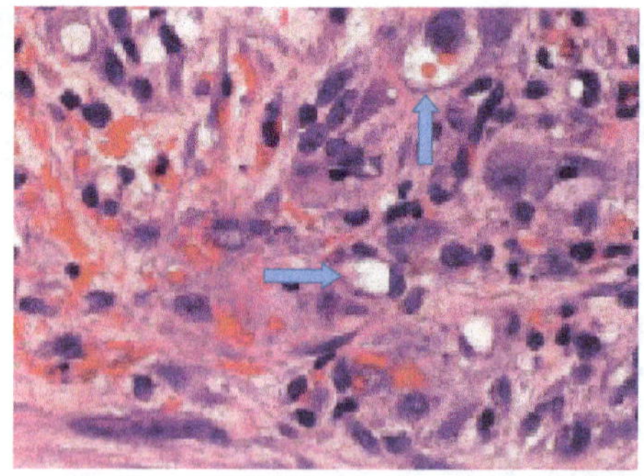

FIGURE 9: Epithelioid cells with pleomorphic nuclei: some with prominent nucleoli and intracytoplasmic vacuolization (arrows) (H&E × 400x).

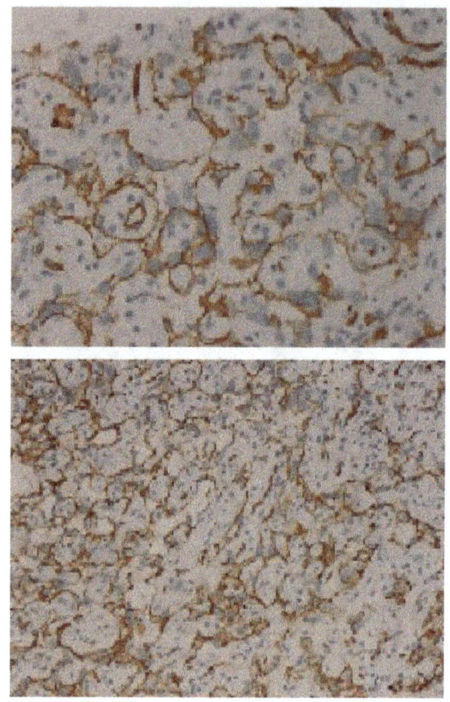

FIGURE 10: The CD34 and CD31 immunohistochemical stain shows positive reactivity in the tumor cells (×200).

Fifty to seventy-six percent (50%-76%) of patients with pulmonary EHE are asymptomatic and are incidentally diagnosed by abnormal chest radiography [1]. EHE may present with nonspecific symptoms such as a cough, dyspnea, pleuritic chest pain, and hemoptysis. Pleural EHE may manifest with pleural effusion, thickening, or pleural tumor; most cases with pleural effusion were serosanguineous in nature [4]. Márquez-Medina et al. reviewed about 22 cases of EHE with pleural effusion, and most of the cases (around 90% of the cases) presented with pleural effusion which was serosanguineous in nature; only 2 of the reviewed cases presented with hemothorax [3, 4].

Pleural epithelioid hemangioendothelioma carries a poor prognosis with a mean survival of 10–12 months. Due to the rarity of this condition, there is still no standardized treatment.

5. Conclusion

Epithelioid hemangioendothelioma is a rare vascular tumor with poor prognosis; a bilateral spontaneous pleural hemothorax may well be the single presentation. Treatment of such condition is not adequate which may require further investigation.

References

[1] A. Sardaro, L. Bardoscia, M. F. Petruzzelli, and M. Portaluri, "Epithelioid hemangioendothelioma: an overview and update on a rare vascular tumor," *Oncology Reviews*, vol. 8, no. 2, 2014.

[2] C. E. Woodall, C. R. Scoggins, A. M. Lewis, K. McMasters, and R. C. Martin, "Hepatic malignant epithelioid hemangioendothelioma: a case report and review of the literature," *The American Surgeon*, vol. 74, no. 1, pp. 64–68, 2008.

[3] H. A. Ali, M. Lippmann, and G. Khaleeq, "Spontaneous hemothorax secondary to epithelioid hemangioendothelioma," *Chest*, vol. 134, no. 4, Supplement 2, p. 61C, 2008.

[4] F. Photowala, U. S. Hatipoglu, and C. Garcia, "An older patient with bilateral non-traumatic haemothoraces," *BMJ Case Reports*, vol. 2012, 2012.

10

Response of Leptomeningeal Metastases in *EGFR*-Mutated Non-Small-Cell Lung Cancer to Afatinib in the Absence of Radiotherapy

Néstor Llinás-Quintero,[1] **David González-Hoyos**,[2] **Andrés Yepes**,[1] **Diego A. Herrera**,[3] **Sebastián Peláez-Arroyave**,[3] **Carlos Caicedo-Zamudio**,[3] **Erick Blanco-Daza**,[4] **and Javier Cuello-López**[1]

[1]*Clinical Oncology Group, Fundación Colombiana de Cancerología-Clínica Vida, Medellín, Colombia*
[2]*School of Medicine, CES University, Medellín, Colombia*
[3]*Diagnostic Imaging Group, CEDIMED, Medellín, Colombia*
[4]*School of Medicine, UPB University, Medellín, Colombia*

Correspondence should be addressed to Néstor Llinás-Quintero; nllinas71@gmail.com

Academic Editor: Francesco A. Mauri

Palliative radiotherapy is currently the medical standard of care for non-small-cell lung cancer (NSCLC) patients with symptomatic CNS and leptomeningeal disease. We report the case of a 62-year-old male patient with EGFR *mutation* (*del*19+) NSLC with symptomatic lymph node, bone, CNS, and leptomeningeal metastases. Taking into account on one hand the response to tyrosine kinase inhibitors (TKIs) and on the other hand the short- to medium-term side effects of radiotherapy and the lack of timely availability in our healthcare system, the patient was treated with afatinib (40 mg daily) and exhibited a rapid response with improvement of neurological symptoms. The patient presented partial response of extracranial, CNS, and leptomeningeal lesions at 3, 6, and 12 months of treatment, currently completing 16 months of progression-free survival despite presenting mild dermatological and gastrointestinal toxicities. Afatinib is an effective and safe option in patients with NSLC EGFR *mutation del*19+ with CNS and leptomeningeal compromise avoiding or delaying radiotherapy and its side effects, especially in countries where there is a lack of access to this kind of therapy.

1. Introduction

Lung cancer is the leading cause of cancer death worldwide [1, 2]. In these patients, central nervous system (CNS) metastases are estimated to occur in 30 to 50% of patients, which carries a poor prognosis of 4.7% in a 5-year relative survival rate, which is even poorer if there is symptomatic leptomeningeal disease [1–3].

Among EGFR-mutant NSCLC patients, leptomeningeal disease occurs in approximately 9% of cases, with a median overall survival of 3 months [4–8]. Thus, treatment goals are improved quality of life and prolonged survival. To date, studies providing evidence on how to best approach these patients are limited; nonetheless, currently used treatment regimens include radiotherapy, intrathecal chemotherapy, and systemic therapy, which—despite achieving various outcomes—carry a poor prognosis [5–7, 9–11].

Treatment of brain metastasis involves whole brain radiation therapy (WBRT), stereotactic radiosurgery (SRS), and surgery. However, with the improvement of systemic therapy, especially for treatment of tumors presenting anaplastic lymphoma kinase (ALK) translocations and epidermal growth factor receptor (EGFR) mutations, cancer control can be achieved. For instance, the third-generation

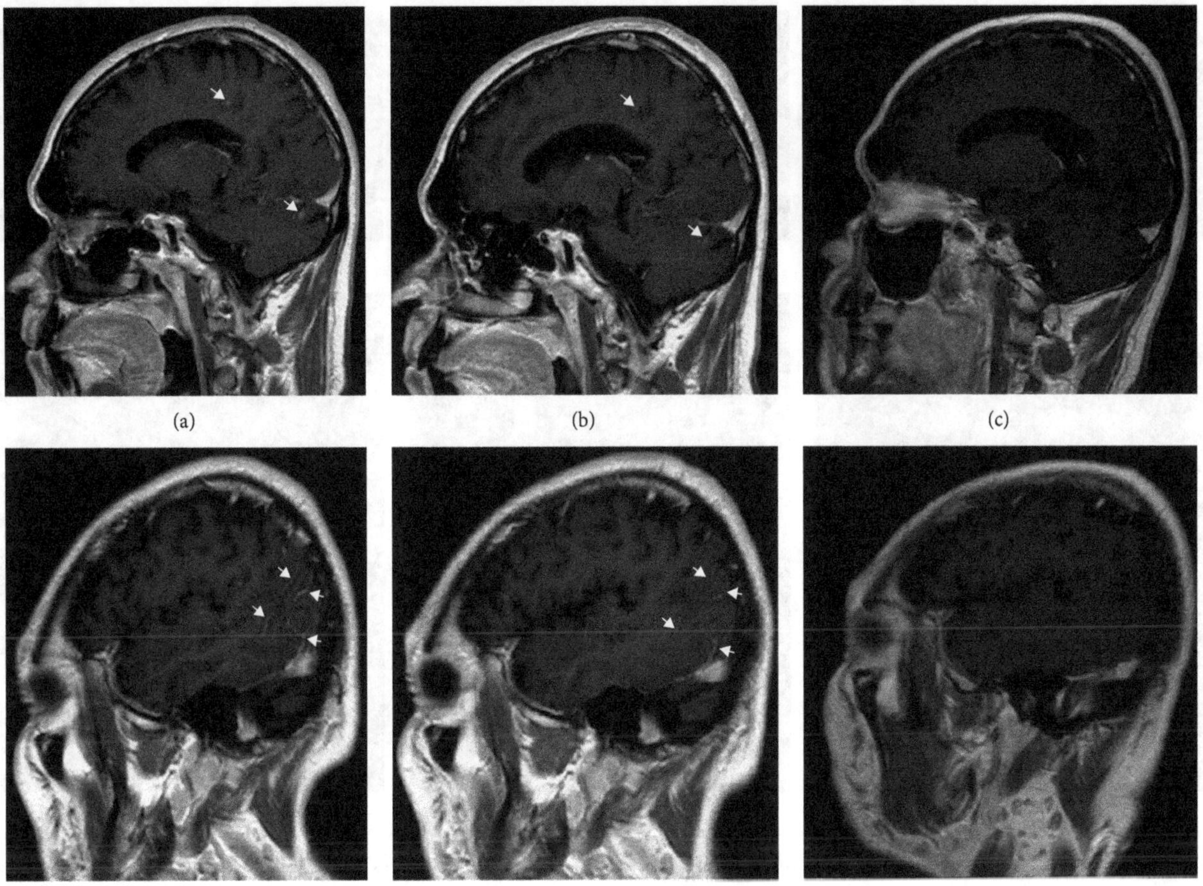

(a) (b) (c) (d) (e) (f)

Figure 1: T1 WI postgadobutrol administration sagittal slices. (a, d) Nodular enhancing lesions between 1 and 4 mm (arrows) at the centrum semiovale and left cerebellar hemisphere. Additional leptomeningeal enhancement was noticed at the pial surface of the left posterior quadrant (arrows). (b, e) Images obtained 7 months later. There is evident reduction in lesion size, and fewer leptomeningeal enhancement is noticed. (c, f) Images obtained 11 months from first study; no lesions or enhancement noted.

EGFR tyrosine kinase inhibitor (EGFR-TKI) osimertinib has been evaluated in prospective trials conducted in patients with brain metastases and showed significant improvement in progression-free-survival (PFS) compared to first-generation EGFR-TKI. However, the cost of treatment has limited the access to this therapy [3, 5, 6, 11–20]. Furthermore, in patients with advanced EGFR-mutant NSCLC, afatinib—a second-generation EGFR-TKI—has demonstrated activity against CNS and leptomeningeal metastases (LM) and to perform superiorly to gefitinib—a first-generation EGFR-TKI [21–24].

2. Case Description

A 62-year-old male with past medical history of hypertension, type 2 diabetes, and fibromyalgia presented to our clinic with complaints of back pain and dyspnea. The chest X-ray showed bilateral micronodular opacities and a nodule in the paramediastinal and aortic regions. Due to worsening of symptoms, a CT scan was performed, and a $35 \times 27 \times 33$ mm speculated mass in the right upper lobe, bilateral mediastinal lymphadenopathies, and bilateral apical diffuse reticulonodular and micronodular opacities were identified. On bronchoscopy, no endobronchial lesions were identified, with a high suspicion of malignancy in aspiration cytology. PET-CT was performed and showed bilateral diffuse pulmonary metastatic disease, lesions in most vertebrae (C2, C6, C7, T2, T4-T6, T8-T12, L1-L5, sacral segments S1 and S2, and both iliac spines), and mediastinal lymph node involvement. A videothoracoscopy-guided segmental lobectomy plus mediastinal lymphadenectomy was performed for pathology confirmation. The pathology report indicated moderately differentiated lung multifocal lepidic-predominant adenocarcinoma, with lymph node involvement and with visceral, pleural, lymphovascular, and border invasion.

The patient was referred to clinical oncology, as he continued presenting symptoms complaining of persistent cough, weight loss, headache, and dyspnea, presenting a NYHA functional class III/IV and poor performance status (Karnofsky Performance Status Scale 70%). Upon physical examination, bibasilar rales and a positive percussion test in the dorsal vertebrae were identified. Laboratory tests showed normal renal, hepatic, and hematologic function. The patient was diagnosed with stage IVB (T2N3M1c) NSCLC adenocarcinoma with bone, mediastinal lymph node, and contralateral lung involvement. A brain MRI showed multiple

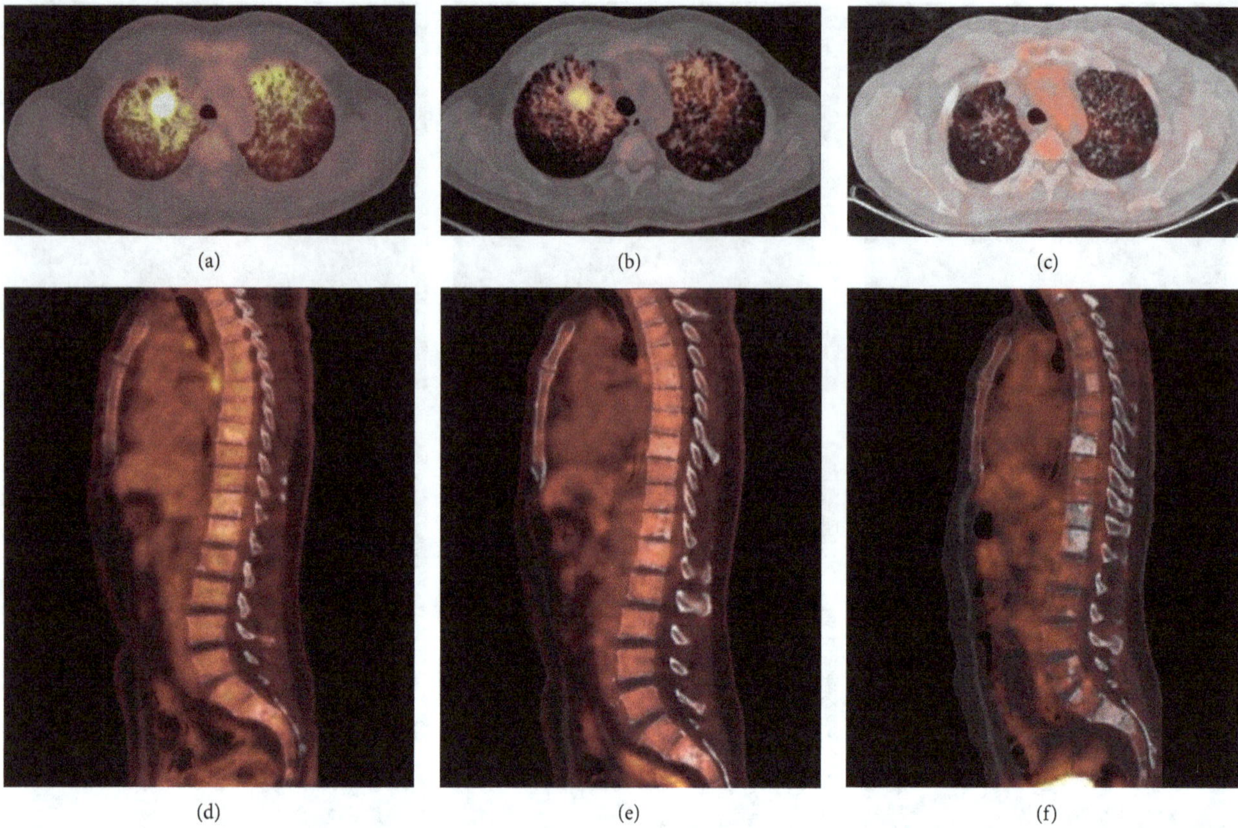

Figure 2: 18-FDG PET CT fusion images: axial and sagittal slices. (a, d) Right upper lobe mass with abnormally increased metabolism with surrounding lymphangitic carcinomatosis on both upper lobes with increased metabolic activity as well. On sagittal slices, multiple mixed type (blastic/lytic) metastatic lesions affecting axial skeleton. (b, e) Images obtained 7 months later showed marked decrease on metabolic activity on both pulmonary and skeletal lesions. (c, f) Images obtained 11 months from first study demonstrate the absence of metabolic activity on both primary site and spinal lesion.

nodular lesions in the brain and cerebellar parenchyma with leptomeningeal enhancement. A spinal MRI confirmed the metastatic involvement in the vertebrae, as indicated by the previous PET-CT scan, but without epidural infiltration. In addition, positive *EGFR* exon 19 deletion was also identified.

Due to the lack of timely access to radiotherapy, and considering its associated side effects, radiation therapy was postponed, and palliative care was initiated with treatment with a tyrosine kinase inhibitor, because of his *EGFR* mutational status. The patient was started on a 40 mg/day dose of afatinib treatment, administered orally, until there was evidence of disease progression or drug tolerance. Additionally, the patient received antiresorptive therapy with intravenous bisphosphonates every month to treat his bone metastasis. Immediately after initiating therapy, the patient exhibited rapid symptom and performance status improvement and was able to tolerate treatment; however, he presented grade 1 gastrointestinal toxicity and grade 2 dermatological toxicity. Follow-up images at 3, 6, and 12 months of treatment showed partial response of extracranial, CNS, and leptomeningeal lesions (Figures 1 and 2). To date, the patient has completed 16 months of treatment, displaying adequate tolerance and partial response to therapy, as well as a preserved quality of life and no evidence of disease progression.

3. Discussion

EGFR mutations are observed in 15% of lung cancer cases and have been associated with metastatic tropism to the brain, as well as to predict sensitivity to tyrosine kinase inhibitors (TKIs) [3, 5, 7, 8, 13, 25]. A retrospective study found a frequency of 7.8% of the lepidic subtypes with 68.8% of them with EGFR mutation [26]. In non-small-cell lung cancer, TKIs have proven efficacy in improvement of progression-free survival, response rate, and quality of life when compared to chemotherapy in patients with an *EGFR* mutation and are included in the current standard of care for patients with symptomatic brain metastasis together with WBRT [3–6, 13, 25–28].

The incidence of leptomeningeal carcinomatosis (LC) in *EGFR*-mutant NSCLC patients is 9%, and while median overall survival (OS) is 3-4.5 months, 44% have prolonged survival of more than 6 months. In a retrospective analysis of patients with LC by NSCLC with *EGFR* mutations, TKI therapy after LC diagnosis was an independent predictive factor of extended survival (median OS 10.0 vs. 3.3 months, HR = 0.218, $p < 0.001$), whereas poor Eastern Cooperative Oncology Group performance status ($p < 0.001$, HR = 3.657) was a predictor of poor survival [29, 30]. In that study, the active treatment with WBRT did not prolong OS for EGFR-mutated patients.

WBRT has been used as a therapeutic strategy in patients with brain and leptomeningeal metastases to relieve symptoms, to reduce bulky or nodular disease, and to correct CSF flow [31]. However, given its short and long-term adverse effects, and the increasing survival with the use of TKIs, even in patients with cerebral involvement, WBRT is being used less in patients with NSCLC with oncodriver gene mutations [6, 27]. Recently, Wang et al. published a meta-analysis that evaluated the role of WBRT as a treatment associated with TKIs in patients with NSCLC with brain metastases and EGFR mutation [10]. This meta-analysis included seven eligible studies for a total of 1086 patients. Compared to TKI alone, upfront WBRT plus TKI showed better PFS (HR = 0.72, 95% CI: 0.53-0.97, $p = 0.028$) and OS (HR = 0.70, 95% CI: 0.53-0.93, $p = 0.015$). Metaregression analyses and subgroup analyses showed that while patients with a limited number of brain metastases (<3) benefited from WBRT as evidenced by improved OS (HR = 0.54, 95% CI: 0.41-0.72, $p \leq 0.001$), patients with more than 3 brain metastases did not show OS benefit by undergoing WBRT [10].

Emerging evidence indicates that second- (afatinib) and third-generation (osimertinib) EGFR TKIs effectively penetrate the blood-brain barrier (BBB) and therefore represent viable treatment options for CNS lesions and can reduce the risk of CNS progression. These agents should be therefore considered as first-line treatment options in patients with *EGFR* mutation-positive NSCLC who have brain metastases and/or LM [7, 8, 32].

Evidence of the activity of afatinib against brain metastases has also been demonstrated by recent risk analyses of the LUX-Lung 3 and 6 studies [24]. In patients with a target brain lesion at the start of afatinib treatment, the risk of CNS progression (34%) was lower than the risk of non-CNS progression (48%). *De novo* CNS progression was observed in only 5% vs. 71% in non-CNS progression of patients after 24 months [13]. A combined analysis of the LUX-Lung 3 and LUX-Lung 6 trials showed benefit in PFS with afatinib as first-line treatment compared with chemotherapy in patients with asymptomatic CNS metastases (8.2 vs. 5.4 months; hazard ratio, 0.50; $p = 0.0297$) [24].

Osimertinib, a third-generation TKI that selectively inhibits both *EGFR*-TKI-sensitizing and *EGFR* T790M resistance mutations, has been approved as first-line treatment for *EGFR* mutation-positive NSCLC and as second-line after *EGFR*-TKI treatment in patients with *EGFR* T790M resistance mutations [16]. Osimertinib has a high bioavailability in the CNS [18]. In the FLAURA study, 556 patients with NSCLC and positive *EGFR* mutation were randomly assigned to osimertinib or standard of care (erlotinib or gefitinib). In this trial, there was a significantly longer PFS in the osimertinib group (18.9 versus 10.2 months; hazard ratio 0.46, 95% CI: 0.37-0.57) [18]. A subanalysis of the FLAURA study in patients with CNS involvement included 128 patients of the 200 that had available brain scans at the baseline. This subanalysis showed that median CNS progression-free survival was not reached with osimertinib (95% CI, 16.5 months to not calculable) and was 13.9 months with standard EGFR-TKIs (95% CI, 8.3 months to not calculable) (hazard ratio, 0.48; 95% CI: 0.26 to 0.86; $p = 0.014$) [19].

In our case, we were unable to provide treatment with osimertinib since it is not currently approved in our country; thus, despite evidence of brain and leptomeningeal metastases, the patient was started on treatment with afatinib, taking into account the evidence on clinical response of *EGFR*-mutated NSCLC without prior radiotherapy. This therapeutic strategy allowed postponing radiotherapy and its side effects. In addition, in some cases, access to radiotherapy can be difficult and delayed, putting the patient's life at risk. The partial response to treatment with improvement of his performance status and an outstanding progression-free survival strongly supports the safety and effectiveness of this therapy. Afatinib is an effective and relatively safe option in patients with *EGFR* mutation *del*19+ with symptomatic CNS and leptomeningeal metastases, especially in countries where the access to radiotherapy is still limited. Additional studies should be conducted to obtain more information on the safety and efficacy of tyrosine kinase inhibitors, especially in patients with CNS and leptomeningeal metastatic involvement.

Acknowledgments

The authors would like to thank Fundación Colombiana de Cancerología-Clínica Vida.

References

[1] N. Howlader, A. Noone, and M. Krapcho, *Surveillance, Epidemiology, and End Results (SEER) Program. SEER Cancer Statistics Review, 1975-2012 (updated August 20, 2015)*, National Cancer Institute, Bethesda, MD, USA, 2016, based on November 2014 SEER data submission, posted to the SEER web site, April 2015.

[2] O. Arrieta, C. Villarreal-Garza, J. Zamora et al., "Long-term survival in patients with non-small cell lung cancer and synchronous brain metastasis treated with whole-brain radiotherapy and thoracic chemoradiation," *Radiation Oncology*, vol. 6, no. 1, p. 166, 2011.

[3] D. E. Dawe, J. N. Greenspoon, and P. M. Ellis, "Brain metastases in non–small-cell lung cancer," *Clinical Lung Cancer*, vol. 15, no. 4, pp. 249–257, 2014.

[4] B. C. Liao, J. H. Lee, C. C. Lin et al., "Epidermal growth factor receptor tyrosine kinase inhibitors for non–small-cell lung cancer patients with leptomeningeal carcinomatosis," *Journal of Thoracic Oncology*, vol. 10, no. 12, pp. 1754–1761, 2015.

[5] N. Chooback, S. Lefresne, S. C. Lau, and C. Ho, "CNS Metastases in epidermal growth factor receptor mutation–positive non–small-cell lung cancer: impact on health resource utilization," *Journal of Oncology Practice*, vol. 14, no. 10, pp. e612–e620, 2018.

[6] W. J. Kelly, N. J. Shah, and D. S. Subramaniam, "Management of brain metastases in epidermal growth factor receptor mutant non-small-cell lung cancer," *Frontiers in Oncology*, vol. 8, p. 208, 2018.

[7] J. Remon, E. Le Rhun, and B. Besse, "Leptomeningeal carcinomatosis in non-small cell lung cancer patients: a continuing challenge in the personalized treatment era," *Cancer Treatment Reviews*, vol. 53, pp. 128–137, 2017.

[8] J. Remon and B. Besse, "Brain metastases in oncogene-

addicted non-small cell lung cancer patients: incidence and treatment," *Frontiers in Oncology*, vol. 8, p. 88, 2018.

[9] J. W. Hyun, I. H. Jeong, A. Joung, H. J. Cho, S. H. Kim, and H. J. Kim, "Leptomeningeal metastasis: clinical experience of 519 cases," *European Journal of Cancer*, vol. 56, pp. 107–114, 2016.

[10] C. Wang, X. Lu, Z. Lyu, N. Bi, and L. Wang, "Comparison of up-front radiotherapy and TKI with TKI alone for NSCLC with brain metastases and EGFR mutation: a meta-analysis," *Lung Cancer*, vol. 122, pp. 94–99, 2018.

[11] Y. Wang, S. Liu, X. Wei et al., "Non-small cell lung cancer leptomeningeal metastases treated with intrathecal therapy plus osimertinib and temozolomide and whole-brain radiation therapy: a case report," *OncoTargets and Therapy*, vol. 11, pp. 4733–4738, 2018.

[12] Y. Ju, S. Sun, J. Wang, and S. Jiao, "Prolonged overall survival of patients with leptomeningeal carcinomatosis from nonsmall cell lung cancer," *Journal of Cancer Research and Therapeutics*, vol. 12, no. 5, p. 126, 2016.

[13] N. Girard, "Optimizing outcomes in *EGFR* mutation-positive NSCLC: which tyrosine kinase inhibitor and when?," *Future Oncology*, vol. 14, no. 11, pp. 1117–1132, 2018.

[14] G. Goss, C. M. Tsai, F. A. Shepherd et al., "CNS response to osimertinib in patients with T790M-positive advanced NSCLC: pooled data from two phase II trials," *Annals of Oncology*, vol. 29, no. 3, pp. 687–693, 2018.

[15] Y. L. Wu, M. J. Ahn, M. C. Garassino et al., "CNS efficacy of osimertinib in patients with T790M-positive advanced non–small-cell lung cancer: data from a randomized phase III trial (AURA3)," *Journal of Clinical Oncology*, vol. 36, no. 26, pp. 2702–2709, 2018.

[16] L. Xie, S. Nagpal, H. A. Wakelee, G. Li, S. G. Soltys, and J. W. Neal, "Osimertinib for *EGFR*-mutant lung cancer with brain metastases: results from a single-center retrospective study," *The Oncologist*, vol. 24, no. 6, pp. 836–843, 2019.

[17] B. C. Cho, B. Chewaskulyong, K. H. Lee et al., "Osimertinib versus standard of care EGFR TKI as first-line treatment in patients with *EGFR*m advanced NSCLC: FLAURA Asian subset," *Journal of Thoracic Oncology*, vol. 14, no. 1, pp. 99–106, 2019.

[18] J. C. Soria, Y. Ohe, J. Vansteenkiste et al., "Osimertinib in untreated EGFR-mutated advanced non–small-cell lung cancer," *The New England Journal of Medicine*, vol. 378, no. 2, pp. 113–125, 2018.

[19] J. Vansteenkiste, T. Reungwetwattana, K. Nakagawa et al., "CNS response to osimertinib vs standard of care (SoC) EGFR-TKI as first-line therapy in patients (pts) with EGFR-TKI sensitising mutation (EGFRm)-positive advanced non-small cell lung cancer (NSCLC): data from the FLAURA study," *Annals of Oncology*, vol. 28, Supplement 10, 2017.

[20] P. N. Aguiar Jr., B. Haaland, W. Park, P. San Tan, A. Del Giglio, and G. de Lima Lopes Jr., "Cost-effectiveness of osimertinib in the first-line treatment of patients with EGFR-mutated advanced non–small cell lung cancer," *JAMA Oncology*, vol. 4, no. 8, pp. 1080–1084, 2018.

[21] A. Tamiya, M. Tamiya, T. Nishihara et al., "Cerebrospinal fluid penetration rate and efficacy of afatinib in patients with EGFR mutation-positive non-small cell lung cancer with leptomeningeal carcinomatosis: a multicenter prospective study," *Anticancer Research*, vol. 37, no. 8, pp. 4177–4182, 2017.

[22] L. Paz-Ares, E. H. Tan, K. O'Byrne et al., "Afatinib versus gefitinib in patients with *EGFR* mutation-positive advanced non-small-cell lung cancer: overall survival data from the phase IIb LUX-Lung 7 trial," *Annals of Oncology*, vol. 28, no. 2, pp. 270–277, 2017.

[23] S. R. Zhang, L. C. Zhu, Y. P. Jiang et al., "Efficacy of afatinib, an irreversible ErbB family blocker, in the treatment of intracerebral metastases of non-small cell lung cancer in mice," *Acta Pharmacologica Sinica*, vol. 38, no. 2, pp. 233–240, 2017.

[24] M. Schuler, Y. L. Wu, V. Hirsh et al., "First-line afatinib versus chemotherapy in patients with non–small cell lung cancer and common epidermal growth factor receptor gene mutations and brain metastases," *Journal of Thoracic Oncology*, vol. 11, no. 3, pp. 380–390, 2016.

[25] A. Diaz-Serrano, P. Gella, E. Jimenez, J. Zugazagoitia, and L. Paz-Ares Rodriguez, "Targeting EGFR in lung cancer: current standards and developments," *Drugs*, vol. 78, no. 9, pp. 893–911, 2018.

[26] Z. Chen, X. Liu, J. Zhao, H. Yang, and X. Teng, "Correlation of EGFR mutation and histological subtype according to the IASLC/ATS/ERS classification of lung adenocarcinoma," *International Journal of Clinical and Experimental Pathology*, vol. 7, no. 11, pp. 8039–8045, 2014.

[27] M. Hochmair, "Medical treatment options for patients with epidermal growth factor receptor mutation-positive non-small cell lung cancer suffering from brain metastases and/or leptomeningeal disease," *Targeted Oncology*, vol. 13, no. 3, pp. 269–285, 2018.

[28] H. Niu, J. Zhou, H. Maan, M. Markman, and J. Niu, "Treatment of leptomeningeal metastases in a patient with non-small cell lung cancer harboring EGFR T790M mutation," *Case Reports in Oncology*, vol. 10, no. 3, pp. 840–845, 2017.

[29] Y. S. Li, B. Y. Jiang, J. J. Yang et al., "Leptomeningeal metastases in patients with NSCLC with *EGFR* mutations," *Journal of Thoracic Oncology*, vol. 11, no. 11, pp. 1962–1969, 2016.

[30] H. Cheng and R. Perez-Soler, "Leptomeningeal metastases in non-small-cell lung cancer," *The Lancet Oncology*, vol. 19, no. 1, pp. e43–e55, 2018.

[31] D. S. Ettinger, D. L. Aisner, D. E. Wood et al., "NCCN Guidelines Insights: non–small cell lung cancer, version 5.2018," *Journal of the National Comprehensive Cancer Network*, vol. 16, no. 7, pp. 807–821, 2018.

[32] M. Hochmair, S. Holzer, and O. C. Burghuber, "Complete remissions in afatinib-treated non-small-cell lung cancer patients with symptomatic brain metastases," *Anti-Cancer Drugs*, vol. 27, no. 9, pp. 914-915, 2016.

11

Reconstruction with Total Scapular Reverse Total Shoulder Endoprosthesis after Radical Tumor Excision

Michael J. Harvey[1] **and Howard G. Rosenthal**[2]

[1]*University of Missouri Kansas City School of Medicine, Kansas City, MO, USA*
[2]*University of Kansas, Sarcoma Center, Overland Park, KS, USA*

Correspondence should be addressed to Michael J. Harvey; mjharveymd@gmail.com

Academic Editor: Jose I. Mayordomo

Malignant musculoskeletal tumors about the shoulder girdle region involving the scapula are fairly rare, but when diagnosed, challenging and complex surgical treatment may be warranted with the primary goal of improving patient survival. These tumors are typically extensive and infiltrative at the time of presentation, requiring radical resection to achieve margins and obtain local tumor control. Historically, forequarter amputation or flail extremity were the mainstays of treatment in these cases. Presently, with recent advances in diagnostics, imaging, adjuvant therapies, and surgical treatment, many patients presenting with malignant tumors involving the scapula are candidates for limb salvage surgery. Reconstruction with endoprosthesis seems to have gained acceptance as the preferred surgical treatment for such lesions, as this intervention has resulted in improved postoperative function and cosmesis, with an acceptable complication rate. We present our experience with recent advancement in these surgical efforts in the form of shoulder girdle reconstruction with total scapular reverse total shoulder prosthesis after radical tumor excision.

1. Introduction

Chondrosarcoma, although a rare malignancy overall, comprises approximately 30% of cancers involving the skeletal system. When these lesions originate about the shoulder girdle region, by the time of presentation they are usually fairly extensive and can involve the rotator cuff and surrounding musculature, glenohumeral joint, and the proximal humerus [1–6]. Unfortunately, this tumor has been found to respond poorly to chemotherapy and radiation therapies, leaving surgical resection as the recommended treatment. Historically, definitive treatment of large chondrosarcomas involving the shoulder girdle region involved flail extremity or forequarter amputation. The results of these procedures could be described as minimally functional and nonaesthetic. More recently, improved outcomes have been reported after scapular reconstruction with prostheses or allograft [7]. Pritsch et al. retrospectively compared outcomes of humeral suspension versus endoprosthetic reconstruction after total scapulectomy and found significantly improved functional and cosmetic results with reconstruction. They recommended that reconstructive efforts be undertaken when feasible [8].

In this manuscript, we describe a surgical technique and discuss a series of three patients in whom a single surgeon (HGR) performed reconstruction with total scapular reverse total shoulder prosthesis after radical excision of chondrosarcoma about the shoulder girdle.

2. Cases

2.1. Case 1. This is a 65-year-old gentleman who was referred from his primary care provider for further evaluation of a right shoulder lesion that was found during routine work-up of atraumatic shoulder pain. After performing appropriate imaging studies and open biopsy, he was diagnosed with a large Grade II chondrosarcoma involving the right scapula and glenohumeral joint (Figure 1(a)). The decision was made to proceed with radical resection of the tumor and reconstruction with total scapular reverse total shoulder replacement prosthesis.

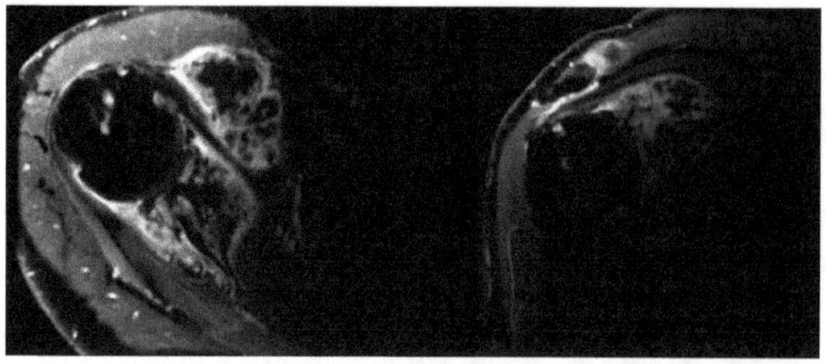

(a)

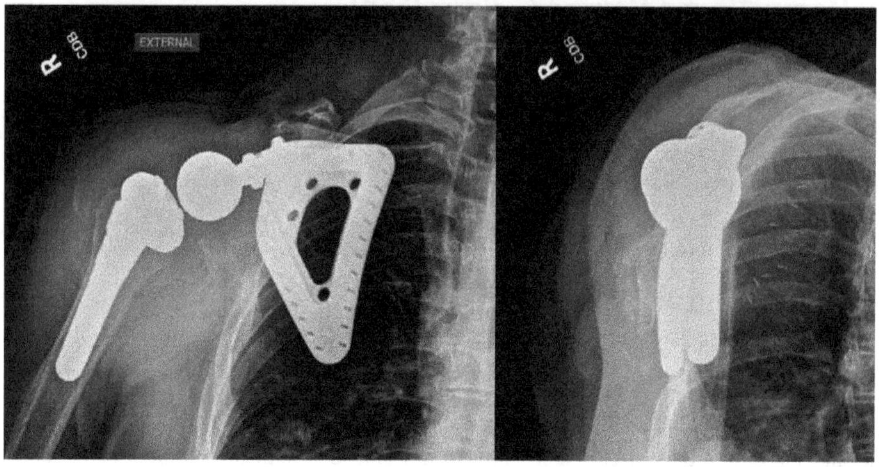

(b)

Figure 1: (a) MRI demonstrating expansive, infiltrative soft tissue malignancy about the scapula and shoulder girdle. (b) Eight-month postoperative radiographs demonstrating well-fixed implants in appropriate alignment.

Postoperatively, this patient's recovery was complicated by persistent wound drainage and prosthetic shoulder dislocation that occurred in physical therapy about six weeks postoperatively. He was brought back to the OR at that time for I&D and open reduction of his shoulder dislocation with antibiotic bead placement. Due to persistent infection, he subsequently underwent repeat irrigation and debridement with removal of deep implants, resterilization and single-stage reimplantation of the custom-made prostheses. This was a final attempt to eradicate infection while retaining the custom made implants. This surgery was performed about 8 weeks after the index reconstruction. During reimplantation, the soft tissue repair about the prosthetic shoulder joint was augmented with semitendinosus allograft.

Subsequently, he progressed well, and by about 8 months postoperatively, he had 5/5 muscle strength about the shoulder and was satisfied with his functional progress and cosmetic outcome (Figure 1(b)).

Unfortunately, about one year postoperatively, he was diagnosed with chondrosarcoma recurrence and evidence of pulmonary metastasis. He eventually underwent forequarter amputation.

2.2. Case 2. This is a 31-year-old male who was referred from his primary care provider for further evaluation of a left shoulder lesion that was found during work-up of atraumatic shoulder pain. After performing appropriate imaging studies, and after formal biopsy, he was diagnosed with low-grade chondrosarcoma with significant involvement of the glenohumeral joint (Figure 2(a)). This patient's index surgery involved intralesional curettage, cryosurgery, grafting, and prophylactic internal fixation of the left glenoid (Figure 2(b)). The patient did well initially, but unfortunately, local recurrence was confirmed with surveillance MRI and biopsy about 9 months after his initial procedure. At this time, his tumor was found to involve a significant portion of the left glenoid with extension into the scapular body. The decision was made to proceed with radical resection of the tumor and reconstruction with total scapular reverse total shoulder replacement prosthesis (Figure 2(c)).

At his first postoperative visit 2 weeks after surgery, the patient was doing well, no longer taking narcotic pain medications, and compliant with full-time shoulder immobilizer use. He was seen one month after surgery and was started on a short course of oral antibiotics for the treatment of peri-incisional cellulitis contributing to delayed wound healing. Although wound healing progressed slowly, his superficial infection resolved and his incision eventually healed. The patient was able to resume range of motion and strengthening therapy with physical therapy about 8 weeks postoperatively. At the four-month postoperative visit, his only complaint was occasional peri-incisional numbness. He had returned to weightlifting and was already able to perform modified push-ups, pull-ups, squats, and deadlift

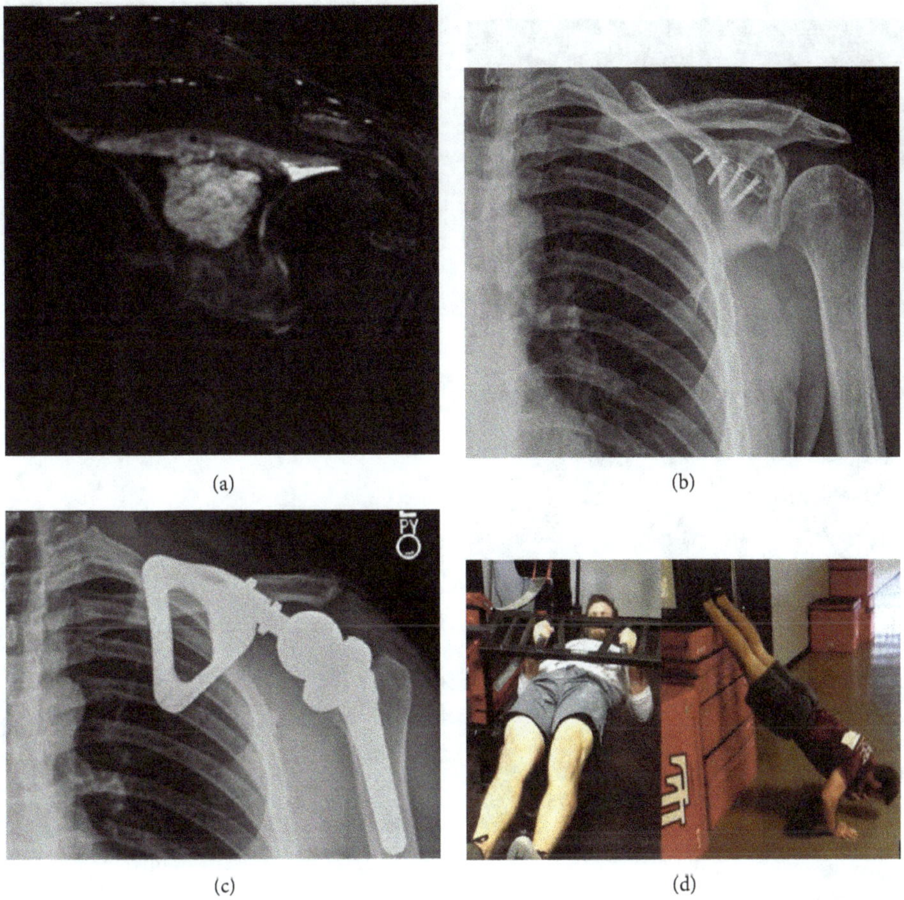

FIGURE 2: (a) MRI demonstrating malignant lesion of the scapula involving the subglenoid region of the shoulder. (b) Shoulder radiograph after index surgery which involved intralesional curettage, cryosurgery, grafting, and prophylactic internal fixation of the left glenoid. (c) Three-year postoperative radiograph after shoulder reconstruction. (d) Patient performing cross-fit activities postoperatively.

exercises (Figure 2(d)). One year postoperatively he had about 80 degrees of active forward elevation of the shoulder and 5/5 strength with shoulder abduction and external and internal rotation. Most recently, he was seen 3 years post-operatively and did not have any evidence of local recurrence. He had continued powerlifting activities and was very pleased with the functional and aesthetic outcome of his surgery.

2.3. Case 3. This is a 44-year-old male who was referred from his primary care provider for further evaluation of a left shoulder lesion that was found during work-up of atraumatic shoulder pain. After performing appropriate imaging studies and biopsy, he was diagnosed with high-grade chondrosarcoma involving the left scapula (Figure 3(a)). The decision was made to proceed with radical resection of the tumor and reconstruction with total scapular reverse total shoulder replacement prosthesis (Figure 3(b)).

Postoperatively, this patient's acute recovery from surgery was unremarkable; at four weeks, he was allowed to discontinue shoulder immobilization and begin physical therapy for range of motion. By his six-week postoperative visit, he had begun strengthening and was allowed to perform activities as tolerated with his left shoulder. He was progressing well until about 6 months postoperatively when he experienced sudden loss of range of motion and mechanical symptoms in the shoulder. Radiographs were obtained which demonstrated dissociation of the morse taper connecting the humeral tray to the stem (Figure 3(c)). He was brought back to the operating room for revision of his humeral component, which consisted of exchange to a larger tray with a retentive polyethylene (Figure 3(d)). At six weeks postrevision surgery, this patient was participating well in therapy and able to perform activities of daily living without significant functional impairment. Most recently, he was seen about 2.5 years after his index reconstructive surgery and was satisfied with his functional and aesthetic outcomes.

3. Surgical Technique

A long incision is made over the anterior aspect of the shoulder above the axillary fold and continued above the top of the shoulder to the posterior side and extended down to the most inferior tip of the scapula. If appropriate, any previous biopsy tracts are to be excised. Deep dissection involves radical tumor excision, taking care to obtain clear margins and avoid contamination. Great care is taken to avoid the lung apex, and to avoid violation of the brachial vessels and brachial plexus within the axillary region. Superiorly, circumferential subperiosteal dissection of the clavicle is performed to expose its lateral third. The lateral third of the clavicle is then

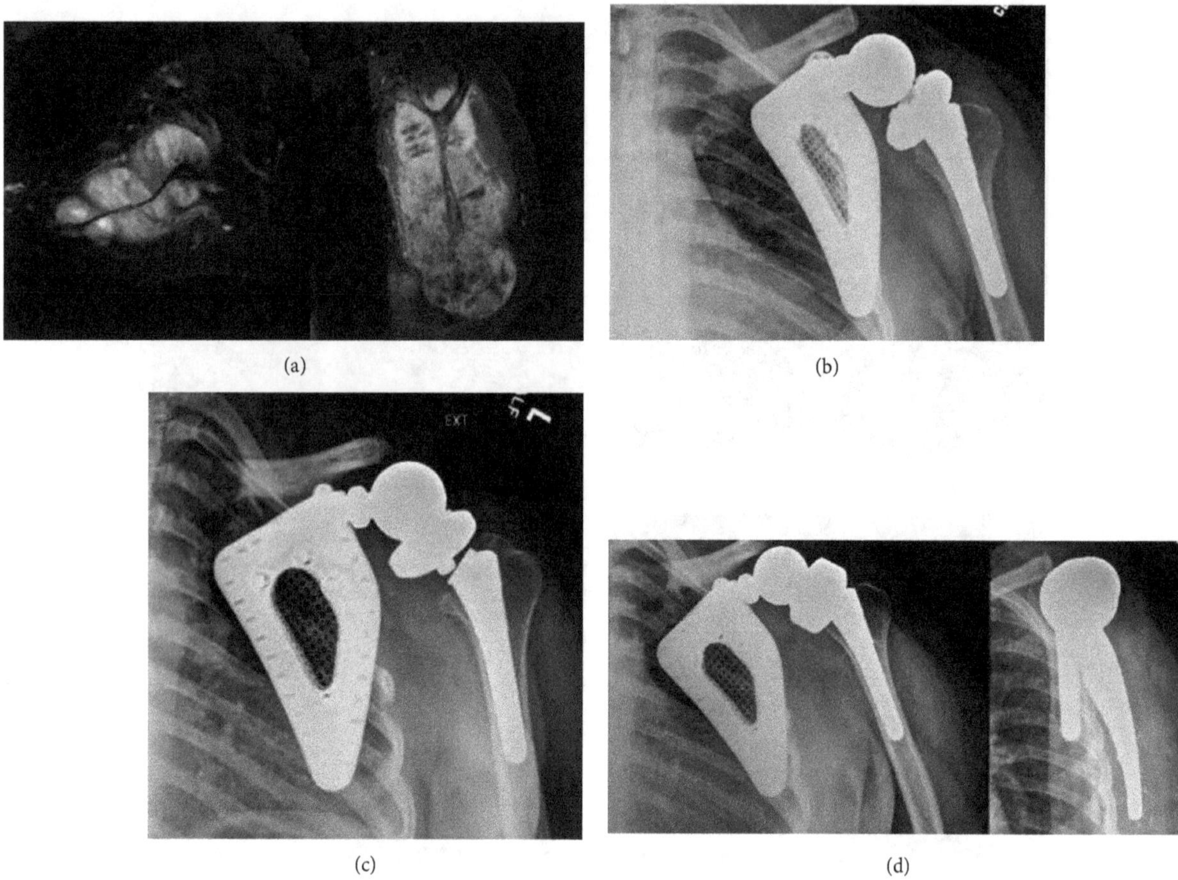

Figure 3: (a) MRI demonstrating expansive, infiltrative soft tissue malignancy about the scapula. (b) Immediate postoperative radiograph. (c) Radiograph demonstrating dissociation of the humeral tray and stem at the Morse taper six months postoperatively. (d) Immediate postoperative radiographs after revision of the humeral component.

osteotomized. Dissection is carried down over the posterior aspect of the scapula, elevating a portion of the supraspinatus and trapezius muscles. Care is taken to maintain the muscles in wide en bloc fashion along the superior aspect of the scapula. At the scapular spine, subperiosteal dissection is carried out to the medial border of the scapula. At this point, the inferior half of the scapula can be identified and the infraspinatus muscle elevated from its origin. The medial scapular border musculature is maintained if possible, to aid in later reconstruction and soft tissue repair. Subperiosteal dissection is then completed to the most inferior and lateral margins of the scapula, exposing entire lateral border, once again taking care to maintain muscle insertions to aid in soft tissue repair.

Attention is then focused on the humerus. Circumferential dissection is carried out to expose the humeral head and proximal humerus. The deltoid muscle is elevated from the acromion, taking care to maintain a cuff of normal tissue on the acromion for later repair. A large deltoid flap is elevated over the top of the humeral head, extending the flap well below the level of the rotator cuff insertion. An anterior capsulotomy is performed, and the rotator cuff tendons are reflected off of their insertion sites. An osteotomy is then performed at the anatomic neck of the humerus. The body of the scapula is then osteotomized, preserving the muscular insertions on the lateral, inferior, and medial borders (Figure 4(b)). The majority of the scapular body is then excised; this includes the superior portion of the body, the acromion, and the coracoid process. It is then possible to elevate the remaining osseous portion of the scapula, and subperiosteal dissection over the anterior aspect of the scapular body can be performed. Once wide en bloc resection of the tumor is completed, frozen sections of margins are reviewed.

Attention can then be focused on reconstruction, starting with the humerus. A reverse total shoulder proximal humerus component is placed in standard press-fit fashion. The final component that we use is a Zimmer-Biomet custom implant designed to receive the sphere on the custom total scapular prosthesis. This implant utilizes a retention-type glenoid and attached glenoid tray for increased stability. After the proximal humerus is reconstructed, the limb is held in anatomic resting position to act as a template for where the scapular prosthesis should be placed.

The scapular prosthesis is then placed and articulated with the glenoid tray on the proximal humerus (Figure 4(a)). If any viable cortical bone is left attached to periscapular musculature including the serratus anterior, levator scapula, rhomboids, and trapezius at the time of our radical resection, drill holes are made in the residual bony true scapular margins. #5 Fiberwire is passed through these holes and through associated holes in the scapular prosthesis to approximate the

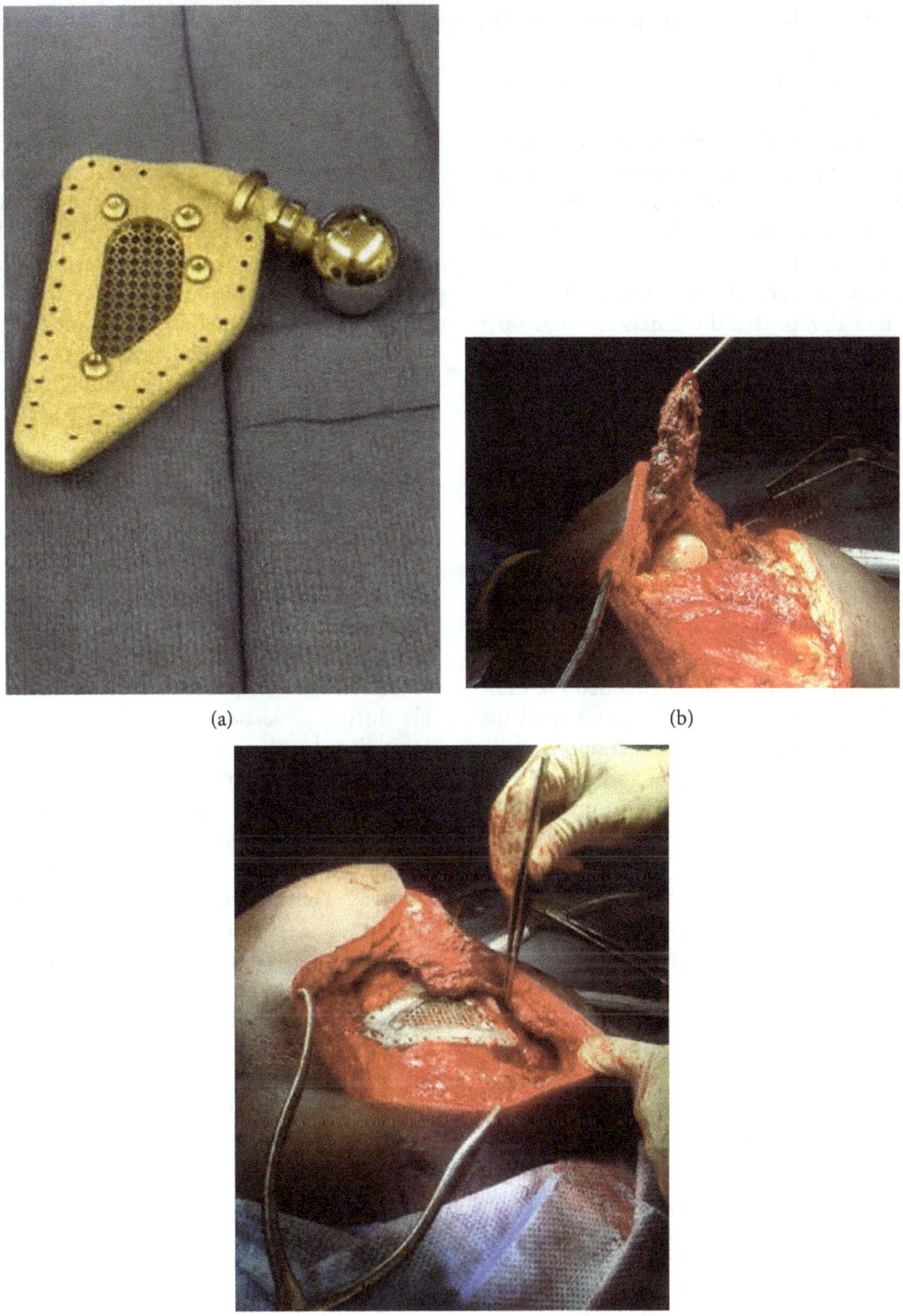

FIGURE 4: (a) Zimmer-Biomet custom total scapula reverse total shoulder prosthesis. (b) Isolation of the periscapular muscle flaps after excision of the scapula. (c) Incorporation of the soft tissue envelope into the scapular prosthesis through preexisting suture holes.

remnant native scapula and associated muscle tissue to the prosthesis, attempting to replicate anatomic positioning. This is performed circumferentially around the prosthesis, and the remaining free muscle flaps are then used to cover the posterior aspect of the prosthesis, and to reconstruct the rotator cuff (Figure 4(c)). Augmentation of the rotator cuff is performed with placement of an acellular dermal matrix allograft over the cuff tissues in 360-degree fashion. The graft is then sewn into the humerus itself, and passed through holes in the scapular prosthesis. The deltoid flap is then brought down and repaired with suture to the anterior shoulder, and into the prosthesis with existing suture holes, thus covering the entire shoulder girdle region and underlying construct. The subdermal and subcutaneous tissues are then approximated over a drain, completing the procedure.

4. Discussion

Historically, definitive treatment of large musculoskeletal malignancies about the shoulder girdle region involved forequarter amputation or flail extremity. The results of these procedures could be described as minimally functional and nonaesthetic. Before the 1970s, high-grade tumors about the shoulder girdle were almost always treated with forequarter amputation. It was not until the 1970s, when the Tickhoff-Linberg procedure was shown to achieve margins and survivorship similar to amputation, that limb salvage surgery was advocated for these tumors. This procedure classically involved en bloc resection of the scapula along with associated shoulder girdle musculature, as well as excision of the lateral clavicle and proximal humerus. Despite this advancement in treatment, patients were still not satisfied with their outcomes [7]. Griffin et al. reported the functional outcomes of patients undergoing total scapulectomy, including the glenohumeral joint, treated with a flail extremity. Seven out of eight patients ended up with a postoperative MSTS rating of poor [8].

Given the less than satisfactory outcomes with flail extremities, modifications to the classic Tickhoff-Lindberg procedure were drafted, including forms of humeral suspension. This typically involved stabilization of the humerus to the lateral clavicle with sutures or wires. Although stability was improved compared to a flail limb, marginal improvements with functionality or cosmesis were noticed. Despite these shortcomings, humeral suspension remained the most popular procedure after shoulder girdle resection until the late 1990s, when a scapular prosthesis was introduced. With a better understanding of endoprosthetic reconstruction, and the availability of custom-made components, improved outcomes have been reported after scapular reconstruction with prostheses [8, 9].

Pritsch et al. retrospectively compared outcomes of humeral suspension versus endoprosthetic reconstruction after total scapulectomy. In their reconstructions, they utilized a total scapula prosthesis from Howmedica Osteonics, combined with a proximal humerus prosthesis, and created an added constraint by reconstructing an artificial joint capsule out of Gore-Tex. They reported significantly improved functional and cosmetic results with reconstruction. They recommended that reconstructive efforts be undertaken when feasible [10].

Puchner et al. compared outcomes between patients treated with either the Tickhoff-Linberg procedure or endoprosthetic reconstruction after scapular resection. They used a custom-made scapula prosthesis from Biomet Orthopaedics coupled with a standard proximal humerus prosthesis. Their patients with endoprostheses reported good oncologic and functional outcomes, with MSTS scores far superior compared to patients who underwent the Tickhoff-Linberg procedure. They attribute their success to improved joint stability, which they believe leads to better function and strength below the level of the shoulder [7].

Mavrogenis et al. published a case report involving a patient with Ewing's sarcoma of the scapula treated with total scapulectomy and reconstruction with total scapula prosthesis and reverse-linked proximal humerus arthroplasty. Their patient was found to have a stable and painless shoulder 12 months postoperatively [11].

Savvidou et al. presented a series of 6 patients treated with total scapulectomy and reconstruction with a custom-made scapular prosthesis with constrained reverse total shoulder after malignant tumor resection. At final mean follow-up of 37 months, 2 patients had passed, leaving 4 patients who all had painless and stable shoulders, and satisfactory elbow, wrist, and hand function [12].

Tang et al. retrospectively reviewed ten patients who underwent total scapulectomy followed by reconstruction with constrained reverse total scapular prosthesis. The implant used was from ChunLi out of China and was comprised of a Co-Cr scapula with a reverse ball and socket hinge linking the proximal humeral prosthesis. At follow-up, they reported one dislocation, 1 infection, and a mean MSTS score of 76.7%. They concluded that constrained scapular prosthetic reconstruction after total scapulectomy for malignant tumors resulted in acceptable functional results and a low complication rate [13].

At our institution, a custom-made Zimmer-Biomet scapular prosthesis is created with a sphere at the reconstructed shoulder joint to accommodate a reverse total shoulder arthroplasty humeral prosthesis. Like any reverse total shoulder replacement, it is critical to evaluate for axillary nerve function and viable deltoid musculature. In the case of concurrent excision of malignancy about the shoulder girdle prior to reconstruction, care must be taken to protect the axillary nerve and preserve as much deltoid muscle as possible during dissection and resection of tumor, while at the same time being cognizant of tumor margins.

Malignant musculoskeletal tumors about the shoulder girdle region involving the scapula are fairly rare, but when diagnosed, challenging and complex surgical treatment may be warranted with the primary goal of improving patient survival. These tumors are typically large and extensive at the time of presentation, requiring radical resection to achieve margins and obtain local tumor control. Historically, forequarter amputation or flail extremity were the mainstays of treatment for this pathology. Presently, with advances in diagnostics, imaging, adjuvant therapies, and surgical treatment, it is reported that about 90% of patients presenting with malignant tumors involving the scapula are candidates for limb salvage surgery [14, 15].

We report on three cases of shoulder girdle sarcoma treated by a single surgeon (H.G.R.) with total scapular reverse total shoulder endoprosthetic reconstruction. Although complications were experienced, which can be expected at a high rate with radical reconstructive tumor surgery, we felt that this was acceptable in light of our functional and cosmetic outcomes, and patient satisfaction. However, we would recommend that such limb-sparing reconstructive procedures be performed only at specialized sarcoma centers by experienced surgeons with the sole focus on musculoskeletal oncology, in order to mitigate potential perioperative risks and complications.

5. Conclusion

Reconstruction with endoprosthesis seems to have gained acceptance as the preferred surgical treatment for extensive malignant musculoskeletal tumors about the shoulder girdle region involving the scapula, as this intervention has resulted in improved postoperative function and cosmesis, with an acceptable complication rate. After performing a literature review and reviewing the results of the three patients included in this case series, we conclude that reconstruction with total scapular reverse total shoulder prosthesis is a viable treatment and reconstructive option after radical excision of malignant lesions about the shoulder girdle region with extensive scapular involvement.

References

[1] R. C. Marcove, "Neoplasms of the shoulder girdle," *The Orthopedic Clinics of North America*, vol. 6, pp. 5415–5452, 1975.

[2] A. N. Papaioannou and K. C. Francis, "Scapulectomy for the treatment of primary malignant tumors of the scapula," *Clinical Orthopaedics and Related Research*, vol. 41, p. 125, 1965.

[3] J. C. Wittig, J. Bickels, F. Wodajo, K. L. Kellar-Graney, and M. M. Malawer, "Constrained total scapula reconstruction after resection of a high-grade sarcoma," *Clinical Orthopaedics and Related Research*, vol. 397, pp. 143–155, 2002.

[4] M. I. O'Connor, F. H. Sim, and E. Y. Chao, "Limb salvage for neoplasms of the shoulder girdle. Intermediate reconstructive and functional results," *The Journal of Bone and Joint Surgery. American Volume*, vol. 78, no. 12, pp. 1872–1888, 1996.

[5] J. Bickels, J. C. Wittig, Y. Kollender, K. Kellar-Graney, I. Meller, and M. M. Malawer, "Limb-sparing resections of the shoulder girdle," *Journal of the American College of Surgeons*, vol. 194, no. 4, pp. 422–435, 2002.

[6] J. C. Wittig, J. Bickels, Y. Kollender, K. L. Kellar-Graney, I. Meller, and M. M. Malawer, "Palliative forequarter amputation for metastatic carcinoma to the shoulder girdle region: indications, preoperative evaluation, surgical technique, and results," *Journal of Surgical Oncology*, vol. 77, no. 2, pp. 105–113, 2001.

[7] S. E. Puchner, J. Panotopoulos, R. Puchner, R. Schuh, R. Windhager, and P. T. Funovics, "Primary malignant tumours of the scapula—a review of 29 cases," *International Orthopaedics (SICOT)*, vol. 38, no. 10, pp. 2155–2162, 2014.

[8] A. M. Griffin, M. Shaheen, R. S. Bell, J. S. Wunder, and P. C. Ferguson, "Oncologic and functional outcome of scapular chondrosarcoma," *Annals of Surgical Oncology*, vol. 15, no. 8, pp. 2250–2256, 2008.

[9] A. Biazzo, M. De Paolis, and D. M. Donati, "Scapular reconstructions after resection for bone tumors: a single-institution experience and review of the literature," *Acta Bio-Medica: Atenei Parmensis*, vol. 89, no. 3, pp. 415–422, 2018.

[10] T. Pritsch, J. Bickels, C. C. Wu, M. H. Squires, and M. M. Malawer, "Is scapular endoprosthesis functionally superior to humeral suspension?," *Clinical Orthopaedics and Related Research*, vol. 456, pp. 188–195, 2007.

[11] A. F. Mavrogenis, D. P. Mastorakos, G. Triantafyllopoulos, V. I. Sakellariou, E. C. Galanis, and P. J. Papagelopoulos, "Total scapulectomy and constrained reverse total shoulder reconstruction for a Ewing's sarcoma," *Journal of Surgical Oncology*, vol. 100, no. 7, pp. 611–615, 2009.

[12] O. D. Savvidou, F. Zampeli, G. Georgopoulos et al., "Total scapulectomy and shoulder reconstruction using a scapular prosthesis and constrained reverse shoulder arthroplasty," *Orthopedics*, vol. 41, no. 6, pp. e888–e893, 2018.

[13] X. Tang, W. Guo, R. Yang, T. Ji, and X. Sun, "Reconstruction with constrained prosthesis after total scapulectomy," *Journal of Shoulder and Elbow Surgery*, vol. 20, no. 7, pp. 1163–1169, 2011.

[14] Q. Yang, J. Li, Z. Yang, X. Li, and Z. Li, "Limb sparing surgery for bone tumours of the shoulder girdle: the oncological and functional results," *International Orthopaedics*, vol. 34, no. 6, pp. 869–875, 2010.

[15] K. Hayashi, M. Karita, N. Yamamoto et al., "Functional outcomes after total scapulectomy for malignant bone or soft tissue tumors in the shoulder girdle," *International Journal of Clinical Oncology*, vol. 16, no. 5, pp. 568–573, 2011.

12

Malignant Phyllodes Tumor in an Adolescent Female: A Rare Case Report and Review of the Literature

Gabriel S. Makar,[1] Michael Makar,[2] Joanna Ghobrial,[3] Kathryn Bush,[1] Ryan Allen Gruner,[4] and Thomas Holdbrook[5]

[1]*Cooper Medical School of Rowan University, 401 Broadway Ave, Camden, NJ 08103, USA*
[2]*Robert Wood Johnson University Hospital, 1 Robert Wood Johnson Pl, New Brunswick, NJ 08901, USA*
[3]*AT Still University School of Osteopathic Medicine, 5850 E Still Cir, Mesa, AZ 85206, USA*
[4]*Cooper University Hospital, Department of Surgery, 1 Cooper Plaza, Camden, NJ 08103, USA*
[5]*Cooper University Hospital, Department of Pathology, 1 Cooper Plaza, Camden, NJ 08103, USA*

Correspondence should be addressed to Gabriel S. Makar; makarg3@rowan.edu

Academic Editor: Jose I. Mayordomo

Primary breast neoplasms are rare in adolescent females, most of which are benign. Phyllodes tumors constitute a remarkably small subset of breast neoplasms (0.3-0.9%) with malignant phyllodes tumors being even more uncommon. Malignant phyllodes tumors tend to progress rapidly though only 1.5% metastasize. They are also associated with a higher rate of recurrence than their benign counterparts, underlying the importance of adequate surgical margins. It is therefore imperative to be able to identify these tumors early allowing for prompt resection and close follow-up. Here, we present the rare case of a 17-year-old female presenting with a rapidly enlarging breast mass, which was ultimately found to be a malignant phyllodes tumor. We further performed a review of the literature to highlight only 22 other cases reported in adolescent females.

1. Introduction

Primary breast neoplasms are extremely rare in adolescent females and most are benign in nature. The incidence of primary breast tumors in females under the age of 20 is approximately 1 in one million [1]. Phyllodes tumors of the breast, previously known as cystosarcoma phyllodes, are rare fibroepithelial tumors that constitute approximately 0.3–0.5% of all breast neoplasms [2, 3]. The incidence for these tumors is remarkably low with an estimated 2.1 per one million women with a higher prevalence among Latina whites [4]. They occur most commonly during the late fifth decade of life in females and are even more rarely do they occur in men [5, 6]. Clinically, these tumors present as palpable, sometimes rapidly enlarging masses of the breast with a median size of approximately 4 cm [7]. Additionally, malignant phyllodes tumors are, on average, larger than their borderline or benign counterparts [6].

Malignant phyllodes tumors account for approximately 6.5-27% of all phyllodes tumors [5, 8–11]. Compared to benign and borderline phyllodes tumors, malignant tumors contain a higher rate of disease recurrence, decreased overall survival, and distant metastasis [5, 10]. Although they are more aggressive, cause-specific survival for these patients was 91%, 89%, and 89%, at 5, 10, and 15 years, respectively [12]. The median age of diagnosis remains similar to benign phyllodes at around 50 years old [12].

Herein, we perform a review of the literature and present the rare case of an adolescent female with a malignant phyllodes tumor.

2. Case Description

A 17-year-old female presented to the emergency department (ED) regarding an enlarging right breast mass. She noticed the mass 1 week prior to presentation. It was associated with mild

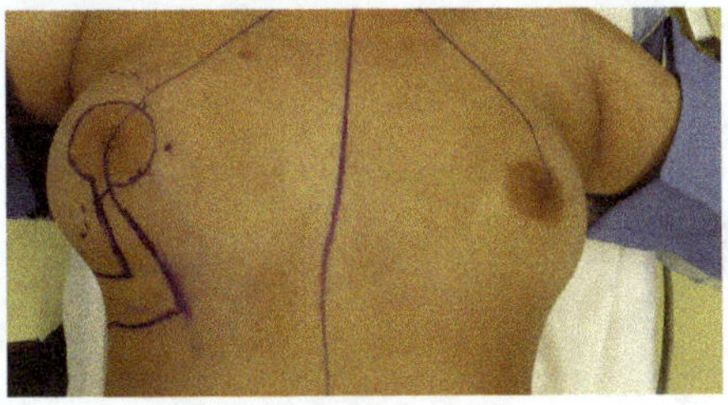

FIGURE 1: Preoperative image capturing prominence of tumor size and breast distortion relative to contralateral breast.

intermittent breast pain and severe periodic episodes of pain rated 10/10. No relieving or exacerbating factors were noted. The patient denied any redness or thickening, nipple discharge, nipple inversion, and any noticeable changes on the contralateral breast. Her breast sizes had not changed relative to one another. She had no previous history of breast biopsies or abnormal breast imaging. She denied additional symptoms including bone pain, rib pain, headache, and shortness of breath and was otherwise in her usual state of health. Her family history was significant only for a maternal aunt with ovarian cancer. The patient underwent menarche at the age of 12. There was no history of use of exogenous hormones to date. Her last menstrual period was approximately 25 days prior to presentation to the ED. Physical exam revealed a large, nontender approximately 15 × 11 cm mass occupying the majority of her right lateral breast (Figure 1). The left breast did not appear to have any masses, inflammatory skin changes, or nipple-areolar complex abnormalities. There was no axillary, infraclavicular, or supraclavicular lymphadenopathy appreciated on exam.

Breast ultrasound at the time of presentation revealed a 11.0 × 7.2 × 5.1 cm complex heterogeneous hypoechoic solid mass, which demonstrated mild internal vascularity on color Doppler flow. The mass was noncompressible with surrounding peripheral fluid. The patient underwent an ultrasound-guided core needle biopsy of the mass, which revealed a fibroepithelial tumor. Final pathology favored phyllodes tumor. The patient was also seen by plastic surgery regarding the anticipated large defect post resection of the tumor. Given the pathological findings, the patient underwent a wide right breast mass excision with a complex closure of the 10 cm wound. Pathologic examination revealed a 12.5 cm malignant phyllodes tumor (Figure 2). Histologic sections of the tumor showed the characteristic leaf-like architecture of phyllodes tumor with areas of prominent hypercellular stroma. The hypercellular stroma displayed marked nuclear pleomorphism and mitotic activity as well as areas of necrosis (Figure 3–5). The tumor was within 0.5 mm of the closest resection margin. Therefore, per the 2019 National Comprehensive Cancer Network guidelines, the patient was sent back to the operating room for reexcision lumpectomy to ensure full 1 cm margins around the malignant tumor. A lateral intercostal artery perforator flap was performed for appropriate wound coverage.

The patient has been doing well since the time of surgery with no current signs of metastasis or local recurrence. Chemotherapy was not currently indicated, and although

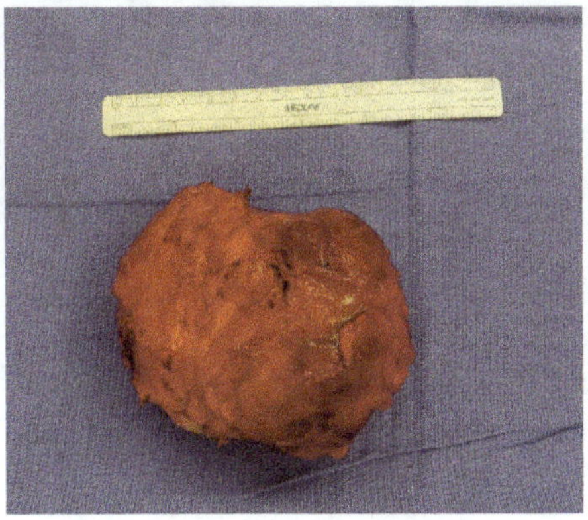

FIGURE 2: Intraoperative image of excised tumor measuring 12.5 cm.

radiation therapy was recommended, the patient refused radiation and opted for close observation [13]. Workup for metastatic and recurrent disease has been negative to date.

We additionally performed a literature review of adolescent females, defined as those 18 years of age or younger, with a confirmed diagnosis of a malignant phyllodes tumor (Table 1). Our report relies predominantly on the review attained from Levêque et al. who reviewed 18 adolescent females with malignant phyllodes tumors and presented a patient of their own (total 19 patients) [14–29]. Our review includes three additional patients for a total of 22 affected adolescent females [30, 31].

3. Discussion

Primary breast neoplasms are uncommon among adolescent females and may be misdiagnosed as a physiologic breast mass, as these are more common in this demographic. Phyllodes tumors constitute a rare subset of breast neoplasms (<1%), with a predilection for women in their late fifth to sixth decade of life and malignant phyllodes tumors account for an even smaller cohort (6.5–27% of all phyllodes tumors). Moreover, malignant phyllodes tumors occur in a population comparable to benign tumors, with rare occurrences in the adolescent population. Our report adds to the scarce literature of adolescent females with malignant phyllodes tumors and provides an overview of these tumors in the adolescent female population.

Phyllodes tumors are fibroepithelial neoplasms of the breast, which can histologically resemble fibroadenomas but typically display distinct stromal hypercellularity, prominent intracanalicular growth pattern, and characteristic leaf-like architecture. The World Health Organization (WHO) classifies phyllodes tumors into benign, borderline, and malignant categories based on the degree of stromal hypercellularity, cytological atypia, mitotic activity appearance of tumor border, and stromal overgrowth [32, 33]. Table 2 contains the current WHO criteria for diagnosis of phyllodes tumors [34]. The intracanalicular growth pattern along with hypercellularity is essential in differentiating fibroadenomas from benign phyllodes tumors, which can at times be difficult. Additionally, progression of fibroadenoma to malignant phyllodes tumors is not unknown as seen in case number 20 (Table 1). In a review of 36 malignant

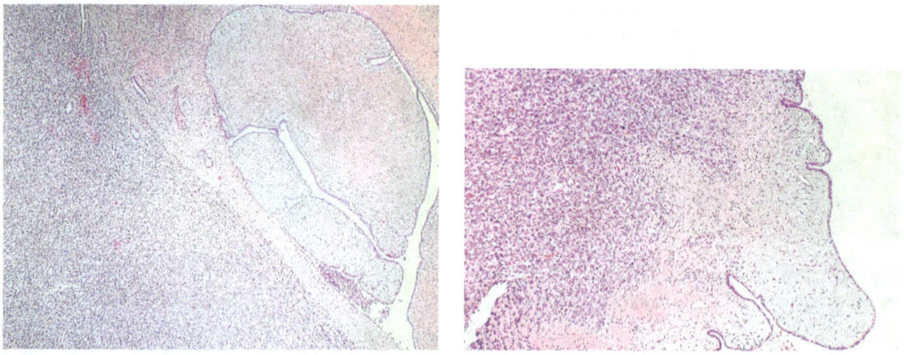

(a) (b)

FIGURE 3: Malignant phyllodes tumor. (a, b) The characteristic leaf-like architecture with epithelium lined clefts is present (right) next to prominent hypercellular stroma (left) (H&E, ×40 (a), ×100 (b)).

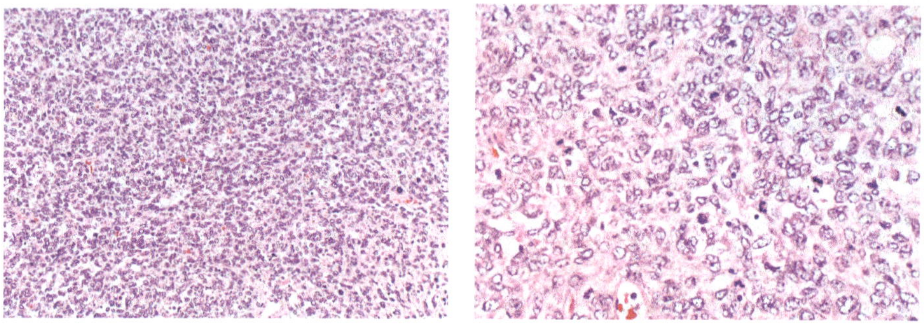

(a) (b)

FIGURE 4: Malignant phyllodes tumor. (a, b) There is marked nuclear pleomorphism and mitotic activity (H&E, ×200 (a), ×400 (b)).

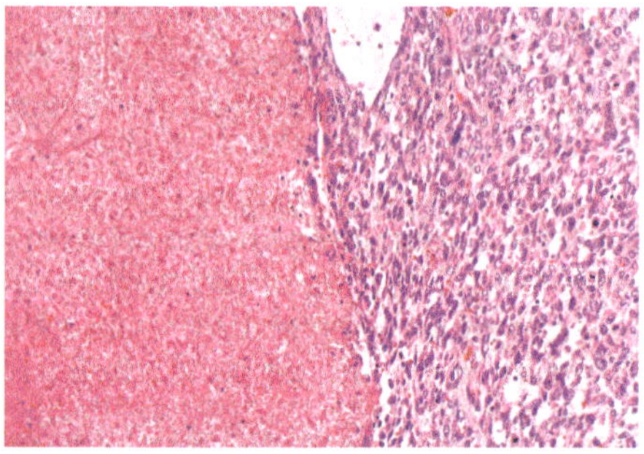

FIGURE 5: Malignant phyllodes tumor. An area of tumor cell necrosis (left) (H&E, ×200).

phyllodes tumors, 11 (30.6%) were given a diagnosis of primary fibroadenomas and experienced recurrence as malignant phyllodes tumors [35]. To properly capture these tumors, the growth rate must be observed closely. Studies suggest growth more than 20% in 6 months may be concerning for phyllodes tumor over fibroadenoma and constitutes surgical excision or biopsy [36, 37].

Formulating a proper diagnosis for patients presenting with breast masses can be stratified based on the patient's age. Less than 10% of phyllodes tumors occur in females younger than 20 years of age [15]. With malignant tumors also being tremendously rare in this population, there is a high likelihood of missing such tumors. These tumors can also be aggressive and rapidly progressive as seen in our case and previous reports [11, 15]. Ample detection of these tumors requires prompt biopsy, as was done in our case, to rule out such aggressive malignancies. After the diagnosis is made, appropriate negative margins must be established to prevent tumor recurrence. For patients with malignant phyllodes tumor, consensus remains that negative margins of 1 to 2 cm be obtained for optimal excision or simple mastectomy if unable to reach such margins [38].

Recurrence rates for benign, borderline, and malignant tumors vary vastly among studies. The literature, in concordance with the work done by the WHO, suggests that recurrence among benign, borderline, and malignant phyllodes tumors is 10–17%, 14–25%, and 23–30%, respectively [32]. Benign phyllodes tumors may be followed closely even with positive margins; however, malignant tumors must have confirmed negative margins given the high rate of recurrence and even death (22%) [32, 39]. Adolescents are said to have a higher rate of recurrence compared to their adult counterparts and therefore should be observed closely with routine follow-up even in light of negative margins [21]. Studies suggest Asian women appear to be at a higher risk of recurrence than non-Asian's [40]. However, a study utilizing the Surveillance, Epidemiology, and End Results Program (SEER) database found that there was no difference in survival among

Table 1: Literature review of malignant phyllodes tumors in adolescent females (part 1).

Case number	Age (years)	Delay (months)	Size (cm)	Treatment	Evolution	Result	Histology	Author
1	16	Short	9 × 8 × 7	Tumorectomy	2 recurrences at 12 months, 18 months, subcutaneous mastectomy +reconstruction	GH at 48 months	NS	Adami et al.
2	14	1.5	7 NS	Tumorectomy	—	GH at 48 months	NS	Azzopardi
3	15	?	8 × 8 NS	Tumorectomy, radiotherapy	2 pregnancies and 2 normal deliveries	GH at 66 months	NS	Rissanen and Holsti
4	17	14	9 right	Mastectomy	—	GH at 35 months	Lipomyxosarcoma	Mollitt et al.
5	16	0.5	7.5 NS	Tumorectomy	2 recurrences at 5 months, 9 months	GH at 37 months	Clear outlines with repression, mitoses 51/10 HPF, atypical aspect 3+, stroma fibrolipochondro sarcoma	Pietruszka and Barnes
6	17	NS	2.5-5 right	Tumorectomy	Adenofibroma at 8 months, tumorectomy	GH at 30 months	NS	Contarini et al.
7	12	6	13 NS	Mastectomy	—	GH at 204 months	NS	Briggs et al. (case 1)
8	18	2	1.5 NS	Tumorectomy	—	GH at 60 months	NS	Briggs et al. (case 2)
9	14	3	6 NS	Tumorectomy	—	Death cause? At 24 months	NS	Briggs et al. (case 3)
10	13	+3.5/2 months	5 NS	Tumorectomy	—	GH at 19 months	Stroma lipofibroma sarcoma	Grigioni et al. (case I)
11	18	+15/2 months	15 NS	Radical mastectomy	Recurrence at 3 months, pulmonary metastasis at 9 months	Death at 10 months	Very aggressive	Grigioni et al. (case 2)
12	18	84	12 × 12 left, nipple discharge	Tumorectomy	2 recurrences at 2 months, 6 months	GH at 42 months	NS	Naryshkin and Redfield
13	12	NS	10 × 12.5 × 15 right, no menarche	Radical mastectomy	—	GH at 12 months	Negative ganglia	Gibbs et al.
14	17	NS	30 axillary adenopathy	Radical mastectomy	—	GH at 96 months	Ganglionic invasion	Long et al.
15	14	4	10 right	Subcutaneous mastectomy and axillary clearing out	Multirecurrences as soon as 1 month, pulmonary and ovarian metastases, radical mastectomy, metastasectomy and exeresis of recurrences, chemotherapy mono then polychemotherapy,	Death at 14 months	Inflammatory reactive axillary ganglia	Hoover et al.

Table 1: Continued.

Case number	Age (years)	Delay (months)	Size (cm)	Treatment	Evolution	Result	Histology	Author
16	18	12	18 × 6 right, orange peel	Tumorectomy	cobaltherapy, surgical castration 3 recurrences at 4 months, 8 months, 19 months tumorectomy then radical mastectomy with radiotherapy, pulmonary metastases at 19 months	Death at 19 months	Almost sarcomatous tumour	Kenda
17	14	4	10 suspect left homolateral axiallty adenopathy	Subcutaneous mastectomy and axillary image radiotherapy, polychemotherapy	Metastases at 2 months (liver, bones, and lungs)	Death at 2 months	Necrosis and haemorrhage, normal epithelium, fibrosarcoma, >10 mitoses/10 HPF, periductular stromal hyper development, 8 reactive ganglia, 2 ganglia, purely stromal metastases	Ogun et al.
18	15	1 NS	Painful mass in left breast	Subcutaneous mastectomy	—	Death at 22 months	NS	Turalba et al.
19	15	4	16 × 6 cm	Enlarged tumorectomy, axillary clearing followed by mastectomy	—	GH at 100 months	Consistent with typical malignant pathology	Levique et al.
20	18	10	3 × 3 cm, right	Lumpectomy with wide local excision followed by simple mastectomy	Recurrence at 1.5 months following lumpectomy and 2 months following mastectomy	Death months following brain metastasis	Spindle cells with slight nuclear variation	Tiwari et al.
21	17	0.25	15 × 11 cm, right	Lumpectomy	—	GH at 2 month	Consistent with typical malignant pathology	Makar et al.

GH: good health; NS: not stated. Table adopted with permissions and additionas from Levêque et al. [14].

TABLE 2: Grading system for phyllodes tumors based on 2012 World Health Organization classification.

Histologic features	Histological type Benign	 Borderline	 Malignant
Stromal cellularity	Mild	Moderate	Marked
Stromal atypia	Mild	Moderate	Marked
Mitosis (per 10 HPF)	<5	9-may	≥10
Stromal overgrowth	Absent	Absent or focal	Present
Tumor margin	Clear	Clear or infiltration	Infiltration

HPF: high-power field. Table adopted with permissions from Zhang and Kleer [34].

white, black, and "other" ethnicities [41]. Further research is necessary to identify the true prevalence and incidence of disease among other ethnicities and in younger populations.

4. Conclusion

Given the unique and uncommon nature of primary breast tumors in adolescent females, appropriate assessment and management must be achieved to prevent misdiagnosing rare, aggressive tumors. It is necessary to be vigilant in the diagnosis and prompt management of rare tumors such as phyllodes tumors, due to the possibility of malignancy and rapid growth. Key features, such as large and rapidly growing mass, can aid in this diagnosis, but biopsy is necessary to characterize the suspect mass. We report the rare case of a rapidly growing malignant phyllodes tumor in an adolescent female.

Disclosure

This study was conducted at Cooper University Hospital, Department of Pathology 1 Cooper Plaza, Camden, NJ, 08103.

References

[1] E. J. Lee, Y.-W. Chang, J. H. Oh, J. Hwang, S. S. Hong, and H.-J. Kim, "Breast lesions in children and adolescents: diagnosis and management," *Korean Journal of Radiology*, vol. 19, no. 5, pp. 978–991, 2018.

[2] M. D. Rowell, R. R. Perry, J. G. Hsiu, and S. C. Barranco, "Phyllodes tumors," *American Journal of Surgery*, vol. 165, no. 3, pp. 376–379, 1993.

[3] M. Reinfuss, J. Mituś, K. Duda, A. Stelmach, J. Ryś, and K. Smolak, "The treatment and prognosis of patients with phyllodes tumor of the breast: an analysis of 170 cases," *Cancer*, vol. 77, no. 5, pp. 910–916, 1996.

[4] L. Bernstein, D. Deapen, and R. K. Ross, "The descriptive epidemiology of malignant cystosarcoma phyllodes tumors of the breast," *Cancer*, vol. 71, no. 10, pp. 3020–3024, 1993.

[5] M. F. Rodrigues, P. T. Truong, E. C. McKevitt, L. M. Weir, M. A. Knowling, and E. S. Wai, "Phyllodes tumors of the breast: the British Columbia Cancer Agency experience," *Cancer Radiothérapie*, vol. 22, no. 2, pp. 112–119, 2018.

[6] O. Hamdy, G. A. Saleh, S. Raafat, A. M. Shebl, and A. Denewer, "Male breast huge malignant phyllodes," *Chirurgia*, vol. 114, no. 4, pp. 512–517, 2019.

[7] S. P. Mishra, S. K. Tiwary, M. Mishra, and A. K. Khanna, "Phyllodes tumor of breast: a review article," *ISRN Surgery*, vol. 2013, Article ID 361469, 10 pages, 2013.

[8] J. P. Bellocq, Ed.G. Magro, "Fibroepithelial tumours," in *World Health Organization Classification of Tumours: Pathology and Genetics of Tumours of the Breast and Female Genital Organs*, J. P. Bellocq, P. Devilee, and , Eds., pp. 99–103, IARC Press, Lyon, 2003.

[9] J. Chang, L. Denham, E. K. Dong, K. Malek, and S. S. Lum, "Trends in the diagnosis of phyllodes tumors and fibroadenomas before and after release of WHO classification standards," *Annals of Surgical Oncology*, vol. 25, no. 10, pp. 3088–3095, 2018.

[10] P. H. Tan, A. A. Thike, W. J. Tan et al., "Predicting clinical behaviour of breast phyllodes tumours: a nomogram based on histological criteria and surgical margins," *Journal of Clinical Pathology*, vol. 65, no. 1, pp. 69–76, 2012.

[11] A. Wada, N. Hayashi, F. Endo et al., "Repeat recurrence and malignant transition of phyllodes tumors of the breast," *Breast Cancer*, vol. 25, no. 6, pp. 736–741, 2018.

[12] O. K. Macdonald, C. M. Lee, J. D. Tward, C. D. Chappel, and D. K. Gaffney, "Malignant phyllodes tumor of the female breast: association of primary therapy with cause-specific survival from the surveillance, epidemiology, and end results (SEER) program," *Cancer*, vol. 107, no. 9, pp. 2127–2133, 2006.

[13] X. Chao, K. Chen, J. Zeng et al., "Adjuvant radiotherapy and chemotherapy for patients with breast phyllodes tumors: a systematic review and meta-analysis," *BMC Cancer*, vol. 19, no. 1, p. 372, 2019.

[14] J. Levêque, B. Meunier, E. Wattier, F. Burtin, J. Y. Grall, and J. Kerisit, "Malignant cystosarcomas phyllodes of the breast in adolescent females," *European Journal of Obstetrics, Gynecology, and Reproductive Biology*, vol. 54, no. 3, pp. 197–203, 1994.

[15] H. O. Adami, L. Hakelius, A. Rismten, and R. Willén, "Malignant, locally recurring cystosarcoma phyllodes in an adolescent female. A case report," *Acta Chirurgica Scandinavica*, vol. 150, no. 1, pp. 93–100, 1984.

[16] J. G. Azzopardi, *Problems in breast pathology*, WB Saunders, London, 1979.

[17] P. M. Rissanen and P. Holsti, "A retrospective study of sarcoma of the breast and the results of treatment," *Oncology*, vol. 22, no. 4, pp. 258–268, 1968.

[18] D. L. Mollitt, E. S. Golladay, E. S. Gloster, and J. F. Jimenez, "Cystosarcoma phylloides in the adolescent female," *Journal of Pediatric Surgery*, vol. 22, no. 10, pp. 907–910, 1987.

[19] M. Pietruszka and L. Barnes, "Cystosarcoma phyllodes: a clin-

icopathologic analysis of 42 cases," *Cancer*, vol. 41, no. 5, pp. 1974–1983, 1978.

[20] O. Contarini, L. F. Urdaneta, W. Hagan, and S. E. Stephenson Jr., "Cystosarcoma phylloides of the breast: a new therapeutic proposal," *The American Surgeon*, vol. 48, no. 4, pp. 157–166, 1982.

[21] R. M. Briggs, M. Walters, and D. Rosenthal, "Cystosarcoma phylloides in adolescent female patients," *The American Journal of Surgery*, vol. 146, no. 6, pp. 712–714, 1983.

[22] W. F. Grigioni, D. Santini, A. Grassigli et al., "A clinicopathologic study of cystosarcoma phyllodes: 22 cases report," *Archives D'Anatomie et de Cytologie Pathologiques*, vol. 30, pp. 303–306, 1982.

[23] G. Naryshkin and E. Redfield, "Malignant cystosarcoma phyllodes of the breast in adolescence, with subsequent pregnancy: report of a case with endocrinologic studies," *Obstetrics & Gynecology*, vol. 23, pp. 140–142, 1964.

[24] B. F. Gibbs Jr., R. D. Roe, and D. F. Thomas, "Malignant cystosarcoma phyllodes in a prepubertal female," *Annals of Surgery*, vol. 167, no. 2, pp. 229–231, 1968.

[25] R. T. Long, A. E. Hesker, and R. E. Johnson, "Surgical management of cystosarcoma phyllodes with a report of 8 cases," *Missouri Medicine*, vol. 59, pp. 1179–1181, 1962.

[26] H. C. Hoover, A. Trestioreanu, and A. S. Ketcham, "Metastatic cystosarcoma phylloides in an adolescent girl: an unusually malignant tumor," *Annals of Surgery*, vol. 181, no. 3, pp. 279–282, 1975.

[27] J. F. Ngala Kenda, "Fatal metastatic cystosarcoma Phylloides in a young woman," *Archives of Surgery*, vol. 118, no. 7, pp. 871-872, 1983.

[28] D. Ogun, O. Gunhan, and H. Goze, "Cystosarcoma phyllodes: a malignant cystosarcoma phyllodes in a 14 year-old girl," *The Turkish Journal of Pediatrics*, vol. 28, pp. 199–203, 1986.

[29] C. I. C. Turalba, A. M. el Mahdi, and L. Ladaga, "Fatal metastatic cystosarcoma phyllodes in an adolescent female: case report and review of treatment approaches," *Journal of Surgical Oncology*, vol. 33, no. 3, pp. 176–181, 1986.

[30] J. Schwartz, A. R. Lentini, and A. Woodworth, "Borderline malignant phyllodes tumor in a 12-year-old: applying oncoplastic principles to adolescents," *The American Surgeon*, vol. 85, no. 5, pp. e252–e253, 2019.

[31] V. Tiwari, V. Mandloi, and H. U. Ghori, "Malignant phyllodes tumor of the breast with isolated brain metastasis: a case report of an intriguing aggressive subtype," *Clinical Cancer Investigation Journal*, vol. 6, no. 3, pp. 167–170, 2017.

[32] S. R. Lakhani, I. O. Ellis, S. J. Schnitt, P. H. Tan, and M. J. Vijvervan de, Eds., *World Health Organization Classification of Tumours of the Breast*, International Agency for Research on Cancer (IARC), Lyon, 2012.

[33] F. A. Tavassoli and P. Devilee, *Pathology and Genetics of Tumours of the Breast and Female Genital Organs. World Health Organization Classification of Tumours*, World Health Organization, Lyon, 2003.

[34] Y. Zhang and C. G. Kleer, "Phyllodes tumor of the breast: histopathologic features, differential diagnosis, and molecular/-genetic updates," *Archives of Pathology & Laboratory Medicine*, vol. 140, no. 7, pp. 665–671, 2016.

[35] M. Abe, S. Miyata, S. Nishimura et al., "Malignant transformation of breast fibroadenoma to malignant phyllodes tumor: long-term outcome of 36 malignant phyllodes tumors," *Breast Cancer*, vol. 18, no. 4, pp. 268–272, 2011.

[36] P. B. Gordon, F. A. Gagnon, and L. Lanzkowsky, "Solid breast masses diagnosed as fibroadenoma at fine-needle aspiration biopsy: acceptable rates of growth at long-term follow-up," *Radiology*, vol. 229, no. 1, pp. 233–238, 2003.

[37] Y. Gao, M. A. Saksena, E. F. Brachtel, D. C. terMeulen, and E. A. Rafferty, "How to approach breast lesions in children and adolescents," *European Journal of Radiology*, vol. 84, no. 7, pp. 1350–1364, 2015.

[38] B. Y. Tan, G. Acs, S. K. Apple et al., "Phyllodes tumours of the breast: a consensus review," *Histopathology*, vol. 68, no. 1, pp. 5–21, 2016.

[39] J. Y. Teo, C. S.-J. Cheong, and C. Y. Wong, "Low local recurrence rates in young Asian patients with phyllodes tumours: less is more," *ANZ Journal of Surgery*, vol. 82, no. 5, pp. 325–328, 2012.

[40] R. Z. Karim, S. K. Gerega, Y. H. Yang et al., "Phyllodes tumours of the breast: a clinicopathological analysis of 65 cases from a single institution," *Breast*, vol. 18, no. 3, pp. 165–170, 2009.

[41] J. C. Gutierrez, N. Housri, L. G. Koniaris, A. C. Fischer, and J. E. Sola, "Malignant breast cancer in children: a review of 75 patients," *The Journal of Surgical Research*, vol. 147, no. 2, pp. 182–188, 2008.

13

Splenectomy for Solitary Splenic Metastasis in Recurrent Papillary Thyroid Cancer: A Case Report and Literature Review

Antonio Maffuz-Aziz,[1] Gabriel Garnica,[1] Silvia López-Hernández,[1] Janet Pineda-Diaz,[2] Javier Baquera-Heredia,[2] and Patricia López-Jiménez[1]

[1]*Department of Surgical Oncology, American British Cowdray Medical Center, Mexico City, Mexico*
[2]*Department of Surgical and Molecular Pathology, American British Cowdray Medical Center, Mexico City, Mexico*

Correspondence should be addressed to Antonio Maffuz-Aziz; tonomaffuz@yahoo.com

Academic Editor: Katsuhiro Tanaka

Thyroid cancer is the most common endocrine malignancy, presenting with 23 500 new cases per year in the United States. About 7-23% of the patients will present recurrent metastases disease during follow-up. The classic variant of papillary carcinoma is less aggressive compared to its other variants like diffuse sclerosing, tall cell or columnar cell, and insular variants, and the sites to which this metastasizes is already well identified. Metastasis to the spleen is an extremely rare manifestation of papillary thyroid cancer. To date, only 3 cases have been reported in the literature. Herein, we present a 52-year-old male, who developed spleen metastases, 2.4 years after total thyroidectomy and central neck dissection followed by radioactive iodine ablation and seven months after treatment with sorafenib for lung metastases. The splenic lesion was detected in surveillance studies. This case highlights that splenic metastasis, although rare, may occur even in a patient with a locoregional and systemic controlled thyroid cancer and that it can be treated safely with surgical resection.

1. Introduction

Thyroid cancer is the leading cause of endocrine cancer and represents 2.1% of all cancer cases worldwide. About 90% are well-differentiated thyroid carcinoma (DTC); papillary cancer is the most common histology [1]. The presence of distant metastases at the time of diagnosis is 4%, and 7-23% during follow-up; in nearly 53% of cases, the relapse is reported in locoregional cancer, 28% in local relapse, and 13% distance metastasis is present; of these, 6% of cases have mixed relapses [2]. It has been reported that a global survival at 10 years is in a range of 25–70% [3].

The most common distant metastasis sites are the lungs and bone with 69.0% and 7.1%, respectively [4]. Rare metastasis site locations are extremely low; they have been identified in sites such as the liver, adrenal gland, central nervous system, kidney, and skin and have been reported in 1.85% of cases [5].

The presentation of spleen metastases of a primary thyroid cancer is even more rare; to date, only 3 cases have been reported [6–8]. In this article, we present a case of splenic recurrence of papillary thyroid cancer and a literature review.

2. Case Presentation

A 52-year-old male presented with dysphonia of 2 months; laryngoscopy was performed identifying right vocal cord paralysis; extension studies identified a tumour dependent on the right thyroid lobe, with oesophageal infiltration and tracheal displacement, with no evidence of cervical lymph nodes. Total thyroidectomy with partial resection of the oesophagus and lymphadenectomy of the central compartment was performed. The pathology report was classic papillary thyroid carcinoma 3.6 cm in tumour size, and mixed pattern, with extra thyroid extension, and 1/7 lymph nodes with metastases. Postoperative iodine-131 dose of 200 mCi was delivered, with subsequent iodine-131 tracing that reported small remnant of functional thyroid tissue in the thyroid bed. He continued hormone replacement therapy and surveillance.

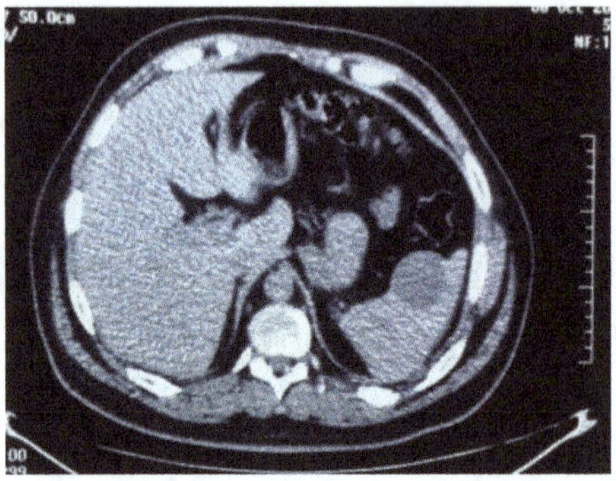

FIGURE 1: Abdominal CT showing cystic lesion in the spleen of 40 mm diameter.

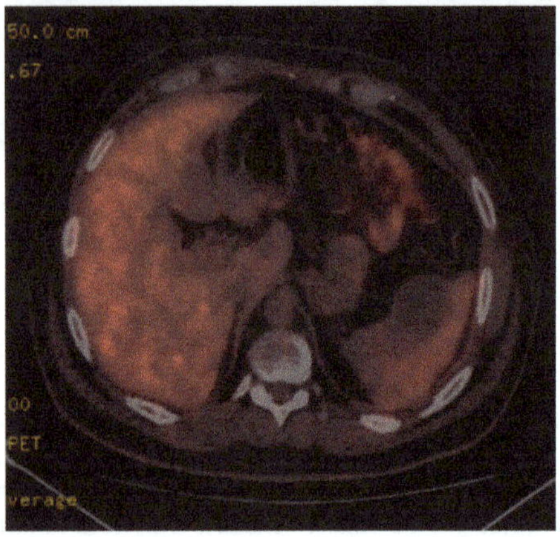

FIGURE 2: PET/CT images show a 40 mm lesion without increased metabolic activity.

At 16 months of surveillance, right basal pulmonary nodule was identified in X-ray; then, whole-body iodine-131 scan and thyroglobulin levels were negative, so 18F-fluorodeoxyglucose-positron emission tomography (18F-FDG PET/CT) was performed which was positive for bilateral pulmonary tumour activity; this being the only place where distant metastasis was found at the time of the study, the spleen was normal. Thoracoscopy was performed, where pulmonary metastases were confirmed secondary to well-differentiated papillary thyroid cancer. Treatment with sorafenib was started, assessing complete pulmonary control after 12 months of treatment.

Seven months after finished sorafenib treatment, and 29 months from initial treatment, 18F-FDG PET/CT was performed, in which there was no evidence of metabolic activity in the lung or in any other organ; however a cystic lesion was found in the spleen 10 mm in diameter without metabolic activity. A control 18F-FDG PET/CT at 6 months showed the lung without evidence of disease, and the splenic lesion grew to a diameter greater than 40 mm; it was observed without metabolic activity (Figure 1). Due to the increment of size and risk of spontaneous rupture, it was decided to perform splenectomy (Figure 2).

Pathology reported a $5.5 \times 5.5 \times 4$ cm semi ovoid tumour, cystic-looking lesion, with serous content, wall cut

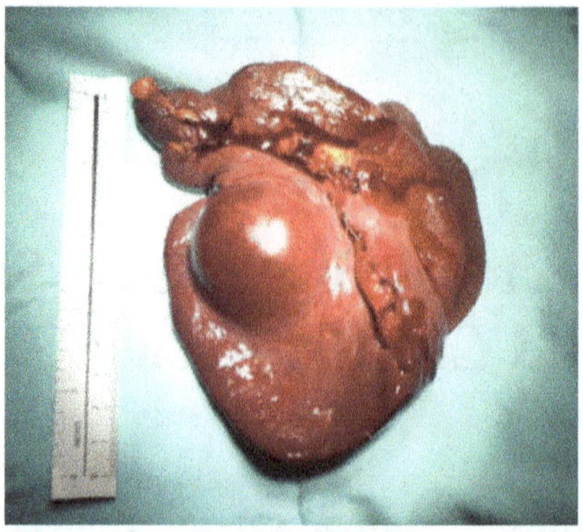

FIGURE 3: Pathology macroscopic picture shows the spleen with a cystic lesion of 5.5 cm.

0.2 cm, with simple papillary formations (Figure 3). In sections with haematoxylin and eosin staining, the neoplastic proliferation cyst is with a papillary growth pattern, and cuboidal cells, nuclear pleomorphism, empty nuclei and abundant nuclear bars are without mitosis (Figure 4). In immunohistochemistry, diffuse cytoplasmic positive thyroglobulin, CK19 diffuse cytoplasmic positive, TTF-1 diffuse nuclear positive, PAX8 diffuse nuclear positive, and CK5/6 negative were observed (Figure 5). The diagnosis was papillary thyroid carcinoma with a cystic pattern, of conventional type, well differentiated, with focal microcalcification and intraluminal xanthomatous response, without extracapsular extension. No areas of tall, columnar, or oncocytic cells were identified. There were no poorly differentiated or anaplastic areas.

3. Discussion

The presence of spleen metastases from solid tumours is extremely rare and generally exists in the context of a multiorgan disease. The presence of isolated spleen metastases has been reported <1% in autopsy studies; however, it is associated in 17 to 61% with metastases in other distant organs [9]. In the present case, spleen metastases present after treating lung metastases. Although the frequency of metastatic lesions of solid organs to the spleen is rare (2.3-7.1%), it is the most common sites of origin in breast (22.9%), lung (20.2%), colorectal (9.4%), ovary (9%), and stomach (6.9%) cancer [10]. The reason why this type of dissemination is rare is still poorly understood; lack of afferent lymphatic vessel, the splenic capsule, the immunological capacity of the spleen parenchyma cells (macrophages and lymphocytes), and the angled and spiral shape of the splenic artery constitute barrier methods for the presence of metastases in this organ [11].

To date, only 3 cases of thyroid metastases to the spleen have been reported. The first case was reported by Paolini et al. [7]; a patient with history of follicular thyroid cancer, which developed lung and spleen metastases; the patient was diagnosed with splenomegaly and infiltration to the diaphragm, colon, pancreas, and stomach. The second case reported was by Mayayo et al. [6]; with poorly differentiated thyroid carcinoma, the patient presented abdominal pain at 6 months of surveillance. Spleen, liver, and pancreas metastases were identified. The diagnosis was made by fine-needle

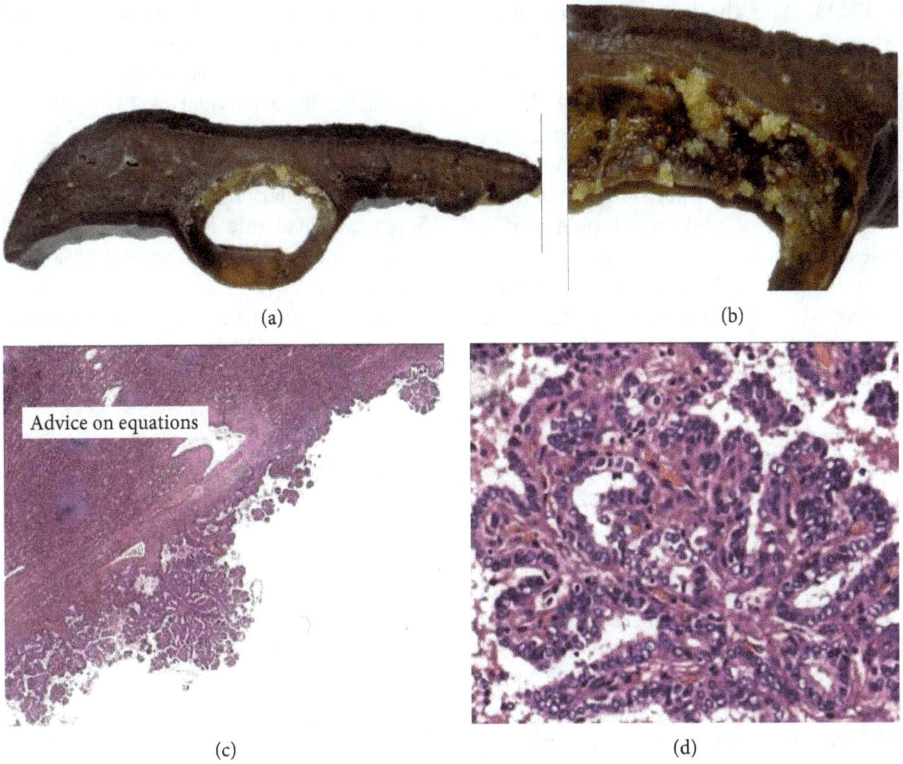

FIGURE 4: (a) Ovoid splenic lesion of cystic appearance, 5.5 cm major axis on the wall. (b) Papillary projections are observed. (c) Photomicrograph in which simple papillae protruding from the cyst wall (haematoxylin and eosin, 4x) are observed. (d). At a higher magnification, cuboidal cells with clear nuclei and bars, characteristic of papillary thyroid carcinoma (haematoxylin and eosin, 20x) are observed.

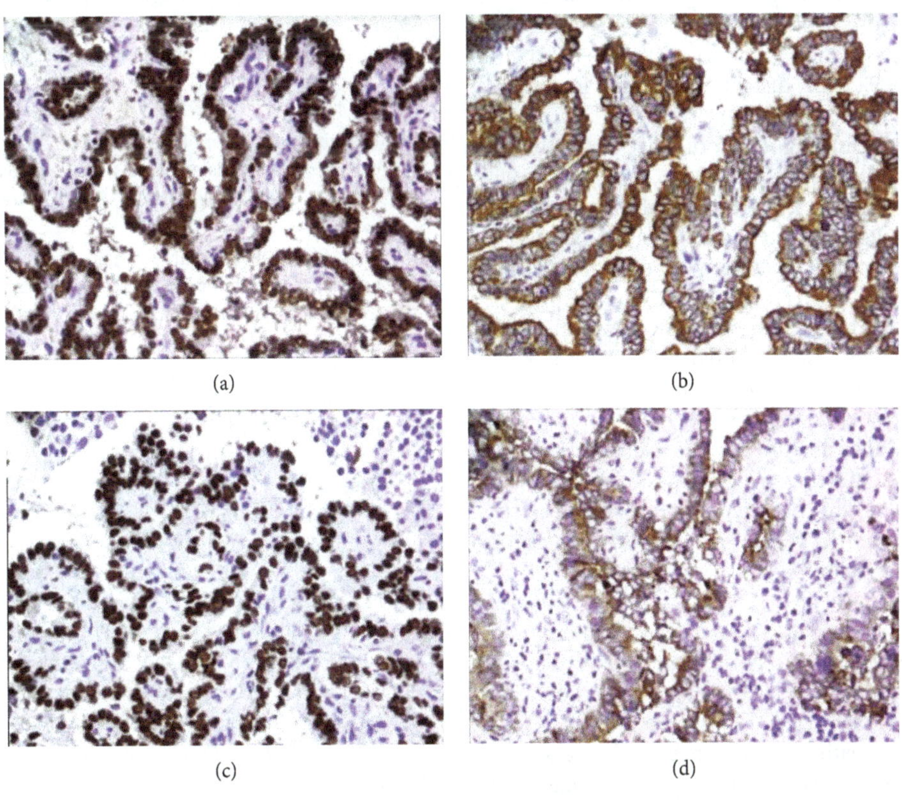

FIGURE 5: Photomicrographs of the immunohistochemical study performed on the splenic lesion. (a) PAX8 diffuse nuclear positive. (b) Diffuse cytoplasmic positive thyroglobulin. (c) TTF-1 diffuse nuclear positive. (d) CK19 diffuse cytoplasmic positive.

aspiration cytology (FNA). And the last case reported by Kand et al. [8] was in a 50-year-old patient with a follicular variant of a papillary carcinoma, who was diagnosed with an iodine-131 uptake study, which was captured at a diffuse level throughout the spleen, in addition to associating bone lesions. The definitive diagnosis was made using FNA as well.

Our patient was diagnosed incidentally in surveillance studies; he had no symptoms of abdominal pain and it seemed only a cystic lesion.

Before 1990, when imaging techniques were not used effectively, splenic metastasis rates were between 2.3% and 7.1% and most of them were found during autopsies or were just encountered coincidentally [10], because they are mostly asymptomatic. Therefore, studies such as 18F-FDG PET/CT currently have an important tool for detection. In a study performed on 68 oncology patients with FDG avid malignancy and solid splenic masses on anatomical imaging, 18F-FDG PET/CT had 100% accuracy in characterizing lesions as benign or malignant. The sensitivity, specificity, positive predictive value, and negative predictive value of 18F-FDG PET/CT in differentiating benign from malignant solid splenic lesions in patients with and without malignant disease are 100%, 100%, 100%, and 100% versus 100%, 83%, 80%, and 100%, respectively. It should however be kept in mind that non-FDG-avid tumours, such as some renal or thyroid cancers, may metastasize to the spleen [12, 13].

Although the information in the literature regarding the relationship between 18F-FDG PET/CT and the diagnosis of metastatic spleen lesions is only for solid tumours, the probable explanation is that most well-differentiated thyroid carcinomas are relatively slow growing and can be 18F-fluorodeoxyglucose negative [14]. Several studies have reported that it has a high sensitivity (up to 85%) and specificity (up to 95%) for distant metastases in patients with well-differentiated thyroid cancer [15].

Use of FNA is a useful diagnosis tool, since a sensitivity of 98.4%, a positive predictive value of 99.2%, and 98.1% accuracy for diagnosis and < 1% of complications have been reported [16], although it is generally avoided because of the risk of intra-abdominal bleeding or dissemination in some cases.

For this reason and based on the clinical evolution that the patient had, which was presented as a growth of the lesion, we decided to perform splenectomy because it was a unique and viable cystic lesion for resection.

Pathologic findings, the presence of isolated epithelial cells or forming three-dimensional groups with round nuclei, with inclusions or bars, are characteristics that should be suspected in a thyroid origin, especially in patients with a history of papillary thyroid carcinoma [6].

The long-term survival after splenectomy in patients with metachronous splenic metastasis from thyroid papillary cancer is unknown because of the limited number of reported cases in the literature; however, based on the data obtained from the study by Madani et al. [17] where they analysed a study of 492 patients with thyroid cancer and rare sites of metastasis, they mention patients with generally aggressive tumours, with a global survival of 60 months and disease-free period of 84 months. Other sites like colorectal carcinoma where the 1-year survival rate was 86.6%, and median survival time is 66.6 months [18], In metastases secondary to melanoma, median overall survival after splenectomy is 11 months, with a survival of 23 months for the subgroup of patients treated for a solitary lesion [19].

Distant metastasis is considered an important prognostic factor in papillary thyroid cancer, which affects survival. The 5-year survival rate is almost 100% for localized papillary, 99% for locoregional cancer and 78% for metastatic papillary thyroid cancer [20].

For patients with only lung metastases, the survival rate at 10 years is 73.6%, which are significantly higher than patients with multiple organ metastases for whom the 10-year survival rate is 34.3% [21].

4. Conclusions

Papillary thyroid cancer is a very common neoplasm; there a lot of information in articles and guides regarding its behaviour and management options. However, on rare behaviour, uncommon site metastases can occur, and its management is not well defined.

References

[1] C. M. Kitahara and J. A. Sosa, "The changing incidence of thyroid cancer," *Nature Reviews. Endocrinology*, vol. 12, no. 11, pp. 646–653, 2016.

[2] R. Cirocchi, S. Trastulli, A. Sanguinetti et al., "Recurrent differentiated thyroid cancer: to cut or burn," *World Journal of Surgical Oncology*, vol. 9, no. 1, pp. 2–5, 2011.

[3] L. Y. Wang, F. L. Palmer, I. J. Nixon et al., "Multi-organ distant metastases confer worse disease-specific survival in differentiated thyroid cancer," *Thyroid*, vol. 24, no. 11, pp. 1594–1599, 2014.

[4] I. Sugitani, Y. Fujimoto, and N. Yamamoto, "Papillary thyroid carcinoma with distant metastases: survival predictors and the importance of local control," *Surgery*, vol. 143, no. 1, pp. 35–42, 2008.

[5] N. S. Fedala, S. Kabour, F. Yaker, L. A. Ali, A. E. M. Haddam, and F. Chentli, "Métastases inhabituelles des carcinomes thyroïdiens différenciés," *Annales d'endocrinologie*, vol. 75, no. 5–6, pp. 360-361, 2014.

[6] E. Mayayo, S. Blázquez, V. Gómez-Aracil, A. Saurí, and S. Martinez, "Spleen metastasis from thyroid carcinoma. Report of a case with diagnosis by fine needle aspiration cytology," *Acta Cytologica*, vol. 47, no. 6, pp. 1116–1118, 2003.

[7] R. Paolini, S. Toffoli, A. Poletti et al., "Splenomegaly as the first manifestation of thyroid cancer metastases," *Tumori*, vol. 83, no. 4, pp. 779–782, 2018.

[8] P. Kand and R. Asopa, "Metastatic involvement of the spleen in differentiated carcinoma of thyroid," *Indian Journal of Nuclear Medicine*, vol. 25, no. 4, pp. 171-172, 2010.

[9] C. A. Schön, C. Görg, A. Ramaswamy, and P. J. Barth, "Splenic metastases in a large unselected autopsy series," *Pathology, Research and Practice*, vol. 202, no. 5, pp. 351–356, 2006.

[10] K. Y. Lam and V. Tang, "Metastatic tumors to the spleen: a 25-year clinicopathologic study," *Archives of Pathology & Laboratory Medicine*, vol. 124, no. 4, pp. 526–530, 2000.

[11] S. S. Lee, L. Morgenstern, E. H. Phillips, J. R. Hiatt, and D. R. Margulies, "Splenectomy for splenic metastases: a changing clinical spectrum," *The American Surgeon*, vol. 66, no. 9, pp. 837–840, 2000.

[12] U. Metser and E. Even-Sapir, "The role of 18F-FDG PET/CT in the evaluation of solid splenic masses," in *Seminars in Ultrasound, CT and MRI*, vol. 27, no. 5pp. 420–425, WB Saunders, 2006.

[13] U. Metser, E. Miller, A. Kessler et al., "Solid splenic masses: evaluation with 18F-FDG PET/CT," *Journal of Nuclear Medicine*, vol. 46, no. 1, pp. 52–59, 2005.

[14] M. W. Saif, I. Tzannou, N. Makrilia, and K. Syrigos, "Role and cost effectiveness of PET/CT in management of patients with cancer," *The Yale Journal of Biology and Medicine*, vol. 83, no. 2, pp. 53–65, 2010.

[15] J. K. Chung, Y. So, J. S. Lee et al., "Value of FDG PET in papillary thyroid carcinoma with negative 131I whole-body scan," *Journal of Nuclear Medicine*, vol. 40, no. 6, pp. 986–992, 1999.

[16] L. Cavanna, A. Lazzaro, D. Vallisa, G. Civardi, and F. Artioli, "Role of image-guided fine-needle aspiration biopsy in the management of patients with splenic metastasis," *World Journal of Surgical Oncology*, vol. 5, no. 1, 2007.

[17] A. Madani, Y. Jozaghi, R. Tabah, J. How, and E. Mitmaker, "Rare metastases of well-differentiated thyroid cancers: a systematic review," *Annals of Surgical Oncology*, vol. 22, no. 2, pp. 460–466, 2015.

[18] T. Okuyama, M. Oya, and H. Ishikawa, "Isolated splenic metastasis of sigmoid colon cancer: a case report," *Japanese Journal of Clinical Oncology*, vol. 31, no. 7, pp. 341–345, 2001.

[19] J. H. W. De Wilt, W. H. McCarthy, and J. F. Thompson, "Surgical treatment of splenic metastases in patients with melanoma," *Journal of the American College of Surgeons*, vol. 197, no. 1, pp. 38–43, 2003.

[20] Cancer.Net, *Thyroid cancer : statistics*, Statistics adapted from the American Cancer Society's (ACS) publications, 2020.

[21] H. J. Song, Z. L. Qiu, C. T. Shen, W. J. Wei, and Q. Y. Luo, "Pulmonary metastases in differentiated thyroid cancer: efficacy of radioiodine therapy and prognostic factors," *European Journal of Endocrinology*, vol. 173, no. 3, pp. 399–408, 2015.

14

High Cervical Intrathecal Targeted Drug Delivery: A Case Report of Refractory Oropharyngeal Cancer Pain

Rajat N. Moman,[1] Julie M. Rogers,[1] and Thomas P. Pittelkow[2]

[1]*Department of Anesthesiology and Perioperative Medicine, Mayo Clinic, Rochester, MN, USA*
[2]*Division of Pain Medicine, Department of Anesthesiology and Perioperative Medicine, Mayo Clinic, Rochester, MN, USA*

Correspondence should be addressed to Thomas P. Pittelkow; pittelkow.thomas@mayo.edu

Academic Editor: Guido Fadda

Introduction. Some patients with head and neck cancers have pain refractory to aggressive multimodal therapies. Herein, we report the use of an intrathecal targeted drug delivery (TDD) system catheter tip placed at C1 for the treatment of recalcitrant oropharyngeal cancer pain. *Case Report.* A patient with recurrent metastatic squamous cell tongue cancer reported severe pain not controlled despite high-dose opioids and nonopioid adjuvants. It was elected to proceed with an intrathecal TDD system with the catheter tip placed at the C1 level. After pump placement, we were able to decrease her daily oral morphine equivalents (OME) from nearly 1000 mg to 300 mg over the course of two months while titrating her TDD from 0.3 mg/day to 0.7 mg/day of intrathecal hydromorphone. Unfortunately, her improvement was limited secondary to aggressive cancer-directed treatments likely contributing to device infection and explant. *Conclusions.* In this patient, high cervical placement of an intrathecal TDD catheter was associated with a decrease in OME. While used in clinical practice on occasion, the use of high cervical TDD placement such as this implantable C1 intrathecal TDD system for cancer-associated pain is underreported in the literature. Further studies on this intervention within this challenging population are warranted.

1. Introduction

Cancer-associated pain is a worrisome problem and is accompanied by numerous psychosocial responses and a diminished quality of life. According to a recent meta-analysis, the prevalence of pain is 66.4% in advanced, metastatic, or terminal cancer and is 55.0% during anticancer treatment [1]. By comparison, a systematic review of pain in patients with head and neck cancer found 50% of patients had pain prior to cancer therapy, 81% had pain during cancer therapy, and 36% had pain 6 months after treatment. Furthermore, the reported intensity of posttreatment pain was often worse than pretreatment pain [2]. It appears that cancer in general, and head and neck cancers in particular, is commonly accompanied by distressing levels of pain.

Given the considerable amount of pain patients with cancer experience, some patients require treatment beyond routine systemic analgesics in the setting of tolerance or side effects with systemic opioids [3], or in the setting of intractable pain. Intrathecal delivery of opioids is an established intervention for patients with poorly treated cancer-related pain [4, 5] and has been associated with lower pain intensity scores and mean morphine equivalent doses [6–9]. The catheter tip is generally placed near to the site of greatest pain, based on the pain physician's clinical judgement. Optimal placement nearest the site of pain may be difficult in patients who experience pain in the head and neck region due to concern for side effects of intrathecal pain medications in the cervical region near critical structures of the brainstem. The literature on implanted intrathecal TDD for head and neck cancer pain focuses on catheter placement outside of the cervical region [10], and, while TDD catheter tips are placed high in the cervical spinal canal in clinical practice, there remains a paucity of literature reporting this technique and associated outcomes. Our report is on the successful use of an implantable intrathecal TDD system catheter tip placed at C1. Intrathecal delivery of analgesics can involve the use of an intrathecal catheter attached to an external infusion

[6, 11] or an implanted pump. Studies of intrathecal opiates have focused on external infusions in patients who are on hospice or patients who have pain from cancer outside of the head and neck area [9]. Our case report focuses on the use of an implanted intrathecal TDD system to improve the quality of life of a patient undergoing cancer-directed treatment for a head and neck cancer who remains hopeful for a cure. Herein, we describe a case of a patient undergoing treatment for recurrent metastatic oropharyngeal squamous cell cancer who is experiencing severe, cancer-associated pain and underwent implantation of an intrathecal TDD system with catheter placement at the C1 level with significant decreases in daily oral morphine equivalents (OME).

2. Case Report

This is a 59-year-old woman with recurrent, metastatic squamous cell tongue cancer who is status post two partial glossectomies, right and left neck dissections, a floor of mouth resection, a neck dissection with radial forearm free flap, tracheostomy, and chemoradiation therapy. She had experienced constant facial pain about the region of the oropharynx, left tongue, and mandible of variable intensity for two years. Additionally, she had prominent nocturnal pain that would awaken her from sleep. She described her pain as throbbing, burning, and sharp in quality. Talking, mucous secretion management, and application of medications for her dental carries all exacerbated her pain. On an 11-point numeric rating scale where 0 is no pain and 10 is the maximal pain imaginable, her average pain intensity was 8/10 and was as high as 10/10. Her level of functioning had declined to the point that her oncologist was unable to offer further chemotherapy treatment. In the setting of her cancer recurrence, she unfortunately struggled with chemical coping and opioid misuse. She had a recent admission to the hospital for a pain crisis during which severe pain limited her oral intake and her ability to communicate verbally. Prior to this admission for her pain crisis, she was on a home regimen of methadone 10 mg every 6 hours, oral morphine 60 mg every 3 hours (600 OME), gabapentin 600 mg three times daily, and venlafaxine 100 mg three times daily. During her admission for a pain crisis, her OME was increased to 2000 mg daily. In addition, a ketamine infusion and lidocaine infusion were initiated to control her intractable pain. Once her pain stabilized, she was transitioned to oral medications and discharged on methadone 15 mg every 6 hours and hydromorphone solution 12 mg per gastric tube every 2 hours (900 OME). Around this time, magnetic resonance imaging of her brain was negative for leptomeningeal metastasis. After discharge, her pain remained a 7/10 and the patient elected to have an intrathecal TDD system placed.

The patient was taken to the operating room. At the time, her last white blood cell count was 6.5×10^9/L. Given her complex airway, she was provided monitored anesthetic care. The patient was placed in a right lateral decubitus position. Previous reports [12] suggest a high cervical entry point; however, in order to reduce the risk of cervical spinal cord injury, a more traditional intrathecal targeted drug delivery approach was undertaken. After gaining intrathecal access at T12/L1 via a left paramedian approach, the catheter was easily advanced to the top of C1 under live fluoroscopy. Her pump was placed in the subcutaneous tissue overlying her left lower abdomen. A hydromorphone infusion was initiated at 300 mcg per day. This medication was chosen over morphine due to its slightly more hydrophobic nature, the anticipated higher flow concentration of CSF within the cervical spine, and, theoretically, a decreased side effect profile [13]. She was admitted to the intensive care unit for cardiopulmonary monitoring initially and remained stable without any event until discharge from general care two days later.

She was seen in follow-up by pain and palliative care physicians as an outpatient over the next eight weeks. During her follow-up, her intrathecal hydromorphone dose was gradually increased to 700 mcg per day by increasing her dose every several days and her systemic use of oral opiates declined to 300 OME with stable pain intensity. During this time, she endorsed being able to use much less of her breakthrough medication and spread her scheduled opioid medications from every two hours to every four hours. Indeed, her pain was so reasonably well controlled that her oncologist planned to resume her treatment. Given the patient's desire to pursue aggressive cancer-directed treatments, her cytotoxic chemotherapy and immune therapy were initiated three days post TDD system placement. Her next white blood cell count check after chemotherapy was started was 3.3×10^9/L. Unfortunately, approximately two months after device implantation, she developed an infection around the reservoir pocket requiring hospitalization and TDD explant.

3. Discussion

This patient had severe unrelenting pain in the setting of recurrent oropharyngeal cancer, which was limiting her ability to receive desired cancer treatment and greatly impacted her quality of life. She additionally struggled with opioid misuse as a means to chemically cope with her terminal diagnosis. Despite aggressive attempts with repeated hospitalizations to treat her pain, she experienced limited effect and the patient and her care team elected to pursue an implantable intrathecal TDD system with the catheter tip placed at the C1 level. As outlined in the guidelines, the catheter tip location, patient goals and performance status, and cerebrospinal fluid dynamics are the most important characteristics to consider when placing an intrathecal catheter [4]. After placement of the intrathecal pain pump and initiation of intrathecal hydromorphone, she did decrease her OME significantly in a controlled fashion while reporting stable pain intensity. In addition to decreasing her OME, she endorsed that her quality of life had improved and she was able to resume chemotherapy shortly after implantation. Our pain assessment focused on the use of an 11-point numeric rating scale where 0 is no pain and 10 is the maximal pain imaginable because of its ease of use and understanding by patients. However, there are other tools that globally assess quality of life of patients with cancer that have been shown to be effective and have been validated for use in patients with cancer [14–16]. One such tool that focuses on the evaluation of patients with head and neck cancer is the

EORTC QLQ-H&N35 evaluation that incorporates mouth pain, swallowing problems, senses, speech, social eating, and social contact, as well as many single scale items. While we did not utilize this measure in our assessment of our patient, this validated tool may have measured the improvements in her quality of life that she reported and may be valuable to include in future prospective assessments [15]. Ultimately, the therapeutic benefit of our patient's intrathecal TDD system was limited secondary to the aggressive nature of her cancer-directed treatments likely resulting in poor wound healing and ultimately infection with device explant. Despite the limited effect in the setting of infection, high cervical placement of an intrathecal pain catheter with an implanted TDD system appears to be an efficacious strategy for treatment of severe, cancer-associated pain.

4. Conclusions

Based on this case report, high cervical intrathecal TDD may be an effective method of treating severe, cancer-associated head and neck pain. In this case, an aggressive chemotherapy regimen may have contributed to limited therapeutic benefit for our particular patient. Experimental studies of TDD are warranted for this often challenging to treat population.

References

[1] M. H. J. van den Beuken-van Everdingen, L. M. J. Hochstenbach, E. A. J. Joosten, V. C. G. Tjan-Heijnen, and D. J. A. Janssen, "Update on prevalence of pain in patients with cancer: systematic review and meta-analysis," *Journal of Pain and Symptom Management*, vol. 51, no. 6, pp. 1070–1090.e9, 2016.

[2] J. B. Epstein, C. Hong, R. M. Logan et al., "A systematic review of orofacial pain in patients receiving cancer therapy," *Supportive Care in Cancer*, vol. 18, no. 8, pp. 1023–1031, 2010.

[3] T. P. Pittelkow, M. A. Bendel, J. J. Strand, and S. M. Moeschler, "Curing opioid toxicity with intrathecal targeted drug delivery," *Case Reports in Medicine*, vol. 2019, Article ID 3428576, 6 pages, 2019.

[4] T. R. Deer, J. E. Pope, S. M. Hayek et al., "The Polyanalgesic Consensus Conference (PACC): recommendations on intrathecal drug infusion systems best practices and guidelines," *Neuromodulation*, vol. 20, no. 2, pp. 96–132, 2017.

[5] T. R. Deer, H. S. Smith, A. Burton et al., "Comprehensive consensus based guidelines on intrathecal drug delivery systems in the treatment of pain caused by cancer pain," *Pain Physician*, vol. 14, no. 3, pp. E283–E312, 2011.

[6] S. E. Brogan, N. B. Winter, and A. Okifuji, "Prospective observational study of patient-controlled intrathecal analgesia: impact on cancer-associated symptoms, breakthrough pain control, and patient satisfaction," *Regional Anesthesia and Pain Medicine*, vol. 40, no. 4, pp. 369–375, 2015.

[7] T. J. Smith and P. J. Coyne, "Implantable drug delivery systems (IDDS) after failure of comprehensive medical management (CMM) can palliate symptoms in the most refractory cancer pain patients," *Journal of Palliative Medicine*, vol. 8, no. 4, pp. 736–742, 2005.

[8] T. J. Smith, P. J. Coyne, P. S. Staats et al., "An implantable drug delivery system (IDDS) for refractory cancer pain provides sustained pain control, less drug-related toxicity, and possibly better survival compared with comprehensive medical management (CMM)," *Annals of Oncology*, vol. 16, no. 5, pp. 825–833, 2005.

[9] T. J. Smith, P. S. Staats, T. Deer et al., "Randomized clinical trial of an implantable drug delivery system compared with comprehensive medical management for refractory cancer pain: impact on pain, drug-related toxicity, and survival," *Journal of Clinical Oncology*, vol. 20, no. 19, pp. 4040–4049, 2002.

[10] P. E. Andersen, J. I. Cohen, E. C. Everts, M. D. Bedder, and K. J. Burchiel, "Intrathecal narcotics for relief of pain from head and neck cancer," *Archives of Otolaryngology - Head & Neck Surgery*, vol. 117, no. 11, pp. 1277–1280, 1991.

[11] L. Baker, J. Balls, C. Regnard, and A. Pridie, "Cervical intrathecal analgesia for head and neck/upper limb cancer pain: six case reports," *Palliative Medicine*, vol. 21, no. 6, pp. 543–545, 2007.

[12] B. J. Crul, R. T. van Dongen, D. G. Snijdelaar, and E. H. Rutten, "Long-term continuous intrathecal administration of morphine and bupivacaine at the upper cervical level," *Anesthesia & Analgesia*, vol. 79, no. 3, pp. 594–597, 1994.

[13] M. Goodarzi, "Comparison of epidural morphine, hydromorphone and fentanyl for postoperative pain control in children undergoing orthopaedic surgery," *Pediatric Anesthesia*, vol. 9, no. 5, pp. 419–422, 1999.

[14] G. Oteri, G. Trifirò, M. Peditto et al., "Treatment of medication-related osteonecrosis of the jaw and its impact on a patient's quality of life: a single-center, 10-year experience from Southern Italy," *Drug Safety*, vol. 41, no. 1, pp. 111–123, 2018.

[15] S. Singer, J. I. Arraras, W. C. Chie et al., "Performance of the EORTC questionnaire for the assessment of quality of life in head and neck cancer patients EORTC QLQ-H&N35: a methodological review," *Quality of Life Research*, vol. 22, no. 8, pp. 1927–1941, 2013.

[16] N. K. Aaronson, S. Ahmedzai, B. Bergman et al., "The European Organization for Research and Treatment of Cancer QLQ-C30: a quality-of-life instrument for use in international clinical trials in oncology," *Journal of the National Cancer Institute*, vol. 85, no. 5, pp. 365–376, 1993.

15

Successful Treatment by Surgery and Lenvatinib of a Patient with Adrenal Metastasis of Papillary Thyroid Cancer

Hajime Nakamura,[1] Kohichi Takada,[1] Kazuyuki Murase,[1] Hiroki Sakamoto,[1] Naotaka Hayasaka,[1] Kazuma Ishikawa,[1] Yuki Ikeda,[1] Makoto Yoshida,[1] Satoshi Iyama,[2] Ko Kobayashi,[3] Tetsuya Shindo,[3] Shintaro Sugita,[4] Koji Miyanishi,[1] Masayoshi Kobune,[2] Naoya Masumori,[3] and Junji Kato[1]

[1]*Department of Medical Oncology, Sapporo Medical University School of Medicine, Japan*
[2]*Department of Hematology, Sapporo Medical University School of Medicine, Japan*
[3]*Department of Urology, Sapporo Medical University School of Medicine, Japan*
[4]*Department of Surgical Pathology, Sapporo Medical University School of Medicine, Japan*

Correspondence should be addressed to Kohichi Takada; ktakada@sapmed.ac.jp

Academic Editor: Katsuhiro Tanaka

Papillary thyroid cancer (PTC) is considered an indolent cancer, but some PTC patients do present with distant metastases and treatment strategies for such patients are not well established. Recently, lenvatinib, an inhibitor of multiple tyrosine kinases, has been introduced to treat patients with advanced PTC but carries a risk of serious adverse events such as hemorrhage. Here, we report a PTC patient with a left adrenal metastasis and lenvatinib-induced hemorrhage who underwent successful surgical resection and was subsequently treated with a lower dose of lenvatinib. The patient has now been in a stable state with no adverse events for nearly two years. This case highlights the importance of surgical resection of metastatic PTC and subsequent lenvatinib therapy, even when the tumor is at an advanced stage.

1. Introduction

Papillary thyroid cancer (PTC) is the most common type of thyroid cancer. PTC is a differentiated thyroid cancer (DTC) considered to be indolent because distant metastases are seen in only a small minority of patients. Standard therapies for metastatic DTC include treatment with radioactive iodine (RAI) [1], but patients who become refractory to this treatment have a poor prognosis [2]. When PTC does metastasize, the sites most frequently infiltrated are the lung and bone [3]. Adrenal metastases are extremely rare, with only a few cases reported [4]. As a result, no treatment strategies are well established for this condition. Lenvatinib, a novel inhibitor of multiple tyrosine kinases, has been approved for treating patients with radioiodine-refractory-(RR-) DTC. Lenvatinib can dramatically suppress DTC but may evoke lethal adverse events such as bleeding [5].

Here, we present a patient with RR-PTC successfully treated by resection of a left adrenal metastasis despite lenvatinib-induced intratumoral hemorrhage. We were able to continue lenvatinib treatment in this patient at a lower dose with no severe adverse effects.

2. Case Presentation

A 70-year-old woman was first diagnosed with PTC at the age of 53. She subsequently underwent a total thyroidectomy together with regional lymph node dissection, followed by iodine-131 (I-131) therapy immediately following the initial diagnosis. The TNM classification at

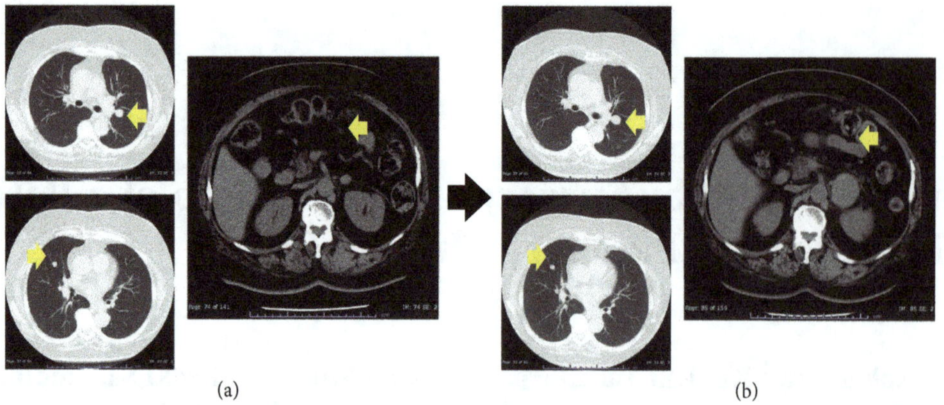

Figure 1: Computed tomography of lung tumors and a left adrenal tumor (arrows). (a) At the time when the left adrenal tumor was initially identified. (b) Six months after the initial diagnosis of the left adrenal tumor.

the first pathological diagnosis was T4aN1aM0. Recurrence did not occur until 10 years after the patient's initial treatment when multiple lung and supraclavicular lymph node metastases were identified during late follow-up. The patient received stereotactic radiotherapy (58 Gy/29 Fr) for the lymph node metastasis and a second course of I-131 therapy. However, metastases in both lung and lymph node gradually progressed despite such therapy. The patient underwent a third round of I-131 therapy three years after the second. Since then, these tumors have remained unchanged for almost 5 years, indicating stable disease (SD).

However, the patient presented with a left adrenal tumor 17 years after her initial treatment for PTC. This grew rapidly over only six months, whereas the lung and supraclavicular lymph node metastases remained stable. We initially considered that the adrenal tumor might not have been a PTC metastasis (Figure 1), but the serum thyroglobulin level rapidly increased as high as 273.83 ng/mL in step with the growth of the tumor (although it had previously remained within the normal range (5.0-30.0 ng/mL) since the first diagnosis). We therefore performed an endoscopic ultrasound-guided fine-needle aspiration (EUS-FNA) for the purpose of histopathological assessment. This revealed that the structure of the tumor was similar to that of the resected PTC. Based on these findings, it was concluded that the left adrenal tumor was indeed a PTC metastasis (Figure 2). Immediately after the EUS-FNA, the patient experienced an intratumoral hemorrhage but recovered quickly with supportive care only. We started 24 mg lenvatinib treatment for advanced RR-PTC five days after the EUS-FNA procedure, but 12 h later, the patient experienced sudden back pain due to intratumoral rebleeding (Figure 3). Although lenvatinib is a promising drug against advanced RR-PTC, it is well-recognized that it carries a risk of adverse bleeding events. To prevent further bleeding and to enable continued lenvatinib treatment, we surgically resected the left adrenal metastasis. Subsequently, the serum thyroglobulin level decreased to within the normal range. We retreated with 8 mg lenvatinib, which has now maintained SD without any serious adverse events for almost two years.

3. Discussion

According to a previous report, distant metastases from PTC are rare, with only 71 of 5,969 resected PTC cases presenting with disease spread [6]. Of these 71 cases, the most frequently affected site was the lung (60 cases) followed by the bone (5 cases). No adrenal metastases were reported in such patients. The most common systemic modality used to treat patients with metastatic DTC is RAI. The survival rate in patients with I-131 uptake was reported to be 56% at 10 years, whereas in patients without I-131 uptake, it was only 10% at that time. The treatment strategy for such patients is not well established [2].

Several multitarget kinase inhibitor drugs have been introduced recently for the treatment of RR-DTC. Sorafenib was first approved for this indication in 2013 after a phase 3 trial showed significant improvement in progression-free survival (PFS) compared to placebo [7]. Lenvatinib treatment also resulted in a significant prolongation of PFS and an improved response rate among patients with RR-DTC [8]. Vandetanib treatment also yielded a significant prolongation of PFS in a phase 3 trial of patients with advanced medullary thyroid carcinoma [9]. Thus, treatment options for RR-DTC are increasing owing to the development of such drugs. However, several well-known distinct adverse events are associated with the use of multitarget kinase inhibitors, of which some may even be fatal, such as hemorrhage with lenvatinib therapy.

In the PTC case described here, surgical resection of a left adrenal metastasis after lenvatinib-induced hemorrhage was performed. Reports of PTC cases with surgical resection of distant metastases are very limited, but long-term survival after the resection of a solitary pancreatic metastasis of thyroid cancer has been reported [10]. Our patient experienced severe back pain when hemorrhage occurred, which seriously compromised her quality of life, such that we considered it impossible to continue lenvatinib

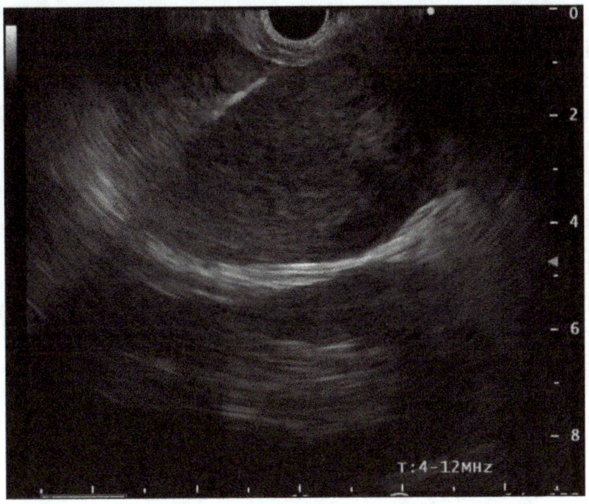

(a)

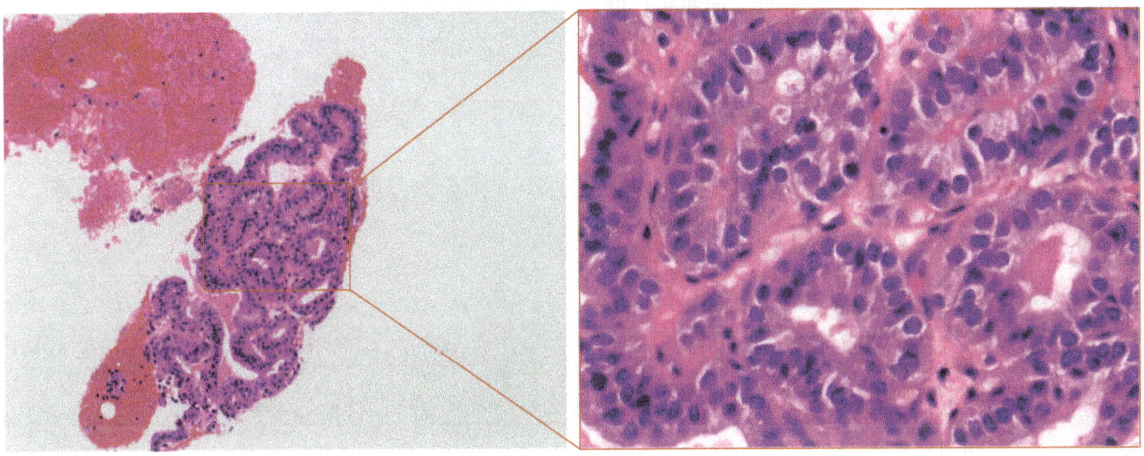

(b)

FIGURE 2: Endoscopic ultrasound-guided fine-needle aspiration (EUS-FNA) procedure and histopathological findings. (a) EUS-FNA was performed on the left adrenal tumor from the posterior wall of the stomach. (b) Histopathological findings showing a papillary structure similar to that of the resected thyroid cancer.

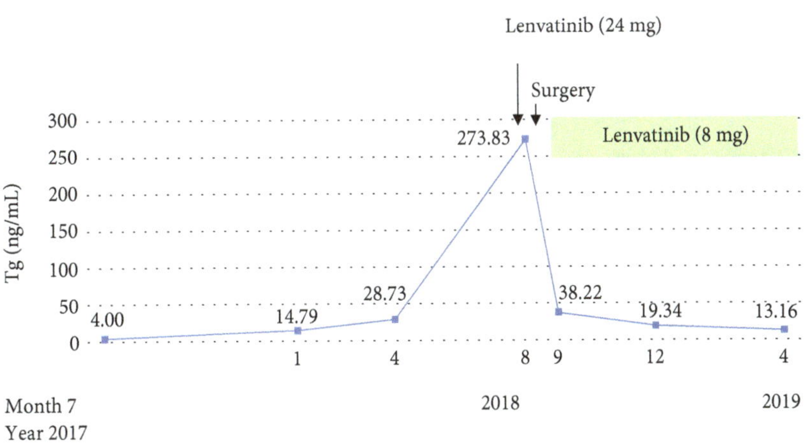

(a)

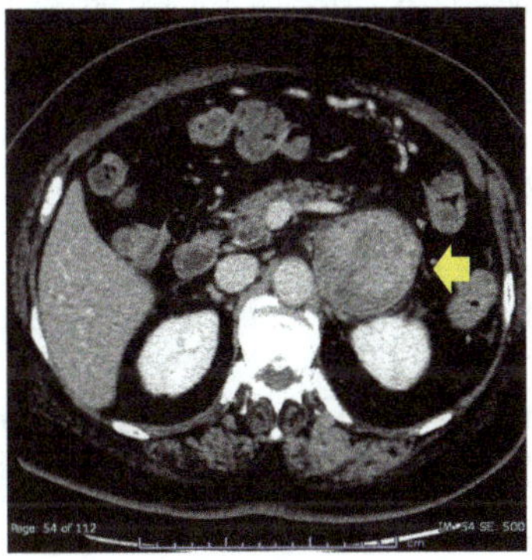

(b)

FIGURE 3: Clinical course of the patient. (a) Serum thyroglobulin level (T) rapidly increased in step with the size of the left adrenal tumor. We initiated 24 mg lenvatinib treatment, but due to uncontrollable intratumoral bleeding, the patient had to undergo surgery. The serum thyroglobulin level immediately decreased after surgery, and the patient was again treated with lenvatinib, now at only 8 mg. (b) Computed tomography findings of intratumoral bleeding of the left adrenal tumor (arrow).

treatment without a risk of rebleeding. However, after surgical resection, the serum thyroglobulin level immediately dropped, and the patient was treated again with 8 mg lenvatinib, which led to a stable condition without serious events for almost two years. Thus, surgical resection of this distant metastasis almost certainly contributed to the patient's long-term survival.

A dose of 8 mg is lower than the recommended initial dose of lenvatinib for RR-DTC. Another successful instance where adverse events of lenvatinib were managed by individualizing the drug schedule in terms of reduced dose and timing, with a significant dose intensity reduction, has also been reported [11]. Our case highlights the efficacy and improved patient safety of a lower dose of lenvatinib for RR-DTC.

Our findings suggest that surgical treatment is an option for rapidly growing metastatic tumors of PTC origin, even at an advanced stage with multiple lung metastases. If a hemorrhage induced by lenvatinib can be managed satisfactorily, lenvatinib administration at a lower dose may be continued for the treatment of metastatic RR-PTC.

References

[1] R. Dadu and M. E. Cabanillas, "Optimizing therapy for radioactive iodine-refractory differentiated thyroid cancer: current state of the art and future directions," *Minerva Endocrinologica*, vol. 37, no. 4, pp. 335–356, 2012.

[2] C. Durante, N. Haddy, E. Baudin et al., "Long-term outcome of 444 patients with distant metastases from papillary and follicular thyroid carcinoma: benefits and limits of radioiodine therapy," *The Journal of Clinical Endocrinology and Metabolism*, vol. 91, no. 8, pp. 2892–2899, 2006.

[3] E. Sampson, J. D. Brierley, L. W. le, L. Rotstein, and R. W. Tsang, "Clinical management and outcome of papillary and follicular (differentiated) thyroid cancer presenting with distant metastasis at diagnosis," *Cancer*, vol. 110, no. 7, pp. 1451–1456, 2007.

[4] N. Batawil, "Papillary thyroid cancer with bilateral adrenal metastases," *Thyroid*, vol. 23, no. 12, pp. 1651–1654, 2013.

[5] M. E. Cabanillas and S. Takahashi, "Managing the adverse events associated with lenvatinib therapy in radioiodine-refractory differentiated thyroid cancer," *Seminars in Oncology*, vol. 46, no. 1, pp. 57–64, 2019.

[6] Y. Ito, H. Masuoka, M. Fukushima et al., "Prognosis and prognostic factors of patients with papillary carcinoma showing distant metastasis at surgery (M1 patients) in Japan," *Endocrine Journal*, vol. 57, no. 6, pp. 523–531, 2010.

[7] M. S. Brose, C. M. Nutting, B. Jarzab et al., "Sorafenib in radioactive iodine-refractory, locally advanced or metastatic differentiated thyroid cancer: a randomised, double-blind, phase 3 trial," *The Lancet*, vol. 384, no. 9940, pp. 319–328, 2014.

[8] M. Schlumberger, M. Tahara, L. J. Wirth et al., "Lenvatinib versus placebo in radioiodine-refractory thyroid cancer," *The New England Journal of Medicine*, vol. 372, no. 7, pp. 621–630, 2015.

[9] S. A. Wells Jr., B. G. Robinson, R. F. Gagel et al., "Vandetanib in patients with locally advanced or metastatic medullary thyroid cancer: a randomized, double-blind phase III trial," *Journal of Clinical Oncology*, vol. 30, no. 2, pp. 134–141, 2012.

[10] M. Hyodo, H. Nagai, N. Sata et al., "Long-term survivor without recurrence after resection of simultaneous solitary pancreatic metastasis from thyroid medullary carcinoma," *Hepato-Gastroenterology*, vol. 50, no. 53, pp. 1687-1688, 2003.

[11] C. Resteghini, L. D. Locati, P. Bossi, C. Bergamini, M. Guzzo, and L. Licitra, "Do not throw the baby out with the bathwater: SELECT a personalized, de-escalated lenvatinib schedule allows response in locally advanced DTC while controlling major drug-related bleeding," *Annals of Oncology*, vol. 28, no. 9, pp. 2321-2322, 2017.

16

Invasive Aspergillosis in a Patient with Stage III (or 3a or 3b) Non-Small-Cell Lung Cancer Treated with Durvalumab

Ashish Gupta,[1] Aung Tun,[2] Katy Ticona,[2] Aam Baqui,[3] and Elizabeth Guevara[1]

[1]*Internal Medicine, The Brooklyn Hospital Center, Brooklyn, New York, NY, USA*
[2]*Hematology Oncology, The Brooklyn Hospital Center, Brooklyn, New York, NY, USA*
[3]*Pathology, The Brooklyn Hospital Center, Brooklyn, New York, NY, USA*

Correspondence should be addressed to Ashish Gupta; ashish@vippllc.com

Academic Editor: Peter F. Lenehan

Durvalumab is a therapeutic monoclonal antibody that blocks the checkpoint inhibitor, programmed death ligand 1 (PD-L1), resulting in T-cell activation and an antitumor response. Durvalumab is approved for patients with unresectable stage III non-small-cell lung cancer (NSCLC) which has not progressed following platinum-based chemoradiotherapy. A 63-year-old man presented to the emergency department with a 15-day history of increasing shortness of breath. Several months previously, he had been diagnosed with a poorly differentiated stage IIIB NSCLC. He had completed six cycles of chemotherapy with paclitaxel and carboplatin and four cycles of immunotherapy with durvalumab 13 days before his emergency hospital admission. Computed tomography (CT) imaging showed a large left-sided loculated hydropneumothorax suggestive of empyema, patchy opacification of the left lung, and a left upper lobe lung mass. Histology of the cell block from the pleural fluid and decorticated lung tissue showed hyphae suggestive of invasive *Aspergillus fumigatus*. Treatment with voriconazole resulted in clinical improvement. To our knowledge, this is the first reported case of pleural aspergillosis in a patient treated with durvalumab. However, the increasing use of immune checkpoint inhibitors in oncology requires increased awareness by clinicians of immune-related adverse events (irAEs) due to opportunistic infection.

1. Introduction

Durvalumab is a therapeutic monoclonal antibody that blocks the checkpoint inhibitor, programmed death ligand 1 (PD-L1), resulting in T-cell activation and an antitumor response [1, 2]. In 2017, durvalumab was approved for patients with unresectable stage III non-small-cell lung cancer (NSCLC) when the disease has not progressed following platinum-based chemoradiotherapy [3]. The approval for durvalumab followed the findings from the PACIFIC phase III clinical trial, which showed that adding durvalumab after chemoradiotherapy for stage III NSCLC resulted in significantly improved progression-free survival (PFS) [1].

In the past decade, the development of targeted therapy and immune therapy for NSCLC has progressed rapidly. Humanized therapeutic monoclonal antibodies that target growth factors, tumor-associated antigens, and immune checkpoint inhibitors are now increasingly used in clinical oncology. Fujita et al. recently reported that patients with NSCLC who received treatment with the anti-programmed cell death protein- (PD-) 1 antibody, nivolumab, were at an increased risk for occult infectious disease, especially patients with a history of diabetes mellitus [4]. The association between the use of immune therapy in oncology, including immune checkpoint blockade, and opportunistic infections has been termed immune-related adverse events (irAEs) [5].

There is a clinical spectrum of pulmonary aspergillosis that develops as a consequence of the interaction between the fungus and the host [6]. More common clinical presentations include invasive aspergillosis that develops in severely immunocompromised patients, chronic pulmonary aspergillosis that affects patients with chronic underlying lung disease, and allergic bronchopulmonary aspergillosis that affects patients with asthma and cystic fibrosis [6]. Pleural aspergillosis is a rare condition that has been reported to be due to *Aspergillus fumigatus*, *Aspergillus flavus*, and *Aspergillus terreus*, but coinfection of the pleural space with bacteria has also been reported [6]. Pleural aspergillosis has also been found in cases following pleural instrumentation and in the presence of a bronchopleural fistula [6]. The current European Organization for Research and Treatment of Cancer (EORTC-MSG) definitions recommend that positive cultures of *Aspergillus* spp. are obtained from lung specimens to confirm the diagnosis of infection [7].

A case is presented of pleural aspergillosis in a patient treated with durvalumab for stage IIIB non-small-cell lung cancer (NSCLC).

2. Case Report

A 63-year-old man who worked as a limousine driver presented to the emergency department of the Brooklyn Hospital Center, New York, with a 15-day history of increasing shortness of breath. Several months previously, he had been diagnosed with a poorly differentiated stage IIIB non-small-cell lung cancer (NSCLC) (squamous cell carcinoma). He had a previous episode of pleural effusion for which he received a thoracentesis. He had also received prednisone 50 mg for 5 days for a COPD exacerbation about a month before the hospital admission. He completed six cycles of chemotherapy with paclitaxel and carboplatin three months previously, before commencing four cycles of immunotherapy with durvalumab, an immune checkpoint inhibitor, which he completed 13 days before his emergency hospital admission.

He had a past medical history of chronic obstructive pulmonary disease (COPD), type 2 diabetes mellitus, hypertension, and chronic hepatitis C treated with sofosbuvir and ledipasvir (Harvoni). He had smoked one pack of cigarettes a week for 40 years and had formerly used alcohol but denied any illicit drug use. His father suffered from gout and hypertension, and his mother had a history of nephrectomy and had a permanent pacemaker.

Laboratory investigations on the day of admission showed reduced hemoglobin (Hb) 11.4 g/dl (normal range, 13.1–15.5 g/dl) and hematocrit 35% (normal range, 39–47%), with basic metabolic panel (BMP) tests within the normal range. An increased white blood cell (WBC) count 15.1×10^9/l (normal range, 4.8 – 10.8×10^9/l) included 87% neutrophils (normal range, 42.4–75.2%), 1.8% lymphocytes (normal range, 20.0–51.0%), and a platelet count of 323×10^9/l (normal range, 130 – 400×10^9/l). On the day following hospital admission, computed tomography (CT) of the chest showed a large left-sided loculated hydropneumothorax suggestive of empyema, patchy opacification in the left greater than the right lobe of the lung along with a left upper lobe lung mass. A pigtail catheter placed percutaneously under CT guidance drained an exudate containing 93% neutrophil polymorphs, which was sent for microbial culture. Intravenous antibiotic treatment commenced with ceftriaxone, which was then changed to vancomycin, piperacillin-tazobactam, and metronidazole, but with limited response. The patient had a persistent air leak and was noted to have a bronchopleural fistula, so on the tenth day after hospital admission, video-assisted thoracoscopic surgery (VATS) was performed.

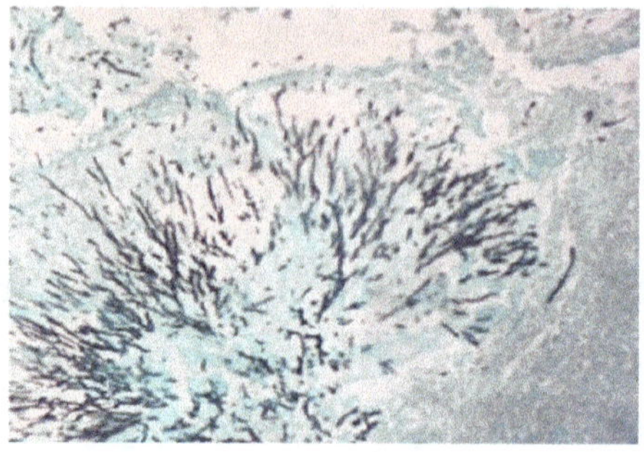

Figure 1: Photomicrograph of the pleural fluid cell block shows *Aspergillus fumigatus*, identified by histochemical staining. The acute angle of the branching hyphae (black) is distinctive (Gomori methenamine silver (GMS)). Magnification ×200.

Two weeks following hospital admission, fungal cultures from the pleural fluid, as well as from decorticated lung tissue, identified *Aspergillus fumigatus* (Figure 1). However, serology did not detect antibodies to *Aspergillus* spp. Treatment for aspergillosis commenced with voriconazole, a triazole antifungal agent. His clinical condition improved, and his WBC count stabilized at 11.1×10^9/l. He was discharged home on linezolid and levofloxacin and a 60-day course of voriconazole.

3. Discussion

Durvalumab, pembrolizumab, and atezolizumab are therapeutic monoclonal antibodies to PD-1/PD-L1 checkpoint inhibitors currently licensed for the treatment of NSCLC [1–3]. This case has demonstrated that with the increasing use of immune checkpoint inhibitors in oncology clinicians should be aware of the association between opportunistic infections and immune therapy or immune-related adverse events (irAEs) due to opportunistic infection [4, 5].

Our patient contracted invasive aspergillosis while receiving durvalumab. However, the patient has COPD, diabetes mellitus, lymphopenia, and recent steroid exposures which are known risk factors for opportunistic infections including invasive aspergillosis (IA). In addition, the patient had a bronchopleural fistula, presumably related to prior thoracocentesis, that may have contributed to the IA in our patient.

Several recent studies have demonstrated the association between the use of immune checkpoint inhibitors and irAEs. The recent findings from a study that included a large cohort of patients with melanoma showed that approximately 7% of patients who received immune checkpoint inhibitors suffered from irAEs associated with severe atypical infection [8]. This study showed that opportunistic infections occurred most commonly in patients treated with infliximab and steroids [8]. The patient presented in this report had completed a course of steroids about a month before his recent hospital admission. The development of acute pulmonary tuberculosis in lung cancer patients following immune checkpoint inhibitor therapy without immunosuppressive treatment has been reported, which suggests the possible role of hypersensitivity, similar to immune reconstitution inflammatory syndrome (IRIS), leading to irAEs associated with opportunistic infection [9].

Fujita et al. retrospectively reviewed 167 patients with NSCLC treated with nivolumab and showed that the prevalence of lung infection was 19.2% (32 cases), of which 25 were bacterial, six were viral, and two cases were fungal [4]. This study showed that patients with NSCLC and a history of diabetes mellitus had a significantly increased prevalence of lung infection (OR, 3.61; 95% CI, 1.14–11.4; $p = 0.028$) [4]. These authors concluded that for patients with NSCLC receiving treatment with the checkpoint inhibitor, nivolumab, there was a significant risk for developing opportunistic infection and that diabetes mellitus was an independent risk factor [4]. The patient presented in this report had a history of diabetes mellitus. On the contrary, immune checkpoint inhibitors are being studied as adjunctive immunotherapy for immunosuppressed patients with IA, particularly AML patients [10].

According to the current European Organization for Research and Treatment of Cancer (EORTC-MSG) definitions, positive cultures of *Aspergillus* spp. from lung specimens, excluding BAL fluid, are recommended to make a proven diagnosis of fungal infection [7]. In this case, fungal organisms were isolated from the pleural fluid as well as from decorticated lung tissue, but no serum antibodies were detected. This finding raises the possibility that fungal organisms may have been a contaminant during the sampling procedure. Also, in immunosuppressed patients these antibodies may be negative. However, the findings from recent studies that have shown that both the *Aspergillus fumigatus*-specific IgM and IgG antibody assays and the galactomannan (GM) assay have limited value for the diagnosis of pulmonary aspergillosis [11]. The radiologic appearance in invasive aspergillosis is varied and nonspecific. It includes bronchial consolidation, centrilobular nodules, and bilateral bronchial dilation [12]. In our case, consolidation was seen which as above is a nonspecific finding. Also, in this case, the patient had a history of thoracocentesis and bronchopleural fistula, which may have been the source of infection.

These previous reports and the findings of this case highlight the importance of obtaining lung or pleural fluid samples for the identification of *Aspergillus fumigatus*, which can be identified directly by light microscopy using appropriate histochemical stains (Figure 1).

4. Conclusion

This report has presented a case of pleural aspergillosis in a patient treated with durvalumab, an immune checkpoint inhibitor, for stage IIIB non-small-cell lung cancer (NSCLC). To our knowledge, this is the first reported case of pleural aspergillosis in a patient treated with durvalumab. However, the increasing use of immune checkpoint inhibitors in oncology requires increased awareness by clinicians of immune-related adverse events (irAEs) due to opportunistic infection.

Longer follow-up and additional studies are required to determine causation between durvalumab treatment and invasive aspergillosis. Nonetheless, our case raises the awareness of opportunistic infections in patients treated with immune checkpoint inhibitors.

Consent

The patient has provided written informed consent to publish this report.

Disclosure

This is an original manuscript that has not been previously published and is not being submitted elsewhere.

Authors' Contributions

All authors have approved the final manuscript.

References

[1] S. J. Antonia, A. Villegas, D. Daniel et al., "Durvalumab after chemoradiotherapy in stage III non-small-cell lung cancer," *The New England Journal of Medicine*, vol. 377, no. 20, pp. 1919–1929, 2017.

[2] A. W. Chalmers, S. B. Patel, and W. Akerley, "Immunotherapy after chemoradiotherapy in stage III non-small cell lung cancer: a new standard of care?," *Journal of Thoracic Disease*, vol. 10, no. 3, pp. 1198–1200, 2018.

[3] Food and Drug Administration (FDA), "IMFINZI® (durvalumab) injection, for intravenous use Initial U.S. Approval," 2017, February, 2019, https://www.accessdata.fda.gov/drugsatfda_docs/label/2018/761069s002lbl.pdf.

[4] K. Fujita, Y. H. Kim, O. Kanai, H. Yoshida, T. Mio, and T. Hirai, "Emerging concerns of infectious diseases in lung cancer patients receiving immune checkpoint inhibitor therapy," *Respiratory Medicine*, vol. 146, pp. 66–70, 2019.

[5] J. M. Michot, C. Bigenwald, S. Champiat et al., "Immune-related adverse events with immune checkpoint blockade: a comprehensive review," *European Journal of Cancer*, vol. 54, pp. 139–148, 2016.

[6] C. Kosmidis and D. W. Denning, "The clinical spectrum of pulmonary aspergillosis," *Thorax*, vol. 70, no. 3, pp. 270–277, 2015.

[7] B. De Pauw, T. J. Walsh, J. P. Donnelly et al., "Revised Definitions of Invasive Fungal Disease from the European Organization for Research and Treatment of Cancer/Invasive Fungal Infections Cooperative Group and the National Institute of Allergy and Infectious Diseases Mycoses Study Group (EORTC/MSG) Consensus Group," *Clinical Infectious Diseases*, vol. 46, no. 12, pp. 1813–1821, 2008.

[8] M. Del Castillo, F. A. Romero, E. Argüello, C. Kyi, M. A. Postow, and G. Redelman-Sidi, "The spectrum of serious infections among patients receiving immune checkpoint blockade for the treatment of melanoma," *Clinical Infectious Diseases*, vol. 63, no. 11, pp. 1490–1493, 2016.

[9] T. Reungwetwattana and A. A. Adjei, "Anti-PD-1 antibody treatment and the development of acute pulmonary tuberculosis," *Journal of Thoracic Oncology*, vol. 11, no. 12, pp. 2048–2050, 2016.

[10] N. Daver and D. P. Kontoyiannis, "Checkpoint inhibitors and aspergillosis in AML: the double hit hypothesis," *The Lancet Oncology*, vol. 18, no. 12, pp. 1571–1573, 2017.

[11] J. Jung, M. Y. Kim, Y. P. Chong et al., "Clinical characteristics, radiologic findings, risk factors and outcomes of serum galactomannan-negative invasive pulmonary aspergillosis," *Journal of Microbiology, Immunology, and Infection*, vol. 51, no. 6, pp. 802–809, 2018.

[12] T. Franquet, N. L. Müller, A. Giménez, P. Guembe, J. de La Torre, and S. Bagué, "Spectrum of pulmonary aspergillosis: histologic, clinical, and radiologic findings," *Radiographics*, vol. 21, no. 4, pp. 825–837, 2001 Jul-Aug.

17

The Three P's: Parotid, PD-L1 and Pembrolizumab

Amanda Wiggins, Zhaohui Arter, and Tamie Kerns

Tripler Army Medical Center, 1 Jarrett White Road, DHCK-DM, Honolulu, HI 96859, USA

Correspondence should be addressed to Amanda Wiggins; amanda.keith8@gmail.com

Academic Editor: Francesco A. Mauri

We present a case of recurrent, platinum-refractory undifferentiated carcinoma of the parotid which was treated with checkpoint inhibitor, Pembrolizumab, and achieved a complete response to therapy. We review the literature of checkpoint inhibitor use in undifferentiated carcinoma of the parotid.

1. Introduction

Immunologic therapy is an emerging treatment modality in oncology, which may provide prolonged survival in numerous malignancies [1]. PD-L1 expression has been found to have both prognostic and treatment utility in the management of metastatic malignancies [2]. We present a patient with one hundred percent PD-L1 expression in an undifferentiated, EBV positive, metastatic carcinoma of parotid origin with near complete remission after treatment with Pembrolizumab.

2. Case Presentation

A previously healthy 52-year-old Samoan woman initially presented to her primary care provider with complaints of otalgia and swelling in the left side of her face for three weeks. She reported no facial weakness, trismus, dysphagia, odynophagia, dental pain, fevers, chills, weight loss, and fatigue. On initial physical exam, a 6 cm nontender, subcutaneous, cystic mass was palpated in the left parotid. The oral cavity showed no deformities or evidence of abnormalities. There was no lymphadenopathy of the anterior or posterior cervical chain, supraclavicular, or axillary lymph nodes. At that time, she was prescribed with antibiotics for presumed sialadenitis with no effect on her symptoms. On the next follow-up visit, she was referred to otolaryngology for further evaluation.

A neck and chest computer topography (CT) scan demonstrated two necrotic left parotid masses measuring 2.5 × 2.8 cm and 2.7 × 2.8 cm, respectively, multiple ipsilateral lymph nodes measuring up to 1.9 cm in diameter, and an asymmetrically enhancing left nasopharynx. A fine needle aspiration (FNA) of an involved local lymph node revealed a nonkeratinizing, undifferentiated carcinoma composed of pleomorphic cells positive for Epstein-Barr virus (EBV). The differential diagnosis based on FNA findings includes primary parotid carcinoma, lymphoepithelial carcinoma, or metastatic nasopharyngeal carcinoma. Blind biopsies of the nasopharynx were negative. PET/CT revealed hypermetabolic activity in the left parotid gland and several local nodes, highly suggestive of a primary parotid neoplasm. Excisional biopsy revealed a nonkeratinizing, undifferentiated carcinoma composed of pleomorphic cells, positive for Epstein-Barr virus (EBV). The results of subsequent excisional biopsy of the parotid gland masses were consistent with previous FNA findings.

The patient was staged as Stage IVa (cT3N2bM0) per AJCC 7th ed. Due to the extension of the parotid disease toward the main trunk of cranial nerve (CN) VII, there was a concern for postoperative CN VII palsy with surgical management. Surgery was therefore deferred, and definitive cisplatin-based concurrent/chemoradiation treatment was initiated. On first surveillance PET/CT, at 12 weeks postconcurrent chemoradiation treatment, she was found to have PET-avid hepatic and bone lesions (Figure 1). A CT-guided portacaval lymph node biopsy confirmed a metastatic disease (Figure 2). IHC staining of the portal cava lymph node demonstrated 100% PD-L1 expression. Next Generation

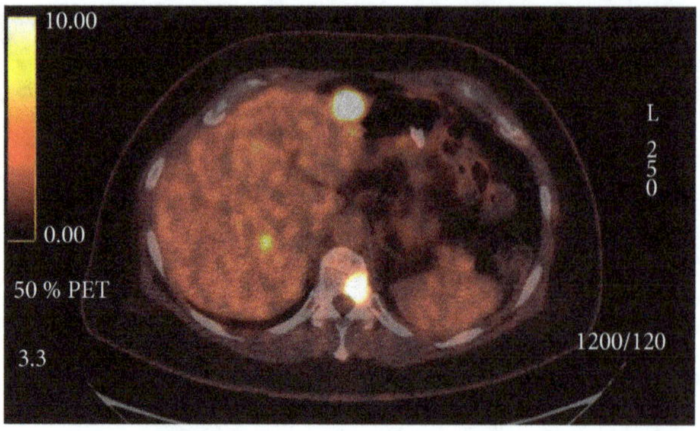

FIGURE 1: PET/CT image prior to immunotherapy.

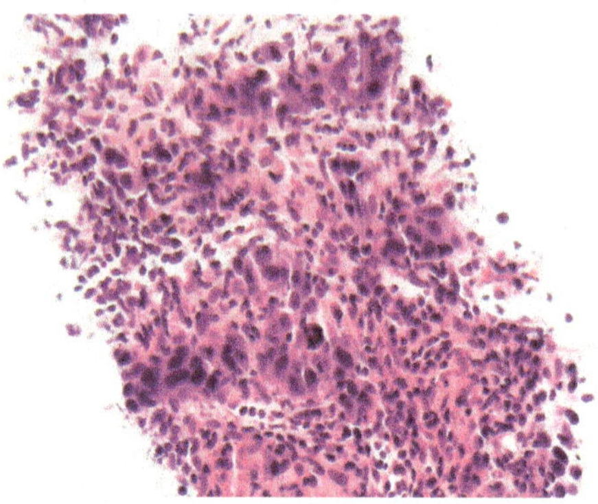

FIGURE 2: Biopsy of metastatic lesion involving the portacaval lymph node.

Sequencing was negative for additional mutations. Pembrolizumab monotherapy resulted in a near complete resolution of her hepatic metastasis and complete metabolic resolution of the left parotid mass, cervical adenopathy, and skeletal lesions on PET/CT following four cycles (Figure 3). Follow-up PET/CT scan found a progression of disease per RECIST v1.1 criteria after seven months of treatment.

3. Discussion

Salivary gland malignancies are uncommon, accounting for 3-6.5% of all head and neck cancers [3]. Undifferentiated salivary gland malignancies, however, are exceedingly rare. Less than 1% of all salivary gland tumors are lymphoepithelial or undifferentiated carcinoma, carrying a poor prognosis [4]. The reported incidence of undifferentiated carcinoma ranged from 1 to 5.5% in all parotid gland malignancies [5]. A literature search for undifferentiated parotid carcinoma returned seldom results; most of these reports were small case series [6–8]. Furthermore, this patient with poorly differentiated parotid carcinoma behaved more like a nasopharyngeal carcinoma (NPC). Traditionally, salivary gland malignancies are slow growing and become metastatic late in the disease process [1]. Conversely, our patient developed metastatic disease early in her course following cytotoxic chemotherapy and local radiation.

Many features of our patient's case mirror previously reported characteristics of NPC, which may suggest a relationship between NPC, salivary carcinomas, and other EBV-associated malignancies. First, ninety-five percent of primary nasopharyngeal carcinomas are poorly differentiated or undifferentiated, nonkeratinizing carcinomas, with the highest incidence in the Asian and Pacific islands [9]. NPC is also well known to be an EBV-associated malignancy and characteristically causes lymphocytic infiltrates surrounding tumors [9]. Finally, the upregulation of PD-L1 expression has been documented in multiple EBV-associated malignancies. While the exact mechanism of PD-L1 upregulation is not well understood, it is suspected to be due to constitutively activated oncogenic pathways [9–11]. In one study, all patients with high tumor PD-L1 expression (PD-L1 expressed in 90-100% of malignant cells) were positive for EBV, similar to our patient [11]. There is conflicting data on the prognostic value of PD-L1 expression in NPC; however, recent studies seem to suggest that a high percentage of PD-L1 expression may be associated with a poor prognosis [12]. Likewise, in other salivary gland malignancies, higher PD-L1 expression has been associated with a more aggressive cancer [13]. In this patient, the similarities between her histology and disease progression bears a striking resemblance to that seen in NPC, suggesting a similar pathophysiology of malignant transformation in undifferentiated primary parotid carcinoma and aggressive behavior.

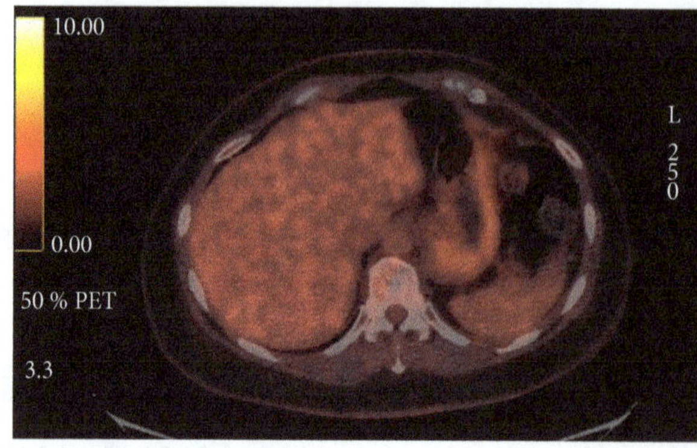

FIGURE 3: PET/CT after 4 cycles of Pembrolizumab.

Targeted immunologic chemotherapy is emerging as a treatment for metastatic malignancies. Research regarding the use of PD-L1 inhibitors in multiple malignancies such as metastatic renal cell carcinoma, lymphoma, breast, colorectal cancer, nonsmall cell lung cancer (NSCLC), urothelial carcinoma, head and neck squamous cell, and melanoma is currently ongoing [10, 14–17]. These studies continue to elucidate the place of Pembrolizumab in various malignancies. For the treatment of recurrent or metastatic head and neck squamous cell cancers, Pembrolizumab was only recently approved in 2016 by the Food and Drug Administration [2]. Published last year, the KEYNOTE-028 was a multicohort, nonrandomized, phase Ib study of advanced salivary gland tumors with PD-L1 expression undergoing treatment with Pembrolizumab [1]. In this study, 46% of patients experienced stable disease with similar adverse events as reported in prior studies.

Additional trials investigating immunotherapy in recurrent and refractory head and neck cancer are now recruiting, for example, a phase-IIb study by Hsu et al. assessing benefit of using PD-L1 inhibitors for treatment of recurrent or metastatic NPC, which was published after the initiation of this patient's treatment [18]. In the 27 patients treated with Pembrolizumab, there was a promising outcome with an objective response rate of 25% per the RESIST v1.1 [18]; however, they could only confidently say that Pembrolizumab would be safe in this population given low power. It is important to note the growing use of targeted therapy has largely been oncologist driven with patients who have poor prognosis and limited therapeutic options, as seen in this case.

As immunotherapies continue to improve and provide significantly longer progression free and overall survival benefit, genetic sequencing and IHC staining should be incorporated into the work-up of a recurrent or metastatic head and neck malignancies.

Still, additional research is needed to fully understand the role of immunotherapies in rare disease types.

Consent

Consent was verbally obtained from the next of kin.

Disclosure

The views expressed in this abstract/manuscript are those of the authors and do not reflect the official policy or position of the Department of the Army, Department of Defense, or the US Government.

Acknowledgments

Peer reviewed internally by Dr. Berenberg, Dr. Murphy, and Dr. Guess. Images were provided by Dr. Kao, MD Tripler radiology.

References

[1] R. B. Cohen, J. P. Delord, T. Doi et al., "Pembrolizumab for the treatment of advanced salivary gland carcinoma: findings of the phase 1b KEYNOTE-028 study," *American Journal of Clinical Oncology*, vol. 41, no. 11, pp. 1083–1088, 2018.

[2] E. Larkins, G. M. Blumenthal, W. Yuan et al., "FDA approval summary: pembrolizumab for the treatment of recurrent or metastatic head and neck squamous cell carcinoma with disease progression on or after platinum-containing chemotherapy," *Oncologist*, vol. 22, no. 7, pp. 873–878, 2017.

[3] K. Harada, T. Ferdous, and Y. Ueyama, "PD-L1 expression in malignant salivary gland tumors," *BMC Cancer*, vol. 18, no. 1, p. 156, 2018.

[4] V. Kumar, A. K. Abbas, and J. C. Aster, *Robbins and Cotran Pathologic Basis of Disease*, Elsevier/Saunders, Philadelphia, PA, USA, 9th edition, 2015.

[5] C. Hatta, T. Terada, J. Okita, M. Kakibuchi, A. Kubota, and M. Sakagami, "Clinicopathological study of undifferentiated carcinoma of the parotid gland," *Auris Nasus Larynx*, vol. 30, no. 3, pp. 273–277, 2003.

[6] K. K. Hui, M. A. Luna, J. G. Batsakis, N. G. Ordóñez, and R. Weber, "Undifferentiated carcinomas of the major salivary glands," *Oral Surgery, Oral Medicine, Oral Pathology*, vol. 69, no. 1, pp. 76–83, 1990.

[7] C. J. R. Stewart, K. MacKenzie, G. W. McGarry, and A. Mowat, "Fine-needle aspiration cytology of salivary gland: a review of 341 cases," *Diagnostic Cytopathology*, vol. 22, no. 3, pp. 139–146, 2000.

[8] J. G. Moore and T. Bocklage, "Fine-needle aspiration biopsy of large-cell undifferentiated carcinoma of the salivary glands: presentation of two cases, literature review, and differential cytodiagnosis of high-grade salivary gland malignancies," *Diagnostic Cytopathology*, vol. 19, no. 1, pp. 44–50, 1998.

[9] W. Fang, J. Zhang, S. Hong et al., "EBV-driven LMP1 and IFN-γ up-regulate PD-L1 in nasopharyngeal carcinoma: implications for oncotargeted therapy," *Oncotarget*, vol. 5, no. 23, pp. 12189–12202, 2014.

[10] B. J. Chen, B. Chapuy, J. Ouyang et al., "PD-L1 expression is characteristic of a subset of aggressive B- cell lymphomas and virus-associated malignancies," *Clinical Cancer Research*, vol. 19, no. 13, pp. 3462–3473, 2013.

[11] A. M. V. Chang, S. I. Chiosea, A. Altman, H. A. Pagdanganan, and C. Ma, "Programmed death-ligand 1 expression, microsatellite instability, Epstein-Barr virus, and human papillomavirus in nasopharyngeal carcinomas of patients from the Philippines," *Head and Neck Pathology*, vol. 11, no. 2, pp. 203–211, 2017.

[12] Y. F. Li, J. W. Ding, L. M. Liao et al., "Expression of programmed death ligand-1 predicts poor outcome in nasopharyngeal carcinoma," *Molecular and Clinical Oncology*, vol. 7, no. 3, pp. 378–382, 2017.

[13] T. Mukaigawa, R. Hayashi, K. Hashimoto, T. Ugumori, N. Hato, and S. Fujii, "Programmed death ligand-1 expression is associated with poor disease free survival in salivary gland carcinomas," *Journal of Surgical Oncology*, vol. 114, no. 1, pp. 36–43, 2016.

[14] J. W. T. Toh, P. de Souza, S. H. Lim et al., "The potential value of immunotherapy in colorectal cancers: review of the evidence for programmed death-1 inhibitor therapy," *Clinical Colorectal Cancer*, vol. 15, no. 4, pp. 285–291, 2016.

[15] M. Reck, D. Rodríguez-Abreu, A. G. Robinson et al., "Pembrolizumab versus chemotherapy for PD-L1-positive non- small-cell lung cancer," *The New England Journal of Medicine*, vol. 375, no. 19, pp. 1823–1833, 2016.

[16] A. Ribas, I. Puzanov, R. Dummer et al., "Pembrolizumab versus investigator-choice chemotherapy for ipilimumab-refractory melanoma (KEYNOTE-002): a randomised, controlled, phase 2 trial," *The Lancet Oncology*, vol. 16, no. 8, pp. 908–918, 2015.

[17] E. Roper, T. Lum, C. E. Palme et al., "PD-L1 expression predicts longer disease free survival in high risk head and neck cutaneous squamous cell carcinoma," *Pathology*, vol. 49, no. 5, pp. 499–505, 2017.

[18] C. Hsu, S. H. Lee, S. Ejadi et al., "Safety and antitumor activity of pembrolizumab in patients with programmed death-ligand 1-positive nasopharyngeal carcinoma: results of the KEYNOTE-028 study," *Journal of Clinical Oncology*, vol. 35, no. 36, pp. 4050–4056, 2017.

18

Readministration of Cancer Drugs in a Patient with Chemorefractory Metastatic Colorectal Cancer

Tetsuro Kawagoe, Go Ikeda, Yu Oshiro, Yuta Maruki, Keiko Kaneko, and Katsuhiko Iwakiri

Division of Gastroenterology, Department of Internal Medicine, Nippon Medical School, Japan

Correspondence should be addressed to Tetsuro Kawagoe; tetsuro@nms.ac.jp

Academic Editor: Ossama W. Tawfik

A 63-year-old woman was admitted to our institution for severe pain in her right lower abdomen caused by the perforation of cecal cancer. She underwent emergency surgery, from which she was diagnosed with cecal carcinoma with liver, lung, and lymph node metastases. As she was taking aspirin to prevent cerebral infarction, anti-vascular endothelial growth factor (receptor) antibody and regorafenib therapy were not used. Thus, we started a modified FOLFOX 6+cetuximab regimen. This first-line treatment initially achieved a partial response (PR), but she then developed progressive disease (PD) after 14 months. We changed the regimen to FOLFIRI, followed by trifluridine/tipiracil, but her progression-free survival periods were 2.7 months and 1 month, respectively. Although we cycled through the available array of standard cancer drugs, the patient showed a good performance status, and some benefit from treatment still seemed plausible. We readministered the 5-fluorouracil oral preparation S-1, which maintained stable disease (SD) for 7 months. After PD emerged, we readministered the anti-epidermal growth factor receptor (EGFR) antibody panitumumab for 7.5 months of SD. Finally, 39 months after her diagnosis, she died from rapidly progressing disease. However, her relatively long survival implies that readministering drugs similar to those used in previous regimens might benefit patients with metastatic colorectal cancer.

1. Introduction

Chemotherapy is usually the first-choice treatment for metastatic colorectal cancer (mCRC). Relatively new cytotoxic agents (such as irinotecan and oxaliplatin) and molecular targeted agents (such as antibodies against vascular endothelial growth factor (receptor) (VEGF (R)) and epidermal growth factor receptor (EGFR)) have extended the median overall survival of patients with mCRC to more than 20 months [1–3]. Guidelines recommend chemotherapy regimens with standard cancer drugs, such as 5-fluorouracil (FU), irinotecan, oxaliplatin, anti-VEGF (R) or anti-EGFR antibodies, regorafenib, and trifluridine/tipiracil [4–6]. More recently, immunotherapy has become available for a minority of patients with microsatellite instability-high tumors [7]. Although patients who have cycled through these standard chemotherapies are usually only treated palliatively, some selected patients can maintain good performance status (PS) and receive further chemotherapies. For such patients, there are limited further chemotherapeutic options. Here, we report a woman with mCRC who benefitted from the reintroduction of S-1, an oral prodrug of 5-FU, and anti-EGFR antibodies after receiving standard 1st-, 2nd-, and 3rd-line chemotherapies.

2. Case Presentation

A 63-year-old woman with a medical history of hypertension and cerebral infarction was admitted to our hospital with severe abdominal pain in October 2012.

Computed tomography (CT) scan of the abdomen and pelvis showed inflammation spread, abscess formation, lymphadenopathy around the cecum, and a huge mass with multiple nodules in the liver (Figures 1(a) and 1(b)). A chest

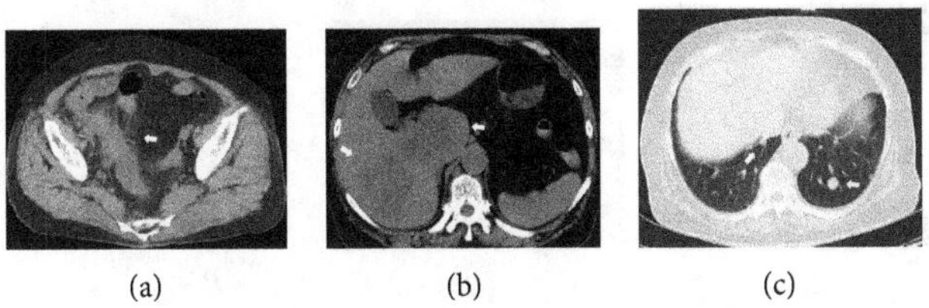

FIGURE 1: Pelvic CT showed inflammation spread and abscess formation around the cecum (a). Abdominal CT showed a huge mass and multiple nodules in the liver (b). Chest CT showed nodules in the lungs (c). Arrows: lesions.

CT also revealed multiple pulmonary nodules (Figure 1(c)). She was clinically diagnosed with intestinal perforation owing to cecal cancer and underwent emergency surgery. She was intraoperatively diagnosed with obstruction of the appendicular root owing to cecal cancer, perforation of the vermiform appendix, intraperitoneal abscess, and lymphadenopathy around the cecum and received an ileocecal resection, D1 lymph node dissection, and a peritoneal wash. After surgery, she was finally diagnosed with moderately differentiated wild-type *KRAS* adenocarcinoma of the cecum (stage: T3N1M1b, per the Union for International Cancer Control criteria). A microsatellite instability (MSI) test was not performed. *RAS* and *BRAF* status were also not investigated. We initiated therapy using cetuximab (500 mg/m^2; 14-day cycle) and the mFOLFOX6 regimen (5-FU 400 mg/m^2 bolus injection; leucovorin (LV) 200 mg/m^2, 46 h continuous infusion with 5-FU 2400 mg/m^2; and oxaliplatin 85 mg/m^2; 14-day cycle) in October 2012. This treatment resulted in 7.75 months of partial response (PR), followed by a stable disease (SD) period of 6.25 months and progressive disease (PD) for a total progression-free survival (PFS) period of 14 months. As a 2nd-line treatment, we started the FOLFIRI regimen (5-FU 400 mg/m^2 bolus injection, LV 200 mg/m^2, 46 h continuous infusion with 5-FU 2400 mg/m^2, and irinotecan 150 mg/m^2; 14-day cycle), but she developed PD after 2.7 months. We started trifluridine/tipiracil (35 mg/m^2 administered twice daily on Days 1–5 and Days 8–12 of a 28-day cycle) as a 3rd-line treatment, but this led to PD after 1 month. As this patient had a history of cerebral infarction and used antiplatelet drugs, anti-VEGF (R) antibody and regorafenib therapies were contraindicated. Hence, at this stage, no new standard cancer drugs could be tried. However, the patient's general condition was still good, and she requested further chemotherapy. Therefore, we readministered the 5-FU oral preparation S-1 (80 mg/m^2, Days 1–28, 42-day cycle), which provided a 7-month SD period (Figure 2). When PD was again confirmed, we administered panitumumab (6 mg/kg once every 2 weeks) as an anti-EGFR antibody rechallenge. The patient achieved SD on this regimen for 7.5 months (Figure 3). Finally, 39 months after her diagnosis, the patient died because of rapid disease progression. While receiving readministered drugs, her PS was well maintained; she suffered no grade ≥ 3 adverse events (per the National Cancer Institute Common Toxicity Criteria, version 4.0; Table 1).

3. Discussion

Although this was a case of unresectable CRC, its treatment can be considered successful because the patient survived for 39 months after diagnosis while maintaining good PS despite being unable to receive anti-VEGF (R) antibody therapy. Because she survived for 14.5 months after cycling through standard cancer regimens, retreatment apparently facilitated her relatively long survival.

Several reports on readministering anticancer drugs [8–16] have suggested that after a washout period, earlier-line drugs that were initially effective but then became ineffective might become effective again [11–15]. Santini et al. reported cetuximab rechallenge to be significantly effective after a cetuximab-free interval with cytotoxic chemotherapy [13]. Their hypothesis is as follows. If the anti-EGFR antibody was initially effective, it would have reduced EGFR-sensitive clonal cells and insensitive clones predominate at the PD stage. Subsequent cytotoxic chemotherapy would reduce the number of insensitive clones, and at the time of PD, sensitive clones would grow and become dominant again. As a result, the anti-EGFR antibody would become active again. Their hypothesis appears to be supported by the result of the CRICKET trial [14], in which rechallenge treatment with cetuximab was demonstrated to be effective, especially in patients without *RAS* mutations in circulating tumor DNA. This hypothesis implies that even if the readministered drug is panitumumab rather than cetuximab, an effect can be expected because both drugs are anti-EGFR antibodies. Panitumumab might also have been effective after cetuximab because panitumumab is a fully human monoclonal antibody (MoAb), whereas cetuximab is a chimeric MoAb consisting of ~30% mouse protein and may have a different sensitivity to cancer. Few reports have investigated the effect of panitumumab after progression on cetuximab in colorectal cancer patients. Marino et al. reported in their retrospective study that treatment with panitumumab after progression on cetuximab was effective because its PR and SD rates were 5% and 25% in 20 patients, respectively, and the median PFS and OS were 5 and 8 months, respectively [15]. In contrast, Wadlow et al. reported no responders to panitumumab treatment after progression on cetuximab and a SD rate of 45% with a median duration of only 1.7 months in their single-arm phase II trial of 20 patients [16]. Because both of these trials were conducted in a small number of patients, and panitumumab treatment after progression on cetuximab was actually effective in our study, it is necessary to identify the type of cases in which panitumumab treatment after progression on cetuximab is effective in the future. S-1 was developed to improve the therapeutic effect of tegafur, an oral fluoropyrimidine, by maintaining high 5-FU concentrations in plasma and tumors with less gastrointestinal toxicity by 5-chloro-4-dihydroxypyridine (CDHP) and potassium oxonate. In this case, the mechanism by which S-1 (as an oral fluoropyrimidine agent) was effective after the 5-FU infusion regimen became ineffective is unclear. Reportedly, the use of the FOLFOX regimen with 5-FU infusion enhances

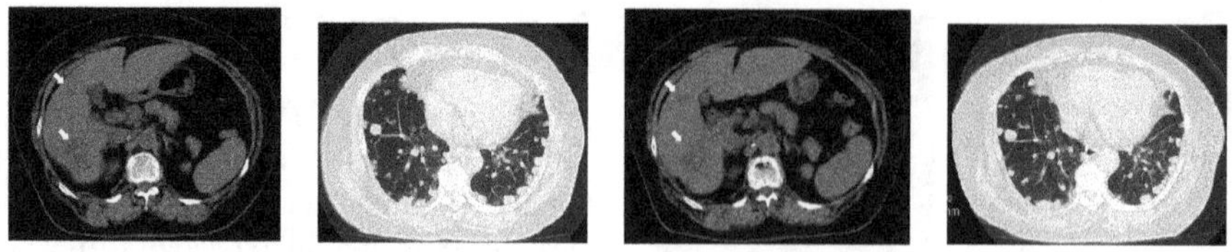

(a) (b) (c) (d)

Figure 2: Abdominal and chest CT before the administration of S-1 (a, b). Stable disease after therapy (c, d). Arrows: lesions in the liver.

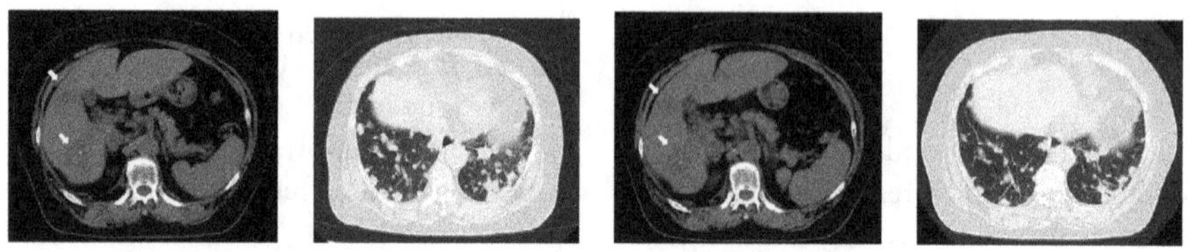

(a) (b) (c) (d)

Figure 3: Abdominal and chest CT before the administration of panitumumab (a, b). Stable disease after therapy (c, d). Pulmonary metastasis was slightly reduced after panitumumab treatment. Arrows: lesions in the liver.

Table 1: Treatment toxicities and performance status.

	mFOLFOX6+Cetu	FOLFIRI	Trifluridine/tipiracil	S-1	Panitumumab
Grade 1/2					
Decreased WBCs	○	○			
Decreased neutrophils		○	○		
Anemia	○	○	○	○	○
Decreased platelets	○			○	
Fever	○		○	○	○
Anorexia	○		○	○	
Dry skin	○				○
Peripheral neuropathy	○	○			
Insomnia	○				
Paronychia	○				○
Fatigue		○	○	○	
Mucositis oral				○	○
Diarrhea				○	
Rash acneiform					○
Grade 3					
Decreased neutrophils	○				
PS	1	1	2	1	1

Cetu: cetuximab; WBC: white blood cells.

dihydropyrimidine dehydrogenase (DPD) activity in tumors [17]. In the present case, S-1 may have maintained high levels of 5-FU in the tumor by suppressing DPD activity enhanced by pretreatment with CDHP.

4. Conclusion

In conclusion, we report a patient with metastatic CRC for whom repeated standard cancer treatments were effective despite prior development of refractory reactions. Why retreatment was effective remains unclear. Further research is needed.

Acknowledgments

We thank Marla Brunker, from Edanz Group (https://en-author-services.edanzgroup.com/), for editing a draft of this manuscript.

References

[1] V. Heinemann, L. F. von Weikersthal, T. Decker et al., "FOLFIRI plus cetuximab versus FOLFIRI plus bevacizumab as first-line treatment for patients with metastatic colorectal

cancer (FIRE-3): a randomised, open- label, phase 3 trial," *The Lancet Oncology*, vol. 15, no. 10, pp. 1065–1075, 2014.

[2] F. Loupakis, C. Cremolini, G. Masi et al., "Initial therapy with FOLFOXIRI and bevacizumab for metastatic colorectal cancer," *The New England Journal of Medicine*, vol. 371, no. 17, pp. 1609–1618, 2014.

[3] H. Baba, Y. Yamada, D. Takahari et al., "S-1 and oxaliplatin (SOX) plus bevacizumab versus mFOLFOX6 plus bevacizumab as first-line treatment for patients with metastatic colorectal cancer: updated overall survival analyses of the open-label, non-inferiority, randomised phase III: SOFT study," *ESMO Open*, vol. 2, no. 1, article e000135, 2017.

[4] T. Watanabe, Japanese Society for Cancer of the Colon, K. M. Rectum et al., "Japanese Society for Cancer of the Colon and Rectum (JSCCR) guidelines 2016 for the treatment of colorectal cancer," *International Journal of Clinical Oncology*, vol. 23, no. 1, pp. 1–34, 2018.

[5] A. B. Benson 3rd, A. P. Venook, L. Cederquist et al., "Colon cancer, version 1.2017, NCCN clinical practice guidelines in oncology," *Journal of the National Comprehensive Cancer Network*, vol. 15, no. 3, pp. 370–398, 2017.

[6] E. Van Cutsem, A. Cervantes, R. Adam et al., "ESMO consensus guidelines for the management of patients with metastatic colorectal cancer," *Annals of Oncology*, vol. 27, no. 8, pp. 1386–1422, 2016.

[7] K. Jeught, H. C. Xu, Y. J. Li, X. B. Lu, and G. Ji, "Drug resistance and new therapies in colorectal cancer," *World Journal of Gastroenterology*, vol. 24, no. 34, pp. 3834–3848, 2018.

[8] G. Tonini, M. Imperatori, B. Vincenzi, A. M. Frezza, and D. Santini, "Rechallenge therapy and treatment holiday: different strategies in management of metastatic colorectal cancer," *Journal of Experimental & Clinical Cancer Research*, vol. 32, no. 1, p. 92, 2013.

[9] A. Hata, N. Katakami, S. Fujita et al., "Panitumumab rechallenge in chemorefractory patients with metastatic colorectal cancer," *Journal of Gastrointestinal Cancer*, vol. 44, no. 4, pp. 456–459, 2013.

[10] A. R. Townsend, S. Bishnoi, V. Broadbridge et al., "Rechallenge with oxaliplatin and fluoropyrimidine for metastatic colorectal carcinoma after prior therapy," *American Journal of Clinical Oncology*, vol. 36, no. 1, pp. 49–52, 2013.

[11] E. Ozaslan, A. O. Duran, O. Bozkurt et al., "Analyses of multiple factors for determination of "selected patients" who should receive rechallenge treatment in metastatic colorectal cancer: a retrospective study from Turkey," *Asian Pacific Journal of Cancer Prevention*, vol. 16, no. 7, pp. 2833–2838, 2015.

[12] C. Yeoh, I. Chau, D. Cunningham, A. R. Norman, M. Hill, and P. J. Ross, "Impact of 5-fluorouracil rechallenge on subsequent response and survival in advanced colorectal cancer: pooled analysis from three consecutive randomized controlled trials," *Clinical Colorectal Cancer*, vol. 3, no. 2, pp. 102–107, 2003.

[13] D. Santini, B. Vincenzi, R. Addeo et al., "Cetuximab rechallenge in metastatic colorectal cancer patients: how to come away from acquired resistance?," *Annals of Oncology*, vol. 23, no. 9, pp. 2313–2318, 2012.

[14] C. Cremolini, D. Rossini, E. Dell'Aquila et al., "Rechallenge for patients WithRASandBRAFWild-Type metastatic colorectal cancer with acquired resistance to first-line cetuximab and Irinotecan," *JAMA Oncology*, vol. 5, no. 3, pp. 343–350, 2019.

[15] A. Marino, C. Caliolo, F. Sponziello et al., "Panitumumab after progression on cetuximab inKRASWild-type metastatic colorectal cancer patients: a single institution experience," *Tumori*, vol. 101, no. 5, pp. 524–528, 2015.

[16] R. C. Wadlow, A. F. Hezel, T. A. Abrams et al., "Panitumumab in patients with KRASwild-type colorectal cancer after progression on cetuximab," *The Oncologist*, vol. 17, no. 1, p. 14, 2011.

[17] H. Baba, M. Watanabe, H. Okabe et al., "Upregulation of ERCC1 and DPD expressions after oxaliplatin-based first-line chemotherapy for metastatic colorectal cancer," *British Journal of Cancer*, vol. 107, no. 12, pp. 1950–1955, 2012.

19

Metastatic Lesion of the Tibia from Renal Cell Carcinoma

Piotr Młodożeniec[1], **Krzysztof Balawender**[1,2] **and Mateusz Zasadny**[1]

[1]*Clinical Department of Urology and Urological Oncology, Municipal Hospital in Rzeszow, Poland*
[2]*Morphological Sciences Department, Institute of Medical Sciences, Medical College of Rzeszow University, Poland*

Correspondence should be addressed to Krzysztof Balawender; balawender82@gmail.com

Academic Editor: Raffaele Palmirotta

Introduction. Renal cell carcinoma is responsible for 3% of all cancers, with the highest incidence occurring in Western countries. Additionally, in patients with osseous metastasis, only 3% occur within the tibia. Rarely, a patient presents with a primary complaint of lower limb pain in advanced metastatic renal cell carcinoma. *Case Presentation.* The patient arrived at the emergency department with a primary complaint of left ankle pain. Ankle X-rays demonstrated a lytic lesion involving the medial malleolus with possible metastatic disease. CT scan confirmed a tumor within the right kidney. The patient was treated with a laparoscopic radical nephrectomy with histopathologic confirmation of clear cell renal cell carcinoma. Biopsy was then performed of the tibial lesion, confirming metastatic clear cell renal cell carcinoma. The tibial lesion was treated with local radiotherapy, and because of the progression of the tibia lesion, a decision was made to amputate the leg. Additionally, the patient was enrolled to sunitinib treatment and was disease free at one year of follow-up. 13 months after diagnosis of cancer, she was suffering a major stroke of the brain that caused her to die. *Conclusion.* The treatment of patients with osseous metastases of renal cell cancer depends on the number of metastases, location of metastases, and overall health of the patient. We performed an overview of available literature and provided a summary regarding the use of cytoreductive nephrectomy, local therapy, target therapy, and bone-targeting agents in the treatment of metastatic renal cell cancer.

1. Introduction

The number of patients diagnosed with oncologic disease has been on the rise. Of all cancers diagnosed, renal cell carcinoma (RCC) makes up 3% of all cases, with the highest incidence occurring in Western countries. In 2018, the European Union recorded 99,200 new cases of RCC and 39,100 kidney cancer-related deaths [1]. Metastatic disease in RCC is not uncommon. The most common sites of RCC metastases are lung (45.2–51.2%), bone (29.5–33.5%) lymph nodes (21.8–41.5%), liver (17–20.3%), adrenal (8.9%), and brain (8.1–9.8%) [2, 3]. In multivariable analyses, young age was an independent predictor for the presence of multiple concomitant metastatic sites (odds ratio: 1.2, $p < 0.001$) [2]. In only 10–20% of patients, bone metastases are found without additional metastatic involvement [2–4]. Most commonly osseous metastases occur in the spinal column (59%), sacrum (39%), and long bones (31%) [4]. At the time of diagnosis of RCC, 31% of patients had a bone metastasis present and 69% developed bone metastasis after RCC diagnosis. Of all patients with RCC bone metastases, 71% had multiple lesions and 29% had a single one [5].

To our knowledge, we report the case of a patient with advanced clear cell renal cell carcinoma (ccRCC) to present solely with manifestations of a bony metastasis. This work has been reported in line with the CARE criteria [6]. We believe this case further elaborates on the presentation of metastatic renal cell carcinoma and adds to the published literature on the topic.

2. Case Presentation

A 59-year-old female presented to the emergency department in September 2019 with a chief complaint of left ankle pain and difficulty walking for 10 days. In physical examination, small swelling and the tenderness of the left medial ankle were found. A patient in an interview with no significant coexisting diseases and injuries accepts medicines for

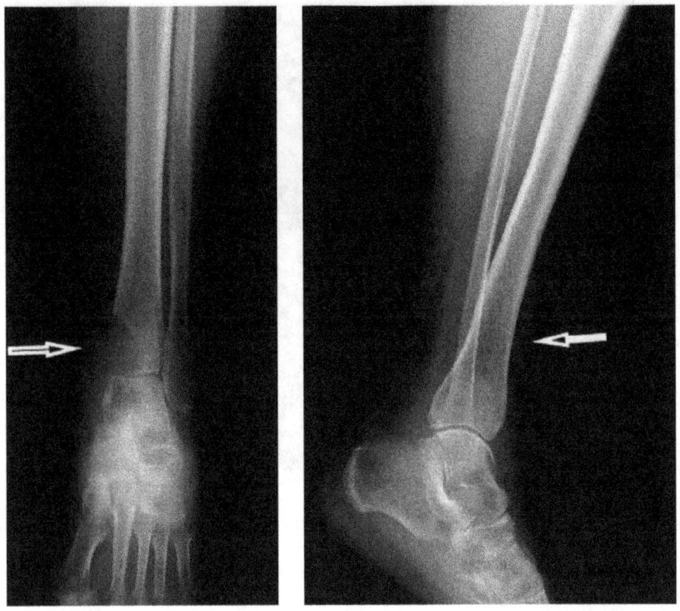

(a) (b)

FIGURE 1: X-ray anteroposterior/lateral view of the leg showing destruction of the distal tibia.

hypertension. Ankle X-rays (anterior-posterior and lateral views) were performed and demonstrated an osteolytic lesion within the medial malleolus and distal tibial metaphysis (Figure 1). Given the clinical picture, metastatic disease was suspected. Therefore, CT scans of the chest, abdomen, and pelvis were performed. A tumor of the right kidney was identified and presumed to be renal cell carcinoma (Figure 2). Surgical treatment of the RCC was undertaken with a laparoscopic radical nephrectomy. The procedure was completed without complication. The histopathologic report confirmed the diagnosis of ccRCC pT1b with angioinvasion with negative surgical margins, WHO/ISUP Grade 2 (Figure 3). Next, an aspiration biopsy of the tibial lesion was performed to confirm the diagnosis of metastatic ccRCC. The biopsy was completed without complication, and histologic diagnosis confirmed a metastasis of ccRCC (CD10+, vimentin+, TTFI−, RCC+, and PAX8+; Figure 3). Decision of immediate local radiotherapy on tibial lesion was taken. After 2 months due to progression of the tibial lesion, a decision was made to amputate the leg above ankle, upon counselling the patient. The patient underwent procedure. Postoperative recovery and rehabilitation were uneventful. Additionally, the patient was considered to be at intermediate risk according to the Memorial Sloan-Kettering Cancer Center (MSKCC) criteria and sunitinib treatment was started at 50 mg daily for two of every three weeks and was disease free at one year of follow-up. 13 months after diagnosis of RCC, she was suffering a major stroke of the brain that caused her to die.

3. Discussion

The predictors of cancer-specific mortality (CSM) in patients with ccRCC metastatic disease at the time of diagnosis are higher cT stage, higher histologic Fuhrman grade, or clinical nodal disease. Despite the fact that clear cell RCC is the most common type of metastatic RCC, sarcomatoid, papillary, and collecting duct type of RCC are associated with higher CSM [3]. Studies have shown the median survival time after diagnosis of skeletal metastasis in RCC to be 12 months [5], 15.8 months [7], and 32 months [8]. Furthermore, the number of bone metastases is inversely associated with overall survival (OS). Patients with 1, 2–5, or >5 bone metastases had a median overall survival of 28 months, 18 months, and 9 months, respectively [9]. The early diagnosis of bony metastases is important in reducing morbidity [10, 11], but formal recommendations do not advise the use of bone scan and/or positron-emission tomography CT in the staging of renal cell carcinoma. These modalities are limited to patients presenting with skeletal-related events (SRE) [12, 13]. The data about tibial metastases in RCC is scarce given the fact that tibial metastases occur in only 3% of all cases of renal cell carcinoma with bone metastases [7].

3.1. Treatment. The first issue of discussion in the treatment of RCC is if cytoreductive nephrectomy (CN) should be conducted. Chandrasekar et al. reported improved CSM with cytoreductive nephrectomy in a large population-based study [3]. Heng et al. further show improved OS with cytoreductive nephrectomy (HR: 0.60; 95% CI, 0.52–0.69; $p < 0.001$) [14]. Conversely, CARMENA, a phase III noninferiority RCT (randomized controlled trail) which found sunitinib alone, was not inferior in regard to OS when compared to CN and sunitinib therapy [15, 16]. European Association of Urology Guidelines 2021 recommends against cytoreductive nephrectomy in MSKCC poor-risk and intermediate-risk patients requiring systemic therapy with vascular endothelial growth factor receptor- (VEGFR-) tyrosine kinase inhibitor (TKI) but suggests cytoreductive nephrectomy in patients with

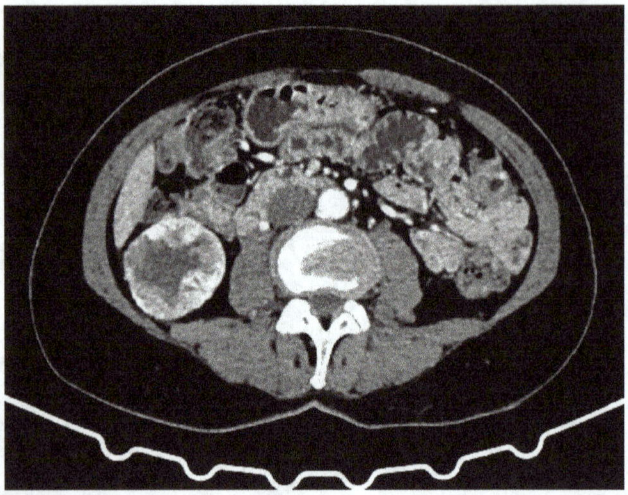

FIGURE 2: Computed tomography showed a solid mass measuring $40 \times 36 \times 30$ mm in the right kidney.

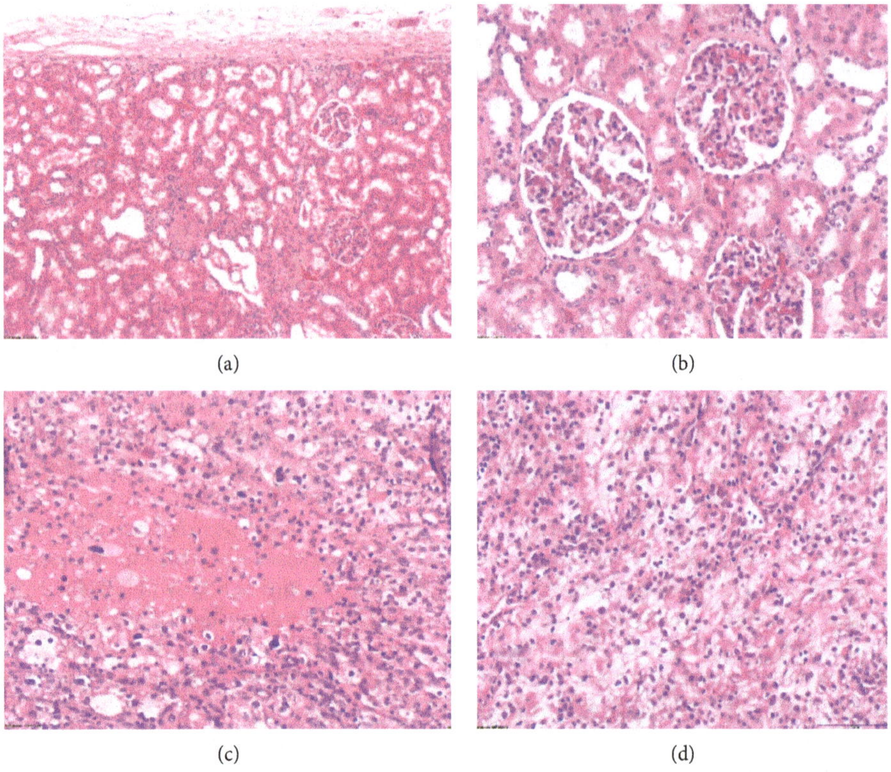

FIGURE 3: (a–d) The micrograph of a clear cell renal cell carcinoma H&E stain. This image demonstrates the optically clear tumor cells with uniform small nuclei without nucleolar ranged in an alveolar pattern. Cells with clear cytoplasm, typically arranged in nests. Nuclear atypia is common. Water-clear or optically clear cells (due to glycogen content) arranged in nests in "chicken wire" vasculatures. Visible subcapsular changes in the area of the kidney cortex. Numerous extravasations are visible in the vascular glomeruli (a, b). Metastasis of renal cell carcinoma. Histological microphotograph showing neoplastic cells with prominent nucleoli. Ankle joint and metastasis of renal cell carcinoma H&E sections (c, d). Scal bar: (a) 200 μm; (b–d) 100 μm. The samples were analyzed morphologically and photographed under an Olympus BX43 light microscope equipped with an Olympus SC50 digital camera.

good renal function who do not require systemic therapy. Additionally, CN is recommended in patients with oligometastases when complete local treatment of the metastases can be achieved.

3.2. Local Therapy. Treatment options for RCC metastases consist of surgery, radiotherapy, and ablation therapy. In the case of a solitary metastatic lesion, resection with tumor-free margins can improved 5-year overall survival significantly from 11% to 31% ($p = 0.028$) [7]. Alt et al. demonstrated that complete surgical resection of multiple RCC metastases was associated with a prolonged median cancer specific survival (CSS) to 4.8 years and, in fact, significantly improved the 5-year CSS rate (49.4%) compared with the rate among patients who did not undergo complete metastasectomy (13.9%) [17]. This benefit of metastatic resection has been confirmed by many other authors [18–20]. Therefore, wide resection with curative intent seems to be the primary approach to solitary or oligometastatic bone metastasis [13]. Patients who are unable to undergo metastasectomy can undergo radiotherapy as an alternative option to help control pain, preserve bone mineralization, and suppress spinal cord compression [21]. Svedman et al. have established in a phase II trial that using SRE for patients with primary and metastatic RCC provides a high degree of local control rate (98%) [22]. High single-fraction (24Gy) stereotactic body radiotherapy has the highest 3-year local relapse-free survival (LRFS) (88%) compered to low single-fractioned (<24Gy) stereotactic body radiotherapy (22%) and hypofractionated radiotherapy (17%) [23]. Radiofrequency ablation (RFA) can be utilized in the palliative treatment of patients with bone metastases for pain relief with a clinical efficiency of 69.7% [24]. Cryoablation is associated with a control-rate per lesion of 82% when used in the setting of bone metastases [25]. Zugaro et al. have shown similar pain relief (64% and 68%) and statistically significant increases in the quality of life ($p = 0.001$) using either technique, radiofrequency ablation, or cryoablation [26]. Chemotherapy however has been shown to be ineffective in the treatment of RCC [27]. Target therapy has become a new hope for patients with RCC metastatic disease. Tyrosine kinase inhibitors (TKIs) can slow the progression of existing bone lesions and reduce the formation of new bone lesions [28, 29]. The first-generation TKIs like sunitinib or sorafenib have improved overall survival (24 months versus 18 months; $p < 0.01$) [30]. Compared with sorafenib, sunitinib significantly decreased formation ($p = 0.034$) and prolonged time to occurrence of new bone lesions ($p = 0.047$) [28]. In the METEOR study, Choueiri et al. reported that treatment with cabozantinib improved median overall survival (21.4 vs. 16.5 months, $p = 0.00026$), progression-free survival (7.4 vs. 3.9 months, $p < 0 \cdot 0001$), and objective response (17% vs. 3%, $p < 0 \cdot 0001$) when compared to the mTOR inhibitor, everolimus [31]. In conclusion, cabozantinib should be used preferentially to treat bone metastases that are not amenable to local therapies [13]. Bisphosphonates (BT) are a group of bone targeting agents that work to decrease osteoclast activity. Before the era of target therapy, zoledronic acid decreased the rate of SREs compared to placebo (37% vs. 74%, $P = 0.0015$) [32]. The use of BT in conjunction with TKIs was not associated with improved OS (13.3 vs. 13.1 months, $p = 0.3801$), improved PFS (5.1 vs. 4.9 months $p = 0.1785$), and decreased rate of SREs compared with nonusers (8.6% vs. 5.8%, $p = 0.191$) [33]. During BT therapy, osteonecrosis of the jaw is possible, so patients should undergo regular dental examinations before and during treatment. Patients treated with zoledronic acid should undergo renal function monitoring [34]. The literature is inconclusive as to whether bone target therapy in addition to target therapy improves clinical outcomes. However, bone-targeting agents should be used to control tumor-associated hypercalcemia, with calcium and vitamin D supplementation [13].

4. Conclusion

Clear cell RCC is the most common type of renal cancer. Metastatic lesions of bone are the 3rd most common site of all metastases with the leg being a rare site of RCC metastases. The median survival time after diagnoses of skeletal metastasis in RCC is 12–32 months. Early diagnosis of bone metastases is important for reducing morbidity. Cytoreductive nephrectomy is not indicated routinely, but only to patients with good renal function who do not require systemic therapy, or to patients with oligometastases when complete local treatment of the metastases can be achieved. Wide resection of metastases with curative intent seems to be the primary approach to solitary or oligometastatic bone metastasis. High single-fraction (24Gy) stereotactic body radiotherapy is the best option in palliative local treatment to patients who are not able to undergo metastasectomy. Chemotherapy is ineffective in the treatment of RCC. In systemic therapy, cabozantinib should be used preferentially to treat RCC with bone metastases. The beneficial effects of adding bone-target agents to TKI therapy in the setting of bone metastasis have not been seen, but in the setting of tumor-associated hypercalcemia, their use is recommended.

Consent

Written informed consent was obtained from the patient for authorization to publish their clinical information in this case report.

References

[1] J. Ferlay, M. Colombet, I. Soerjomataram et al., "Cancer incidence and mortality patterns in Europe: estimates for 40 countries and 25 major cancers in 2018," *European Journal of Cancer*, vol. 103, pp. 356–387, 2018.

[2] M. Bianchi, M. Sun, C. Jeldres et al., "Distribution of metastatic sites in renal cell carcinoma: a population-based analysis," *Annals of Oncology*, vol. 23, no. 4, pp. 973–980, 2012.

[3] T. Chandrasekar, Z. Klaassen, H. Goldberg, G. S. Kulkarni, R. J. Hamilton, and N. E. Fleshner, "Metastatic renal cell carcinoma: Patterns and predictors of metastases–A contemporary population-based series," *Urologic Oncology*, vol. 35, no. 11, pp. 661.e7–661.e14, 2017.

[4] F. Ruatta, L. Derosa, B. Escudier et al., "Prognosis of renal cell carcinoma with bone metastases: experience from a large cancer centre," *European Journal of Cancer*, vol. 107, pp. 79–85, 2019.

[5] D. Santini, G. Procopio, C. Porta et al., "Natural history of malignant bone disease in renal cancer: final results of an Italian bone metastasis survey," *PLoS One*, vol. 8, no. 12, article e83026, 2013.

[6] D. S. Riley, M. S. Barber, G. S. Kienle et al., "CARE guidelines for case reports: explanation and elaboration document," *Journal of Clinical Epidemiology*, vol. 89, pp. 218–235, 2017.

[7] A. Fottner, M. Szalantzy, L. Wirthmann et al., "Bone metastases from renal cell carcinoma: patient survival after surgical treatment," *BMC Musculoskeletal Disorders*, vol. 11, no. 1, p. 145, 2010.

[8] P. Bonnevialle, J. Descamps, L. Niglis et al., "Surgical treatment of tibial metastases: retrospective, multicenter, observational study of 25 patients," *Orthopaedics & Traumatology, Surgery & Research*, vol. 106, no. 6, pp. 1039–1045, 2020.

[9] F. Ruatta, L. Derosa, L. Albiges et al., "Prognosis of renal cell carcinoma with bone metastases: experience in 300 consecutive patients," *Journal of Clinical Oncology*, vol. 35, 6_suppl, p. 463, 2017.

[10] S. C. Chen and P. L. Kuo, "Bone Metastasis from Renal Cell Carcinoma," *International Journal of Molecular Sciences*, vol. 17, no. 6, p. 987, 2016.

[11] R. J. Motzer, J. Bacik, L. H. Schwartz et al., "Prognostic factors for survival in previously treated patients with metastatic renal cell carcinoma," *Journal of Clinical Oncology*, vol. 22, no. 3, pp. 454–463, 2004.

[12] S. Koga, S. Tsuda, M. Nishikido et al., "The diagnostic value of bone scan in patients with renal cell carcinoma," *The Journal of Urology*, vol. 166, no. 6, pp. 2126–2128, 2001.

[13] V. Grünwald, B. Eberhardt, A. Bex et al., "An interdisciplinary consensus on the management of bone metastases from renal cell carcinoma," *Nature Reviews. Urology*, vol. 15, no. 8, pp. 511–521, 2018.

[14] D. Y. Heng, J. C. Wells, B. I. Rini et al., "Cytoreductive nephrectomy in patients with synchronous metastases from renal cell carcinoma: results from the International Metastatic Renal Cell Carcinoma Database Consortium," *European Urology*, vol. 66, no. 4, pp. 704–710, 2014.

[15] B. Bhindi, E. J. Abel, L. Albiges et al., "Systematic review of the role of cytoreductive nephrectomy in the targeted therapy era and beyond: an individualized approach to metastatic renal cell carcinoma," *European Urology*, vol. 75, no. 1, pp. 111–128, 2019.

[16] A. Méjean, A. Ravaud, S. Thezenas et al., "Sunitinib alone or after nephrectomy in metastatic renal-cell carcinoma," *The New England Journal of Medicine*, vol. 379, no. 5, pp. 417–427, 2018.

[17] A. L. Alt, S. A. Boorjian, C. M. Lohse, B. A. Costello, B. C. Leibovich, and M. L. Blute, "Survival after complete surgical resection of multiple metastases from renal cell carcinoma," *Cancer*, vol. 117, no. 13, pp. 2873–2882, 2011.

[18] C. Kwak, Y. H. Park, C. W. Jeong, S. E. Lee, and J. H. Ku, "Metastasectomy without systemic therapy in metastatic renal cell carcinoma: comparison with conservative treatment," *Urologia Internationalis*, vol. 79, no. 2, pp. 145–151, 2007.

[19] G. Petralia, M. Roscigno, R. Zigeuner et al., "450 Complete metastasectomy is an independent predictor of cancer-specific survival in patients with clinically metastatic renal cell carcinoma," *European Urology Supplements*, vol. 9, no. 2, p. 162, 2010.

[20] A. F. Fares, D. V. Araujo, V. Calsavara et al., "Complete metastasectomy in renal cell carcinoma: a propensity-score matched by the International Metastatic RCC Database Consortium prognostic model," *Ecancermedicalscience*, vol. 13, 2019.

[21] R. McDonald, K. Ding, M. Brundage et al., "Effect of radiotherapy on painful bone metastases: a secondary analysis of the NCIC clinical trials group symptom control trial SC.23," *JAMA Oncology*, vol. 3, no. 7, pp. 953–959, 2017.

[22] C. Svedman, P. Sandström, P. Pisa et al., "A prospective phase II trial of using extracranial stereotactic radiotherapy in primary and metastatic renal cell carcinoma," *Acta Oncologica*, vol. 45, no. 7, pp. 870–875, 2006.

[23] M. J. Zelefsky, C. Greco, R. Motzer et al., "Tumor control outcomes after hypofractionated and single-dose stereotactic image-guided intensity-modulated radiotherapy for extracranial metastases from renal cell carcinoma," *International Journal of Radiation Oncology • Biology • Physics*, vol. 82, no. 5, pp. 1744–1748, 2012.

[24] N. Tanigawa, Y. Arai, K. Yamakado et al., "Phase I/II study of radiofrequency ablation for painful bone metastases: Japan Interventional Radiology in Oncology Study Group 0208," *Cardiovascular and Interventional Radiology*, vol. 41, no. 7, pp. 1043–1048, 2018.

[25] C. S. Gardner, J. E. Ensor, K. Ahrar et al., "Cryoablation of bone metastases from renal cell carcinoma for local tumor control," *The Journal of Bone and Joint Surgery. American Volume*, vol. 99, no. 22, pp. 1916–1926, 2017.

[26] L. Zugaro, M. di Staso, G. L. Gravina et al., "Treatment of osteolytic solitary painful osseous metastases with radiofrequency ablation or cryoablation: a retrospective study by propensity analysis," *Oncology Letters*, vol. 11, no. 3, pp. 1948–1954, 2016.

[27] R. J. Amato, "Chemotherapy for renal cell carcinoma," *Seminars in Oncology*, vol. 27, no. 2, pp. 177–186, 2000.

[28] S. L. Wood and J. E. Brown, "Skeletal metastasis in renal cell carcinoma: current and future management options," *Cancer Treatment Reviews*, vol. 38, no. 4, pp. 284–291, 2012.

[29] J. Żołnierek, P. Nurzyński, P. Langiewicz et al., "Efficacy of targeted therapy in patients with renal cell carcinoma with pre-existing or new bone metastases," *Journal of Cancer Research and Clinical Oncology*, vol. 136, no. 3, pp. 371–378, 2010.

[30] S. Kalra, J. Verma, B. J. Atkinson et al., "Outcomes of patients with metastatic renal cell carcinoma and bone metastases in the targeted therapy era," *Clinical Genitourinary Cancer*, vol. 15, no. 3, pp. 363–370, 2017.

[31] T. K. Choueiri, B. Escudier, T. Powles et al., "Cabozantinib versus everolimus in advanced renal cell carcinoma (METEOR): final results from a randomised, open-label, phase 3 trial," *The Lancet. Oncology*, vol. 17, no. 7, pp. 917–927, 2016.

[32] A. Lipton, A. Colombo-Berra, R. M. Bukowski, L. Rosen, M. Zheng, and G. Urbanowitz, "Skeletal complications in patients with bone metastases from renal cell carcinoma and therapeutic benefits of zoledronic acid," *Clinical Cancer Research*, vol. 10, no. 18, pp. 6397S–6403S, 2004.

[33] R. R. McKay, X. Lin, J. J. Perkins, D. Y. Heng, R. Simantov, and T. K. Choueiri, "Prognostic significance of bone metastases and bisphosphonate therapy in patients with renal cell carcinoma," *European Urology*, vol. 66, no. 3, pp. 502–509, 2014.

[34] S. A. North, Canadian Kidney Cancer Forum 2015, N. Basappa et al., "Management of advanced kidney cancer: Canadian Kidney Cancer Forum consensus update," *Canadian Urological Association Journal*, vol. 9, no. 5-6, pp. 164–170, 2015.

20

Annexin A2 Expression in the Aerogenous Spread of Pulmonary Invasive Mucinous Adenocarcinoma with Gastric Lineage

Kazumori Arai,[1] **Tomohiro Iwasaki**,[1] **Chinatsu Tsuchiya**,[1] **and Akihiro Sonoda**[2]

[1]*Department of Pathology, Shizuoka General Hospital, 4-27-1 Kitaando, Aoi-ku, Shizuoka 420-0881, Japan*
[2]*Department of Clinical Research, Shizuoka General Hospital, Japan*

Correspondence should be addressed to Kazumori Arai; m-arai@ny.tokai.or.jp

Academic Editor: Constantine Gennatas

Spread through air spaces (STAS) is a unique form of lung cancer progression associated with a worse prognosis. However, the mechanisms underlying STAS and the associated proteins remain unclear. Annexin A2 (ANX A2), which is a membrane-binding protein involved in cell adhesion, is known to promote cancer invasion. In this report, we describe the immunohistochemical analysis of ANX A2 expression in an invasive mucinous adenocarcinoma (IMAC) resected from a 63-year-old man in whom the tumor cells had detached from the alveolar wall and exhibited STAS. At the detachment site, we observed cytoplasmic ANX A2 positivity on the basal side and in the exfoliative gap, as well as reduced collagen IV positivity expression. This biomarker pattern suggested an IMAC with gastric lineage. We hypothesize that ANX A2 is secreted from the basal sides of tumor cells and induces tumor cell detachment by degrading the basement membrane. A further comparison of this case with an IMAC with nongastric lineage suggested the following probabilities: (1) ANX A2 likely contributes to STAS in a manner that is dependent on its subcellular localization. (2) Both the subcellular localization of ANX A2 and the detachment site depend on tumor cell characteristics, including the biomarker immunophenotype.

1. Introduction

Spread through air spaces (STAS) is a unique form of lung cancer progression from the primary tumor site via the airways [1, 2]. This new category is included in the definition of lung adenocarcinoma (AC) invasion, along with stromal (including vascular) and pleural invasion [1]. STAS is also considered the origin of aerogenous metastasis (AM) [1, 2]. Although STAS has elicited great interest in the field of lung cancer [3–7], its status as either a true invasive form or a technical artifact of sample processing remains controversial [3]. However, recent reports have provided evidence that favors STAS as a true invasive pattern and have demonstrated a significant association with a worse prognosis [4–7]. Furthermore, STAS is associated with a higher risk of locoregional recurrence, thus preventing limited resection [4–6]. The inhibition of STAS is an important research issue, but the underlying pathogenic mechanisms remain unclear. We believe that the ability to inhibit STAS will depend on an understanding of the protein(s) involved in the processes of tumor cell detachment into alveolar spaces and adhesion to the alveolar wall.

Invasive mucinous AC (IMAC) frequently progresses via STAS/AM [8]. Recently, we reported the expression of annexin A2 (ANX A2), which is a Ca^{2+}/membrane-binding protein in a case of IMAC with STAS/AM [9]. To the best of our knowledge, our report was the first to indicate the involvement of this protein in STAS/AM. In the reported case, tumor cell detachment occurred at the tip of a villous-shaped tumor component that had projected into the alveolar spaces [9]. In contrast to our previous report, other researchers described tumor cell detachment from the basement membrane (BM) of the alveolar wall as a common origin of STAS/AM from IMAC [10, 11].

ANX A2 is expressed in various cells and is involved in cell adhesion, cell proliferation, and cell polarity within the cytoplasm and plasma membranes [12, 13]. This protein is also expressed in various cancers, including lung cancer, and extracellular membrane-bound ANX A2 acts as a plasminogen activator to promote angiogenesis and cancer cell

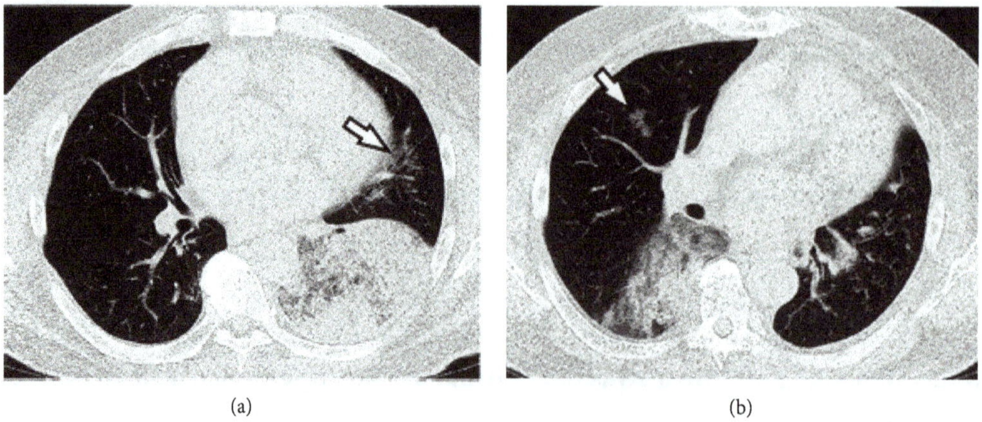

FIGURE 1: Axial CT images. (a) A chest CT image obtained 7 days after the initial visit shows a large infiltrative shadow, as well as a small infiltrative shadow that is suspected to be a skip lesion (arrow). (b) A chest CT image obtained 2 months after left lobectomy shows an infiltrative shadow with a skip lesion (arrow) in the right lung.

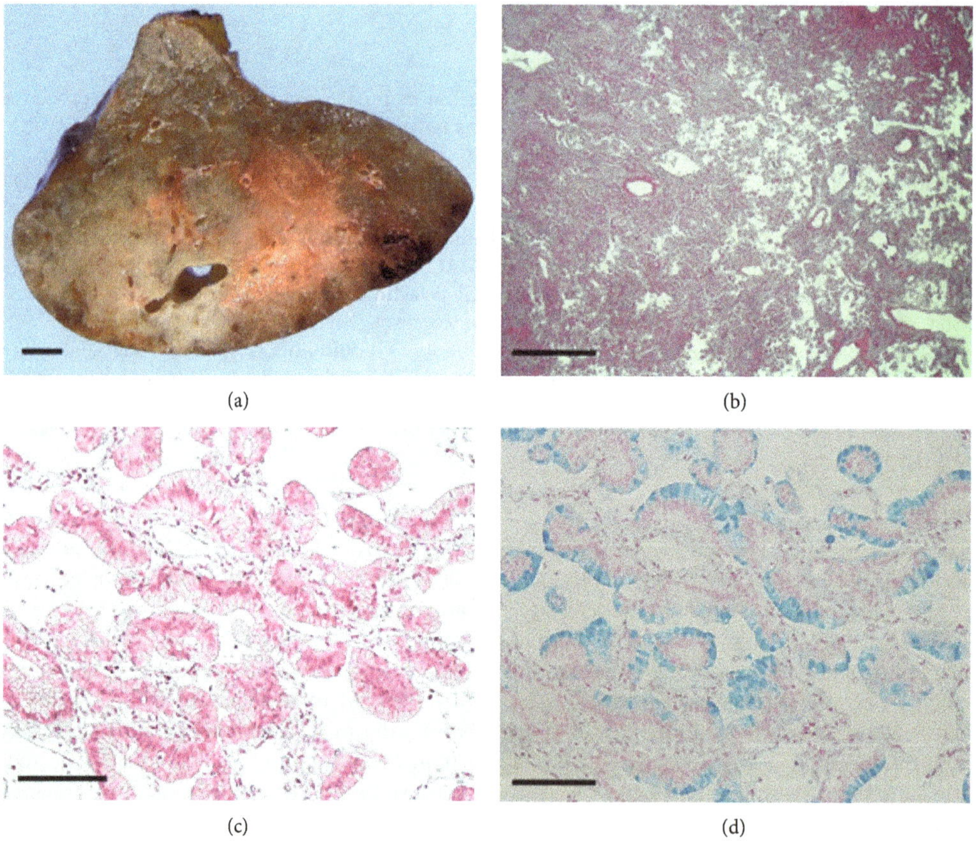

FIGURE 2: Left lung cancer I. (a) Gross view showing an ill-defined tumor with a diffuse pneumonia-like consolidation. Scale bar: 1 cm. (b) The tumor cells exhibit lepidic or papillary growth, with detached tumor cells scattered in the alveolar spaces. Hematoxylin and eosin (H&E) staining, scale bar: 2 mm. (c) Columnar tumor cells with intracytoplasmic vacuoles are shown in a monolayer arrangement. H&E stain, scale bar: 200 μm. (d) Multiple mucin-producing tumor cells are visible. Alcian blue stain, scale bar: 200 μm.

invasion in the stroma [14, 15]. The other functions of ANX A2 in cancer are currently under investigation [15]. We hypothesized that ANX A2 may also be involved in the STAS/AM of lung AC and that the observed discrepancies in IMAC detachment sites would result from differences in ANX A2 expression or subcellular localization. In the current report, we immunohistochemically examined the expression of ANX A2 in a case of IMAC in which tumor cell detachment occurred from the alveolar wall, consistent with previous reports [10, 11].

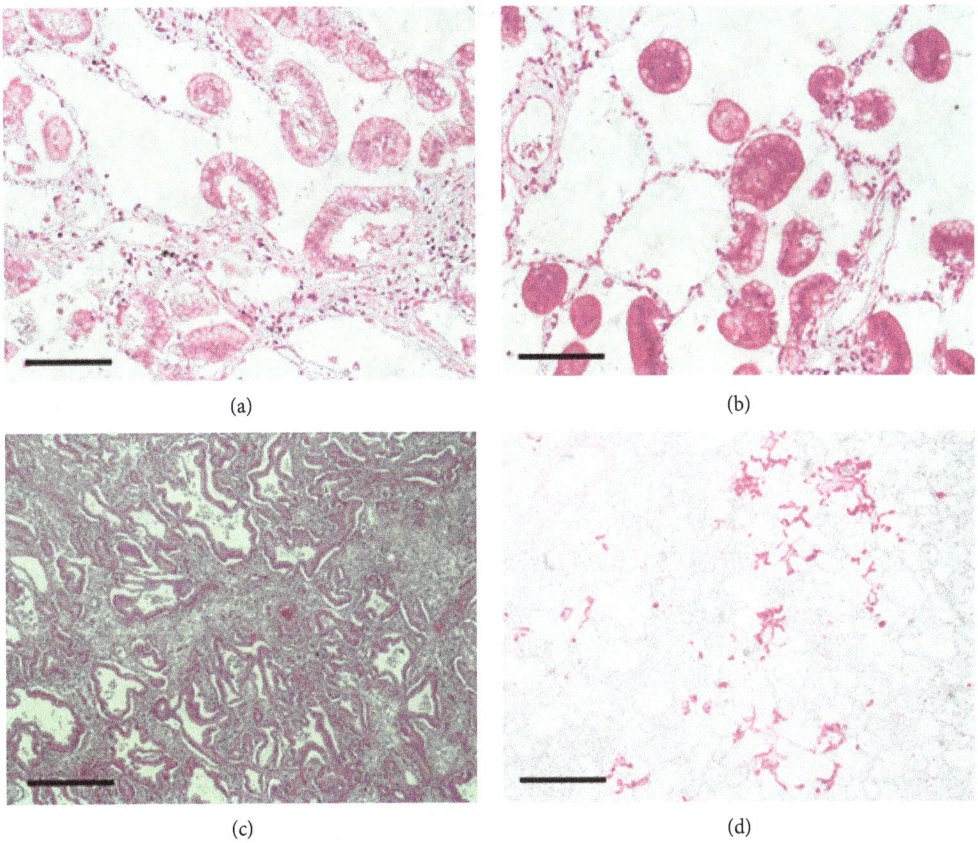

Figure 3: Left lung cancer II. (a) Small groups of tumor cells that detached from the alveolar wall. Only a slight inflammatory cell infiltration is visible. H&E stain, scale bar: 200 μm. (b) Detached tumor cells with a micropapillary pattern float within the alveolar spaces. H&E stain, scale bar: 200 μm. (c) The invasive component exhibits glandular or papillary growth. H&E stain, scale bar: 1 mm. (d) Many scattered tumor cell aggregates that detached from the primary tumor are visible within the air spaces and on the alveolar wall. The latter aggregates exhibit lepidic or papillary growth that is suggestive of microscopic aerogenous metastases. H&E stain, scale bar: 2 mm.

2. Case Presentation

The subject of this case study provided written informed consent for the publication of the case details. A 63-year-old man with no history of smoking presented with fever, cough, and mucinous sputum. Chest computed tomography (CT) revealed a large infiltrative shadow that is approximately 10 cm in size in the lower lobe of the left lung. No enlargement of the hilar or mediastinal lymph nodes was observed. The differential diagnosis was challenging, and pneumonia or IMAC was suspected [16]. Seven days later, chest CT demonstrated the expansion of the shadow and a small infiltrative shadow suggestive of a skip lesion (Figure 1(a)). The patient was then hospitalized immediately. Full-body CT did not reveal any metastatic lesions in the right lung or extrapulmonary organs. Considering that a transbronchial lung biopsy revealed a mucus-producing AC, the patient underwent thoracoscopic lobectomy with no adjuvant therapy.

Two months postoperatively, a follow-up chest CT revealed an infiltrative shadow with an approximate diameter of 6 cm and a skip lesion in the lower lobe of the right lung (Figure 1(b)). A right lung biopsy revealed an AC that shared cell morphologic features with the left lung tumor. The comprehensive clinical course led to a clinical suspicion that the right lung tumor was an AM from the left lung tumor [17]. No metastatic lesion was detected in the left lung. The patient did not undergo surgery for the right lung tumor and instead received various chemotherapy regimens for 30 months, including 11 cycles of paclitaxel, carboplatin, and bevacizumab; 10 cycles of pemetrexed; and 16 cycles of docetaxel. However, no distinct therapeutic effect was observed, and CT revealed a further enlargement of the shadow. The patient developed right pleuritis carcinomatosa at 31 months after the start of chemotherapy and died of respiratory failure 36 months after surgery. An autopsy was not performed.

In addition to a routine pathological analysis, tissue from the left-sided tumor was subjected to immunohistochemical analyses to detect the expression of various proteins, including ANX A2 and collagen IV. Immunohistochemistry was performed using Leica Bond-Max (Leica Biosystems, Australia) and a previously described ANX A2 antibody and staining protocol [9]. A mouse antihuman collagen IV antibody (clone CIV 22, DAKO, USA) was used as the primary antibody at a dilution ratio of 1 : 25 after a 5 min treatment with proteinase K. Only routine immunohistochemistry was performed on the right lung tumor because of the small amount of available tissue.

Macroscopically, the resected tumor was ill-defined and gelatinous with a diffuse pneumonia-like consolidation

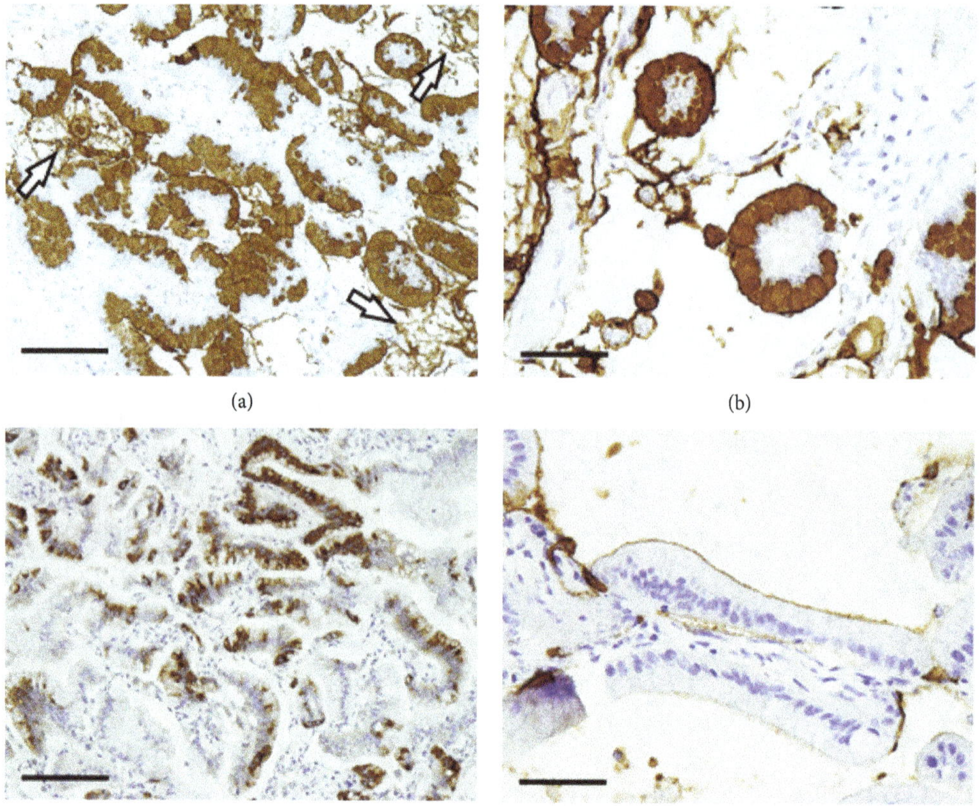

(a) (b) (c) (d)

FIGURE 4: Immunostaining of mucin glycoproteins in the left lung tumor. (a) Diffuse cytoplasmic positivity is visible in the lepidic or papillary component, and positive staining is present in the alveolar spaces (arrows). MUC 5AC immunostain, scale bar: 200 μm. (b) Floating tumor cells exhibit the same positive reaction. MUC 5AC immunostain, scale bar: 100 μm. (c) Some tumor cells exhibit cytoplasmic positivity. MUC 6 immunostain, scale bar: 200 μm. (d) In some cells, positive staining is visible on the cell surfaces but not in the cytoplasm. MUC 1 immunostain, scale bar: 100 μm.

(Figure 2(a)). Histopathologically, the majority of the tumor cells were columnar, contained varying amounts of intracytoplasmic mucins, and exhibited lepidic or papillary growth in a single-layer arrangement (Figures 2(b)–2(d)). Small groups of tumor cells had detached from the alveolar wall and were scattered diffusely (Figure 3(a)). Tumor cell aggregates floating within the alveolar spaces were round-shaped but had apical–basal polarity (Figure 3(b)). The apical surface of the tumor cells was located at the outer edge of the aggregates but naturally lacked central fibrovascular cores (Figure 3(b)), corresponding to the micropapillary pattern of the three morphological patterns of STAS [6].

Slight neutrophil and macrophage infiltration was observed at the detachment site. No desmoplastic reaction was observed.

Invasive foci with a maximum diameter of 2.2 cm were observed in the tumor. These foci had a glandular or papillary structure (Figure 3(c)) and greatly reduced levels of intracytoplasmic mucins. However, the nonmucinous component accounted for <10% of the tumor. Lymphatic and vascular permeation and pleural invasion were not observed. Many scattered tumor cell aggregates that had detached from the main tumor were observed within the air spaces and on the alveolar wall. The latter aggregates exhibited lepidic or papillary growth that is suggestive of microscopic AMs (Figure 3(d)) [2]. Tumor cell detachment was also often observed in the larger foci.

In the left lung tumor, the majority of tumor cells were positive for MUC 5AC (Figures 4(a) and 4(b)) and CK7 (data not shown). Abundant positive MUC 5AC staining was also observed in the alveolar spaces (Figures 4(a) and 4(b)). Some tumor cells exhibited intracytoplasmic positivity for MUC 6 (antibody clone CLH 5, Abnova, Taiwan; Figure 4(c)). Additionally, some tumor cells exhibited a positive MUC 1 reaction at the cell surface but not in the cytoplasm (Figure 4(d)), in contrast to our previously reported case [9]. The tumor cells were negative for MUC 2, CK20, TTF-1, Napsin A, CDX2, and ALK (data not shown). The clone and manufacturer of each antibody, except MUC6, have been described elsewhere [9]. The immunohistochemical results of the right lung tumor were similar to those of the left lung tumor.

As shown in Figures 5 and 6 (5(a), 5(c), 6(a), and 6(b) show ANX A2 staining), granular cytoplasmic ANX A2 positivity was observed on the basal sides of tumor cells exhibiting lepidic or papillary growth (Figure 5(a)), whereas no positive signal was detected at the cell–cell borders. Some tumor cells also exhibited weak ANX A2 positivity near the cell surfaces. A similar expression pattern was observed in the detached tumor cells, and positive expression was also

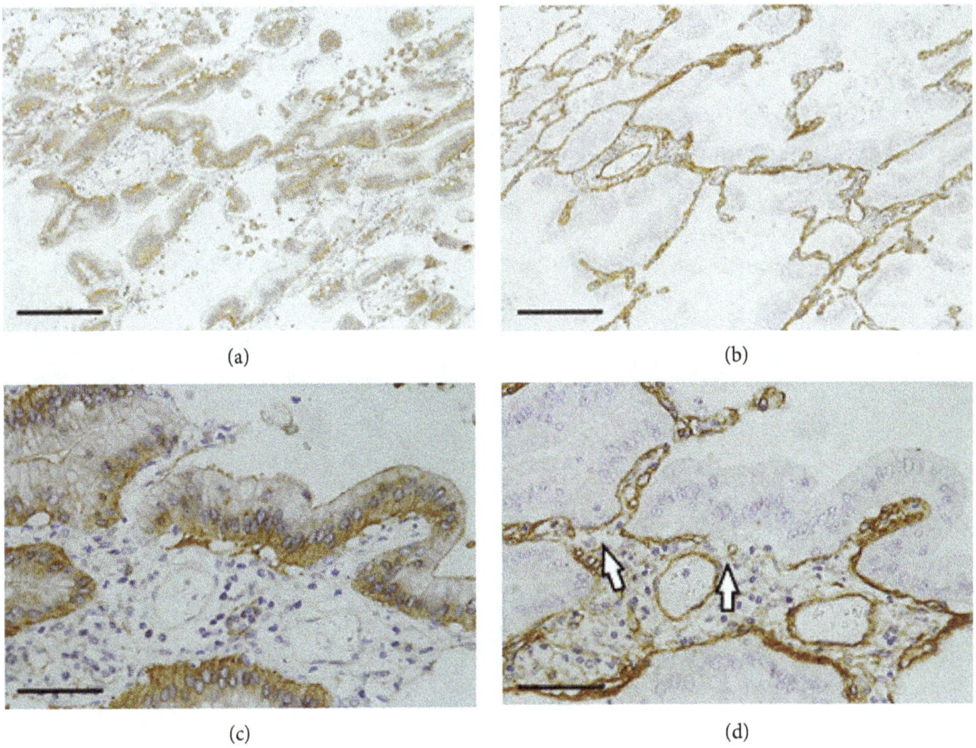

FIGURE 5: ANX A2 and collagen IV immunostaining of the lepidic or papillary component of the left lung tumor. (a) Tumor cells exhibit cytoplasmic ANX A2 positivity on the basal side. ANX A2 immunostain, scale bar: 400 μm. (b) A linear positive collagen IV reaction corresponding to the basement membrane is seen on the surfaces of both alveolar and vessel walls. Collagen IV immunostain, scale bar: 400 μm. (c) Detached tumor cells also exhibit cytoplasmic ANX A2 positivity on the basal side but not at the cell–cell borders. Positive staining is also observed in the exfoliative gap. ANX A2 immunostain, scale bar: 100 μm. (d) Weak or no collagen IV positivity is visible at the detachment site (arrows). Collagen IV immunostain, scale bar: 100 μm.

observed in the exfoliation gap (Figure 5(c)). Noticeably, weaker ANX A2 positivity was observed in the tumor cells floating within the alveolar spaces (Figure 6(a)). In the invasive component, stronger cytoplasmic positivity on the basal side was observed relative to that observed in the lepidic or papillary growth component (Figure 6(b)), and membranous positivity was observed on the cell–cell borders (Figure 6(b)).

As shown in Figures 5 and 6 (5(b), 5(d), and 6(c) show collagen IV staining), the lepidic or papillary area exhibited linear positive collagen IV staining corresponding to the BM, which was detected in both the surfaces of the alveolar and vessel walls (Figure 5(b)). However, either weak positivity or no signal was observed at the detachment site (Figure 5(d)). In the invasive area, the desmoplastic stroma exhibited positive staining for collagen IV (Figure 6(c)), thus suggesting the presence of cancer-associated fibroblasts and neogenic collagen [18, 19]. No positive reactions were observed in the tumor cells irrespective of invasiveness.

In an analysis of the AM, no positive reaction to ANX A2 beyond weak staining near the cell surface was observed in the minute foci (i.e., tumor cells that had newly adhered to the alveolar wall; Figure 7(a)). However, the staining patterns in larger foci became similar to those observed in the lepidic or papillary growth component of the primary lesion (Figure 7(b)). Similar findings were observed at the detachment site. Regarding collagen IV, the same findings as those of lepidic or papillary growth component of primary lesion were seen. Similar findings were also observed at the detachment site (data not shown).

3. Discussion

ANX A2 expression in the STAS/AM of the present tumor differed slightly from that in our previously reported case [9], particularly with regard to the following four points. (1) At the tumor cell detachment site, ANX A2 positivity was observed in the cytoplasm on the basal side and in the exfoliative gap. (2) No positive staining of the cell–cell borders was observed in any component, except the invasive component. (3) No distinct ANX A2 positivity was observed in either the tumor cell aggregates floating within alveolar spaces or the minute foci of AM. (4) No ANX A2 positivity was observed in the intracytoplasmic mucus. These discrepancies are likely attributable to differences in the cellular characteristics and growth patterns between the tumors. In the present case, both the mucin immunophenotype and negative immunostaining for TTF-1 and CDX 2 suggest an IMAC with gastric lineage [20–22]. The IMAC with gastric lineage was first reported as a mucinous bronchioloalveolar carcinoma, with cell morphology mimicking the mucous cells of gastric pyloric mucosa and with its mucin immunophenotype [21, 22]. Recently, Sonzogni et al. have classified the lineage of IMACs based on their immunophenotype, histology, and genetic alterations [20]. The IMAC with gastric

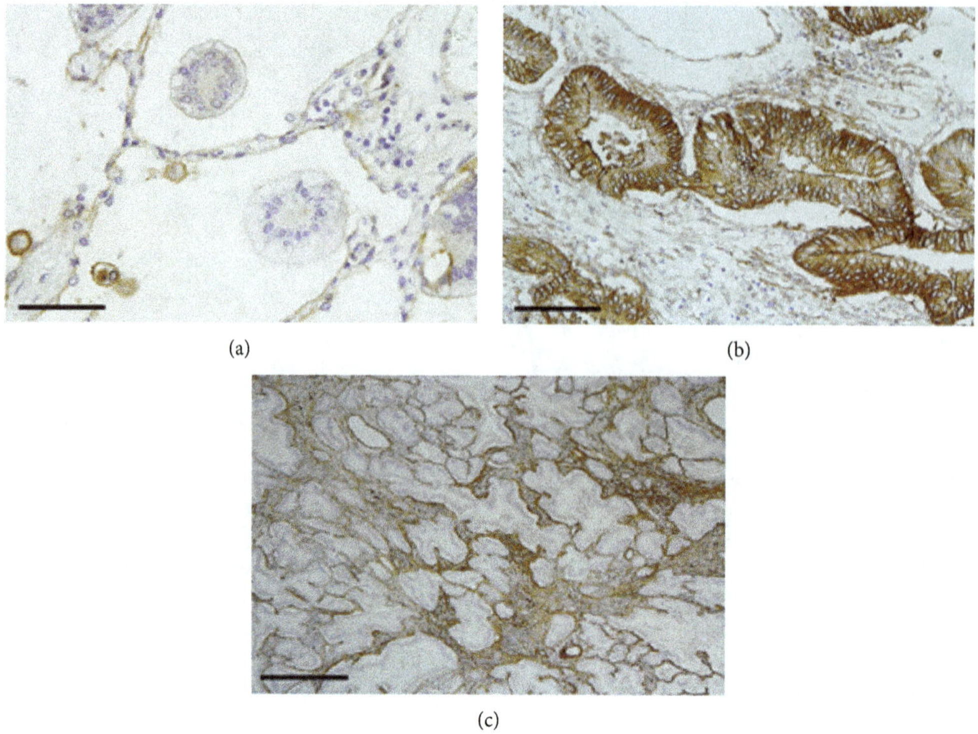

FIGURE 6: Floating tumor cells (a) and invasive components (b and c) of the left lung tumor. (a) No distinct ANX A2 positivity is visible in the floating tumor cells within alveolar spaces. ANX A2 immunostain, scale bar: 100 μm. (b) Stronger cytoplasmic ANX A2 positivity is observed on the basal side, and positive staining is visible at the cell–cell borders. ANX A2 immunostain, scale bar: 200 μm. (c) The desmoplastic stroma exhibits positive collagen IV staining, particularly around the tumor cells. Collagen IV immunostain, scale bar: 1 mm.

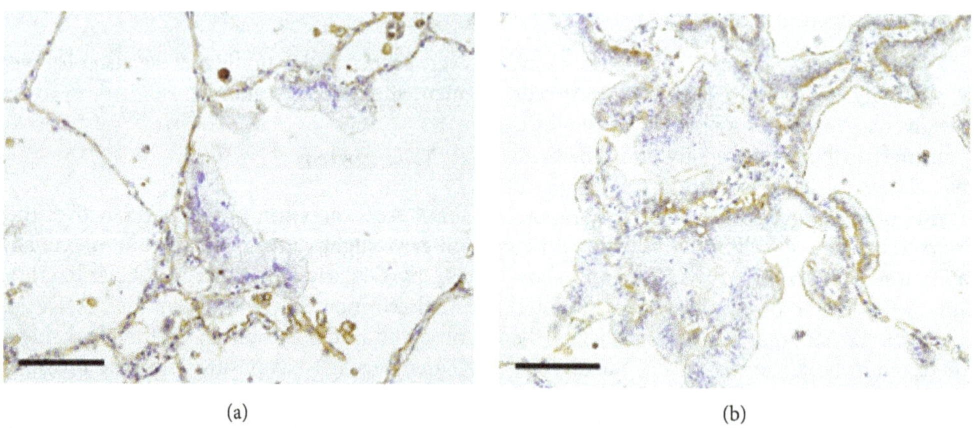

FIGURE 7: ANX A2 immunostaining of microscopic aerogenous metastases in the left lung. (a) No distinct positivity is visible in the minute foci. Scale bar: 200 μm. (b) Basal-side cytoplasmic positivity is detected in the larger metastatic foci. Scale bar: 200 μm.

lineage is characterized by expressions of both membranous MUC 1 and cytoplasmic MUC 6 and is suggested to be derived from the distal terminal bronchiole [20]. In contrast, our previously reported case was negative for subsequent MUC 6 immunostaining (data not shown) and showed non-typical immunohistochemical results for any of the classification by Sonzogni et al. [9, 20]. If the previous case is categorized, it is considered to exhibit characteristics of the pancreatobiliary type in terms of the classification of the intraductal papillary mucinous neoplasms of the pancreas, particularly given the intracytoplasmic expressions of both MUC 1 and MUC 5AC in the AC [9, 23].

ANX A2 moves inside the cell according to its roles [13]. Cytoplasmic ANX A2 is involved in cytoskeleton remodeling, exocytosis, and endocytosis [13]. In addition, a part of ANX A2 binds to the extracellular surface-membrane or is secreted [13]. This protein is expressed aberrantly in various cancers [14, 15] and may also be secreted [14]. A recent report further suggested that secreted ANX A2 contributes to the proteolysis of the extracellular matrix [24]. In the present tumor, we observed reduced collagen IV staining at the detachment site, thus leading us to consider that the ANX A2 secreted from the basal sides of tumor cells might induce cell detachment by degrading the BM [13–15, 24]. Therefore, in IMAC, the detachment site of the tumor cells and the subcellular localization of ANX A2 might differ depending on the immunophenotype of the detected biomarkers [9, 20].

Indistinct membranous ANX A2 positivity in contact with the alveolar wall suggests poor capacity of IMAC for stromal invasion [1, 9, 25]. However, we observed more intense cytoplasmic ANX A2 expression in the invasive component in the present IMAC case, thus suggesting that this protein is involved in stromal invasion [9, 12, 13]. Therefore, we presume (1) that whether IMAC tumor cells detach into alveolar spaces or infiltrate toward the stroma depends on the amount of secreted ANX A2, (2) that the stromal invasion of IMAC requires a stronger cytoplasmic expression of ANX A2, and (3) that extracellular membrane-bound ANX A2 enhances the aggressiveness of stromal invasion in AC [14, 15, 25, 26].

We note that weaker ANX A2 positivity was observed at the cell–cell borders in the detachment site, even in our previously reported case [9]. The expression of ANX A2 at the cell–cell borders is possibly related to the adhesions between tumor cells and the suppression of tumor cell detachment [9, 12, 13]. In other words, little or no expression of ANX A2 at the cell–cell borders might facilitate tumor cell detachment. Thus, we presumed that the lepidic or papillary component of the present tumor harbors a high capacity for detachment [9, 12, 13]. Nevertheless, the small groups of detached tumor cells showed a micropapillary pattern without the original monolayer arrangement. It has been suggested that tumor cells forming a micropapillary pattern acquire resistance to anoikis (cell detachment-induced apoptosis) and facilitate anchorage-independent growth [27]. Therefore, the morphological change of detached tumor cells is considered to be a defense reaction against the loss of interaction with the BM [11, 27]. It has been known that ANX A2 is released extracellularly during various stresses, including hypoxia [13], which is consistent with the findings that tumor cell aggregates floating within the alveolar spaces do not show a distinct ANX A2-immunopositivity.

Some reports have suggested that neutrophils and tumor-associated macrophages and fibroblasts promote STAS/AM [28, 29]. In the present case, we did not notice a particular infiltration of any of those cell types into the tumor. Although we agree that the tumor microenvironment is an important factor in STAS/AM, the present case suggests that the tumor cells can induce STAS/AM directly.

In this case, we consider that ANX A2 was only weakly involved in mediating the adhesions between tumor cells and in the anchoring of floating tumor cells to the alveolar wall. Conversely, abundant MUC 5AC was detected within and outside the tumor cells. In an IMAC with gastric lineage, MUC 5AC is thought to play a major role in the formation of contacts with the alveolar wall [30]. We assume that upon attaching to the alveolar wall, the round-shaped tumor cell aggregates stretch to form a monolayer along the alveolar wall in a manner independent of ANX A2.

It remains unclear whether the right lung tumor originated as a second primary lesion or was caused by an AM of the left lung tumor [17, 31, 32]. A similarly rapid clinical course was also reported in a previous case of multifocal IMAC [32]. Given that we did not genetically confirm monoclonality between the tumors and could not detect a recurrence in the ipsilateral lung, the right tumor might instead have been another lesion of multifocal IMAC.

This report had some additional limitations. Particularly, we analyzed only two cases, including our previously reported case. Moreover, our analysis lacked a functional assay and an immunohistochemical investigation of various BM matrices. Further investigations are needed to confirm our suppositions.

In conclusion, our findings from this case suggest the following points. (1) ANX A2 plays a dual role in tumor progression and suppression according to its subcellular localization. (2) The subcellular localization of ANX A2 depends on the characteristics of the tumor cell, including the biomarker immunophenotype and tumor cell growth pattern. (3) In the gastric lineage, ANX A2 secretion induces tumor cell detachment by degrading the BM. (4) The expression of ANX A2 (or lack thereof) at the cell–cell borders influences the detachment site.

Ethical Approval

Ethical approval for this study was provided by the ethics committee of Shizuoka General Hospital.

Consent

Written informed consent to publish the case details was obtained from the patient.

Acknowledgments

The authors would like to thank Enago (http://www.enago.jp/) for providing the English language review. This report received no specific grant from any funding agency in the public, commercial, or nonprofit sector.

References

[1] W. D. Travis, E. Brambilla, A. P. Burke, A. Marx, and A. G. Nicholson, *World Health Organization Classification of Tumours of the Lung, Pleura, Thymus and Heart*, International Agency for Research on Cancer Press, Lyon, 2015.

[2] A. Gaikwad, C. A. Souza, J. R. Inacio et al., "Aerogenous metastasesa potential game changer in the diagnosis and management of primary lung adenocarcinoma," *American Journal of Roentgenology*, vol. 203, no. 6, pp. W570–W582, 2014.

[3] H. Blaauwgeers, P. A. Russell, K. D. Jones, T. Radonic, and E. Thunnissen, "Pulmonary loose tumor tissue fragments and spread through air spaces (STAS): Invasive pattern or artifact? A critical review," *Lung Cancer*, vol. 123, pp. 107–111, 2018.

[4] T. Eguchi, K. Kameda, S. Lu et al., "Lobectomy is associated with better outcomes than sublobular resection in spread through air spaces (STAS)-positive T1 lung adenocarcinoma: a propensity score-matched analysis," *Journal of Thoracic Oncology*, vol. 14, pp. 87–98, 2018.

[5] K. Kadota, Y. Kushida, S. Kagawa et al., "Limited resection is associated with a higher risk of locoregional recurrence than lobectomy in stage I lung adenocarcinoma with tumor spread through air spaces," *The American Journal of Surgical Pathology*, vol. 43, no. 8, pp. 1033–1041, 2019.

[6] K. Kadota, J. Nitadori, C. S. Sima et al., "Tumor spread through air spaces is an important pattern of invasion and impacts the frequency and location of recurrences after limited resection for small stage I lung adenocarcinomas," *Journal of Thoracic Oncology*, vol. 10, no. 5, pp. 806–814, 2015.

[7] D. Chen, Y. Mao, J. Wen et al., "Tumor spread through air spaces in non-smal cell lung cancer: a systematic review and meta-analysis," *The Annals of Thoracic Surgery*, vol. 108, no. 3, pp. 945–954, 2019.

[8] Y. J. Cha and H. S. Shim, "Biology of invasive mucinous adenocarcinoma of the lung," *Translational Lung Cancer Research*, vol. 6, no. 5, pp. 508–512, 2017.

[9] K. Arai and M. Hirose, "Annexin A2 expression in aerogenous metastasis of pulmonary invasive mucinous adenocarcinoma: a case report including immunohistochemical analysis," *Case Reports in Oncological Medicine*, vol. 2019, 7 pages, 2019.

[10] P. N. Ohori, S. A. Yousem, J. Griffin et al., "Comparison of extracellular matrix antigens in subtypes of bronchioloalveolar carcinoma and conventional pulmonary adenocarcinoma: an immunohistochemical study," *The American Journal of Surgical Pathology*, vol. 16, no. 7, pp. 675–686, 1992.

[11] K. Kodama, G. Ishii, S. Miyamoto et al., "Laminin 5 expression protects against anoikis at aerogenous spread and lepidic growth of human lung adenocarcinoma," *International Journal of Cancer*, vol. 116, no. 6, pp. 876–884, 2005.

[12] J. K. Hitchcock, A. A. Katz, and G. Schäfer, "Dynamic reciprocity: the role of annexin A2 in tissue integrity," *Journal of Cell Communication and Signaling*, vol. 8, no. 2, pp. 125–133, 2014.

[13] A. K. Grindheim, J. Saraste, and A. Vedeler, "Protein phosphorylation and its role in the regulation of annexin A2 function," *Biochimica et Biophysica Acta*, vol. 1861, no. 11, pp. 2515–2529, 2017.

[14] N. A. Lokman, M. P. Ween, M. K. Oehler, and C. Ricciardelli, "The role of annexin A2 in tumorigenesis and cancer progression," *Cancer Microenvironment*, vol. 4, no. 2, pp. 199–208, 2011.

[15] M. V. Christensen, C. K. Hødall, K. M. Jochumsen, and H. EVS, "Annexin A2 and cancer: a systematic review," *International Journal of Oncology*, vol. 52, no. 1, pp. 5–18, 2017.

[16] K. Shimizu, R. Okita, S. Saisho, A. Maeda, Y. Nojima, and M. Nakata, "Clinicopathological and immunohistochemical features of lung invasive mucinous adenocarcinoma based on computed tomography findings," *OncoTargets and Therapy*, vol. 10, pp. 153–163, 2017.

[17] Y. Liu, H. L. Zhang, J. Z. Mei et al., "Primary mucinous adenocarcinoma of the lung: a case report and review of the literature," *Oncology Letters*, vol. 14, no. 3, pp. 3701–3704, 2017.

[18] Y. Soini, P. Pääkkö, and H. Autio-Harmainen, "Genes of laminin B1 chain, alpha 1 (IV) chain of type IV collagen, and 72-kd type IV collagenase are mainly expressed by the stromal cells of lung carcinomas," *The American Journal of Pathology*, vol. 142, no. 5, pp. 1622–1630, 1993.

[19] R. M. Bremnes, T. Dønnem, S. al-Saad et al., "The Role of Tumor Stroma in Cancer Progression and Prognosis: Emphasis on Carcinoma-Associated Fibroblasts and Non-small Cell Lung Cancer," *Journal of Thoracic Oncology*, vol. 6, no. 1, pp. 209–217, 2011.

[20] A. Sonzogni, F. Bianchi, A. Fabbri et al., "Pulmonary adenocarcinoma with mucin production modulates phenotype according to common genetic traits: a reappraisal of mucinous adenocarcinoma and colloid adenocarcinoma," *The Journal of Pathology: Clinical Research*, vol. 3, no. 2, pp. 139–151, 2017.

[21] T. Honda, H. Ota, K. Ishii, N. Nakamura, K. Kubo, and T. Katsuyama, "Mucinous bronchioloalveolar carcinoma with organoid differentiation simultating the pyloric mucosa of the stomach: clinicopathologic, histochemical, and immunohistochemical analysis," *American Journal of Clinical Pathology*, vol. 109, no. 4, pp. 423–430, 1998.

[22] H. Ota, M. Hayama, J. Nakayama et al., "Cell lineage specificity of newly raised monoclonal antibodies against gastric mucins in normal, metaplastic, and neoplastic human tissues and their application to pathology diagnosis," *American Journal of Clinical Pathology*, vol. 115, no. 1, pp. 69–79, 2001.

[23] V. M. Castellano-Megias, C. Ibarrola-de Andres, G. Lopez-Alonso, and F. Colina-Ruizdelgado, "Pathological features and diagnosis of intraductal papillary mucinous neoplasm of the pancreas," *World journal of gastrointestinal oncology*, vol. 6, no. 9, pp. 311–324, 2014.

[24] S. Maji, P. Chaudhary, I. Akopova et al., "Exosomal annexin II promotes angiogenesis and breast cancer metastasis," *Molecular Cancer Research*, vol. 15, no. 1, pp. 93–105, 2017.

[25] C. H. Luo, Q. Q. Liu, P. F. Zhang, M. Y. Li, Z. C. Chen, and Y. F. Liu, "Prognostic significance of annexin II expression in non-small cell lung cancer," *Clinical & Translational Oncology*, vol. 15, no. 11, pp. 938–946, 2013.

[26] E. Tristante, C. M. Martínez, S. Jiménez et al., "Association of a characteristic membrane pattern of annexin A2 with high invasiveness and nodal status in colon adenocarcinoma," *Translational Research*, vol. 166, no. 2, pp. 196–206, 2015.

[27] K. Kamiya, Y. Hayashi, J. Douguchi et al., "Histopathological features and prognostic significance of the micropapillary pattern in lung adenocarcinoma," *Modern Pathology*, vol. 21, no. 8, pp. 992–1001, 2008.

[28] M. Wislez, M. Antoine, N. Rabbe et al., "Neutrophils promote aerogenous spread of lung adenocarcinoma with bronchioloalveolar carcinoma features," *Clinical Cancer Research*, vol. 13, no. 12, pp. 3518–3527, 2007.

[29] X. Qiu, D. Chen, Y. Liu et al., "Relationship between stromal cells and tumor spread through air spaces in lung adenocarcinoma," *Thoracic Cancer*, vol. 10, no. 2, pp. 256–267, 2019.

[30] S. Yamazoe, H. Tanaka, T. Sawada et al., "RNA interference suppression of mucin 5AC (MUC5AC) reduces the adhesive and invasive capacity of human pancreatic cancer cells," *Journal of Experimental & Clinical Cancer Research*, vol. 29, no. 1, pp. 53–58, 2010.

[31] A. Warth, S. Macher-Goeppinger, T. Muley et al., "Clonality of multifocal nonsmall cell lung cancer: implications for staging and therapy," *The European Respiratory Journal*, vol. 39, no. 6, pp. 1437–1442, 2012.

21

Response to Dabrafenib and Trametinib of a Patient with Metaplastic Breast Carcinoma Harboring a BRAF V600E Mutation

Takuji Seo,[1] Emi Noguchi,[1] Masayuki Yoshida,[2] Taisuke Mori,[2] Maki Tanioka,[1] Kazuki Sudo,[1] Akihiko Shimomura,[1] Kan Yonemori,[1] Yasuhiro Fujiwara,[1] and Kenji Tamura[1]

[1]*Department of Breast and Medical Oncology, National Cancer Center Hospital, 5-1-1, Tsukiji, Chuo-ku, Tokyo 104-0045, Japan*
[2]*Department of Pathology and Clinical Laboratories, National Cancer Center Hospital, 5-1-1, Tsukiji, Chuo-ku, Tokyo 104-0045, Japan*

Correspondence should be addressed to Emi Noguchi; enoguchi@ncc.go.jp

Academic Editor: Ossama W. Tawfik

Background. Metaplastic breast carcinomas are rare and carry poor prognoses. They are also more aggressive than other breast cancers and are known for their resistance to chemotherapy. Prolonged treatment with dabrafenib and trametinib is a therapy for malignant melanoma that improves the progression-free survival and overall survival. Such molecular-targeted therapies are also being developed for cancers with BRAF mutation, a driver of malignant melanoma. *Case Presentation.* A 57-year-old woman with metaplastic breast cancer and chemotherapy-refractory massive pleural effusion. After contained anthracycline regimen failure, her breast cancer progressed to an advanced stage. We ordered next-generation sequencing- (NGS-) based tumor molecular profiling from core needle biopsy of the breast. The NGS report indicated the presence of a BRAF V600E mutation. After initiation of dabrafenib and trametinib, her symptom and the pleural effusion were decreased. The first assessment of CT scans showed a decreased pleural effusion and shrunken subcutaneous lesions. Approximately 2 weeks later, a new lesion appeared. She died from 12 weeks after initiation of dabrafenib and trametinib treatment. *Conclusion.* To the best of our knowledge, this is the first report of BRAF mutation breast cancer treated with dabrafenib and trametinib and it heralds the possibility of targeted therapy for rare breast cancers.

1. Introduction

Metaplastic breast carcinoma is a rare subtype of breast cancer that consists of cells that have undergone metaplasia, a differentiation from glandular to nonglandular squamous or mesenchymal components [1]. It accounts for 0.2%–5% of all breast cancers. Metaplastic carcinoma is usually negative for hormone receptors and human epidermal growth factor receptor 2 (HER2) and is classified as triple negative breast cancer (TNBC) [2–5]. Due to its rarity and the lack of randomized trials, the treatment approach is usually extrapolated from those for other subtypes of breast cancer. Anthracyclines and taxanes have been the mainstay of chemotherapy for decades. However, patients with metaplastic breast carcinoma are often resistant to these conventional chemotherapies, and their prognosis is poor [4–6].

The BRAF gene encodes a serine-threonine protein kinase that plays an important role in the RAS-RAF-MAPK pathway. BRAF mutations are present in many tumor types including cutaneous melanomas (50%), thyroid cancer (20%–50%), colorectal cancer (10%), non-small-cell lung cancer (2%–4%), and hairy cell leukemia (>90%) [7]. The somatic point mutation of BRAF exon-15 (V600E) is the most common mutation among the BRAF gene mutations [7]. BRAF inhibitor monotherapy is usually not long lasting due to the development of acquired resistance and the reactivation of the mitogen-activated protein kinase (MAPK) pathway [8]. Therefore, a combination therapy with a BRAF and a MEK inhibitor would be expect to delay the development of MAPK-driven acquired resistance. Phase III studies on the combination of a BRAF inhibitor (dabrafenib) and a MEK inhibitor (trametinib) in untreated patients with BRAF V600E/V600K-mutated metastatic melanomas demonstrated a prolongation of both the progression-free survival (PFS) and the overall survival (OS) compared to monotherapy with a BRAF inhibitor (vemurafenib or dabrafenib) [9–11]. BRAF inhibition has also been assessed in BRAF-mutant nonmelanoma cancers and is expected to provide new therapeutic options.

We present here the first report of a patient with a BRAF V600E mutation and metastatic metaplastic breast carcinoma that was resistant to anthracycline chemotherapy and was treated with a combination therapy of dabrafenib and trametinib.

2. Case Presentation

A previous healthy 57-year-old woman presented to the local hospital with complaints of swelling and right breast pain. Physical examination identified a 5.2 × 4.0 cm induration and redness of the skin in the upper inner quadrant of the right breast with lymphadenopathy. Mammography and ultrasonography revealed no definite tumor, but thickening of the parenchyma was observed throughout the mammary gland. Magnetic resonance imaging revealed a mass enhancement in the upper lesion of the right breast and a tumor invading the pectoralis major muscle. Histopathological examination of the core needle biopsy specimen showed round, pleomorphic, or spindle sarcomatoid cells with myxoid stroma. The differential diagnoses included metaplastic carcinoma with melanocytic differentiation or malignant melanoma. Estrogen and progesterone receptors (ER/PgR) and HER2 expression by immunohistochemistry (IHC) were all negative. The tumor was also negative for pan-cytokeratin (AE1/3), desmin, epithelial membrane antigen (EMA), HHF35, and S100 and positive for CK7 (focal) and melan A (diffuse, strong). From these negative markers, the pathologist ruled out sarcoma and malignant melanoma, and the final pathological diagnosis was metaplastic breast cancer. We cannot show the pictures of the immunohistochemistry results because these tests were performed prior to her referral to our hospital. The patient was tentatively diagnosed as having breast cancer (T4dN3bM0, Stage IIIC) and received 2 cycles of FEC (fluorouracil 500 mg/m^2, day 1, epirubicin 100 mg/m^2, day 1, cyclophosphamide 500 mg/m^2, day 1; every 3 weeks). However, a computed tomography (CT) scan showed progressive disease (PD) of the breast tumor mass and lymph nodes.

She was referred to our hospital for further treatment. We performed again a biopsy of the breast tumor. Histopathological examination showed a poorly differentiated carcinoma negative for ER, PgR, HER2, gross cystic disease fluid protein, and GATA-binding protein 3 (GATA3) (Figures 1(a)–1(c)). We excluded a diagnosis of malignant melanoma based on the following IHC findings: positive for pankeratin AE1/3 (Figure 1(d)) and negative for CK8, SOX10 (Figure 1(e)), S100 (Figure 1(f)), melan A, CD45, and desmin. Therefore, she was diagnosed as presenting a metaplastic carcinoma with melanocytic differentiation. We checked gene mutation using the tissue sample obtained from prior hospital, which was ineffective for chemotherapy. A targeted next-generation sequencing (NGS) using the NCC Oncopanel System [12] identified genomic alterations including BRAF p.V600E, PIK3CA p.H1047R, CDKN2A p.R58X, and TP53 p.W146X mutations (Table 1). The NCC oncopanel covered 114 gene alternations, along with rearrangements and fusions of 12 oncogenes. Tumor progression after chemotherapy is eligible for NGS using NCC oncopanel in our institute. In this case, we analyzed the tumor sample after anthracycline- and taxane-based chemotherapy. We confirmed the BRAF V600E mutation using a real-time PCR gene mutation assay (THxID™ BRAF kit).

She underwent palliative radiotherapy to the right breast with a total dose of 30 Gray in 10 fractions; however, the breast mass increased in size and new metastases in the sacrum, causing pleural effusion, appeared. Thoracotomy tube was inserted into the right chest to control pleural effusion. We confirmed an approval by the institutional committee for off-label drug use and started the patient on treatment with dabrafenib at 150 mg BID and trametinib at 2 mg QD after obtaining the patient's informed consent [10]. After a single dose of dabrafenib and trametinib, she experienced grade 1 fever (Common Toxicity Criteria for Adverse Event ver. xx), which we controlled by withdrawing drug administration for a day. The swelling and pain in the right breast improved remarkably after the initiation of dabrafenib and trametinib. A chest X-ray at the 1-week follow-up showed the right pleural effusion had decreased in size (Figure 2(a)). We removed thoracotomy tube without pleurodesis three days after combination therapy. Following 2 weeks of dabrafenib and trametinib administration, a CT scan showed a decrease in pleural effusion and a reduction in the size of the axillary lymph nodes. There was a general improvement in conditions, and we discharged the patient (Figure 3). After 6 weeks of treatment, a CT scan showed further reduction in the size of the tumors in the right breast, axillary lymph nodes, and pleura (Figure 4). The right chest pleural effusion did not increase, and she did not have dyspnea after treatment initiation. However, a new subcutaneous tumor appeared in the right abdominal wall at this time. To confirm the diagnosis of the newly recognized lesion and to monitor whether additional genetic alterations had occurred, we carried out a biopsy of the new subcutaneous tumor after 7 weeks of treatment. The histopathological findings and NGS results were the same as the ones in the primary breast tumor. After 8 weeks of treatment, we observed disease progression with increased pleural effusion and skin metastases in the abdominal wall. The treatment with dabrafenib and trametinib was discontinued and the patient received palliative care. The patient died from breast cancer 12 weeks after the initiation of the dabrafenib and trametinib treatment.

3. Discussion

To the best of our knowledge, this is the first case report of a patient with a BRAF-V600E-mutant breast cancer treated

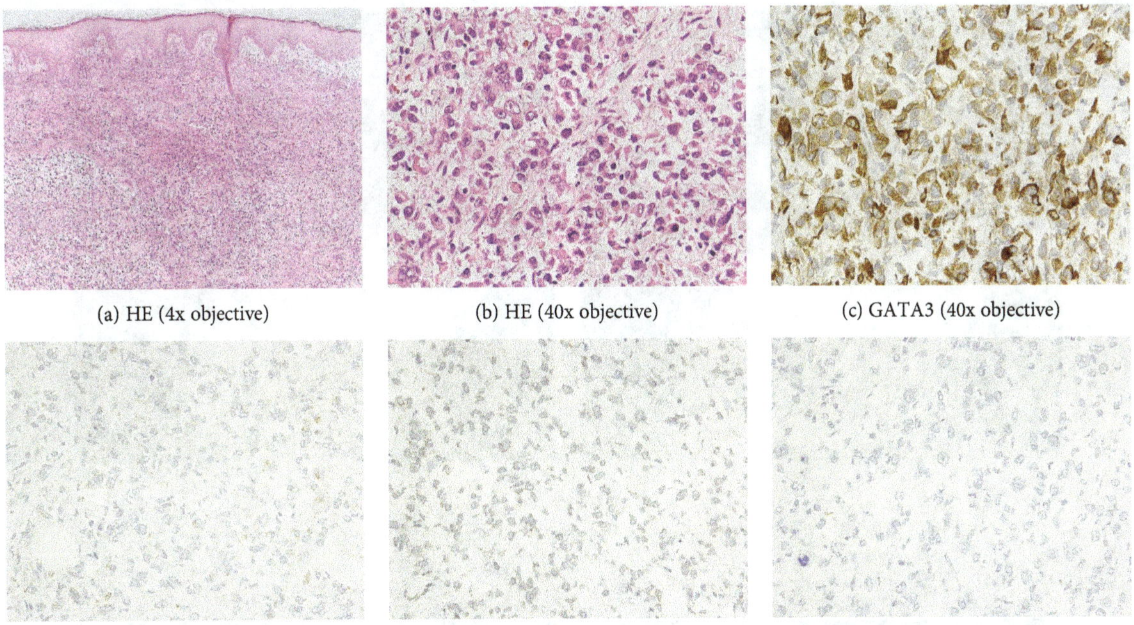

(a) HE (4x objective) (b) HE (40x objective) (c) GATA3 (40x objective)

(d) AE1/AE3 (40x objective) (e) SOX10 (40x objective) (f) S100 (40x objective)

Figure 1: HE and IHC of histopathology. Histopathology of biopsy of the breast. (a) and (b) show HE staining. Poorly differentiated malignant cells invading stromal areas. (c) shows an IHC positive for AE1/3, which rules out sarcoma. (d)–(f) show negative IHCs for GATA3, SOX100, and S100. These results exclude malignant melanoma.

Table 1: The result of NGS.

Genes	CDS	Amino acid
PIK3CA	Exon21:c.A3140G	p.H1047R
BRAF	Exon15:c.T1799A	p.V600E
CDKN2A	Exon2:c.C172T	p.R58X
TP53	Exon5:c.G438A	p.W146X

with dabrafenib and trametinib. Even though our patient was refractory to conventional chemotherapy and had a rapidly progressing cancer, she experienced a partial response and we observed dramatic primary tumor shrinkage within 2 weeks following the initial treatment of dabrafenib and trametinib. The patient underwent repeated genomic testing at progression to identify mechanisms of acquired resistance, but we found no additional gene alterations.

During the last two decades, molecular profiling for targeted therapy in breast cancer has been studied but still presents a challenge, especially in cases with metaplastic carcinoma. Microarray-based gene expression profiling has demonstrated that most of metaplastic carcinomas are classified as basal-like molecular subtypes [13]. In a study, researchers classified a subgroup of metaplastic carcinomas as claudin-low subtypes [14] (claudin-low is a molecular subtype), but they identified most of the claudin-low tumors as basal-like before assigning them a specific molecular subtype. In view of reports of epidermal growth factor receptor (EGFR) gene amplification and overexpression in metaplastic carcinoma [15, 16], therapeutics targeting EGFR have been studied, but data supporting the efficacy of EGFR-targeted therapy in metaplastic carcinoma have not been obtained.

Breast cancer genomes have been investigated to introduce precision medicine into the clinical practice. The Cancer Genome Atlas data showed that TP53, PIK3CA, and GATA3 are the most often mutated genes in breast cancer [17]. Genomic profiling of metaplastic carcinoma also demonstrated that the most common alterations are in TP53 and PIK3CA [18, 19]. Of note, the frequency of BRAF mutations in breast cancer is extremely small. Albanell et al. reported that comprehensive genomic profiling of 10,428 metastatic breast cancer cases identified 135 (1.3%) BRAF alterations: amplifications (0.6%), mutations (0.5%), and rearrangements (0.2%), respectively [20]. In a report by the same group, among 115 BRAF-mutated cases with known hormone receptor and HER2 statuses, 63 (55%) were TNBCs [21].

The efficacy of BRAF inhibitors against BRAF-mutant solid tumors has been studied [22, 23]. In a phase I study investigating the efficacy of dabrafenib against solid tumors, twenty-eight patients with BRAF-mutant colorectal cancer, non-small-cell lung cancer, ovarian cancer, or thyroid cancer showed partial responses in cases with nonmelanoma tumors [22]. A phase II trial on dabrafenib and trametinib for V600E-mutated anaplastic thyroid cancer showed a highly objective response rate (69%) [23]. A phase II basket trial on dabrafenib and trametinib for patients with various nonmelanoma cancers harboring BRAF V600E mutations is underway (NCT02034110).

Our patient developed resistance to BRAF and MEK inhibitors relatively sooner than has been reported for nonmelanoma tumors [22, 23].

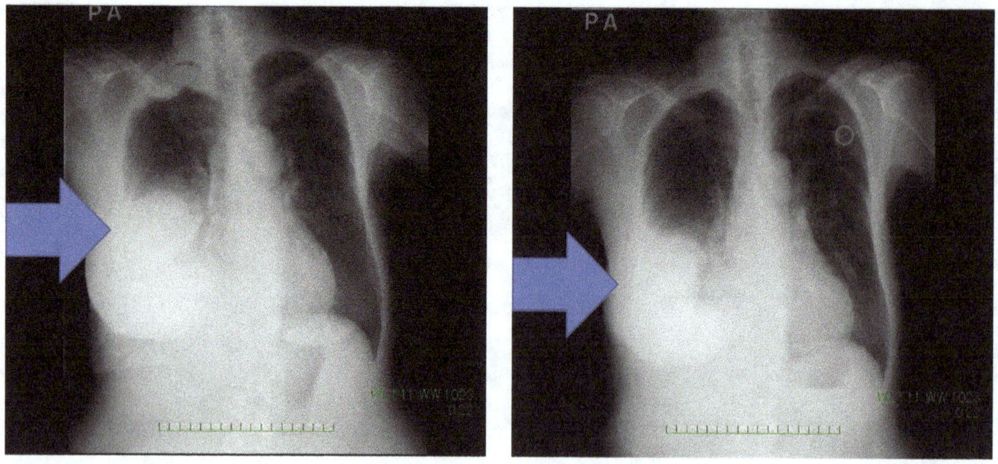

(a) (b)

Figure 2: (a) CXR before dabrafenib and trametinib initiation. (b) 1 week after treatment. Arrow shows pleural effusion.

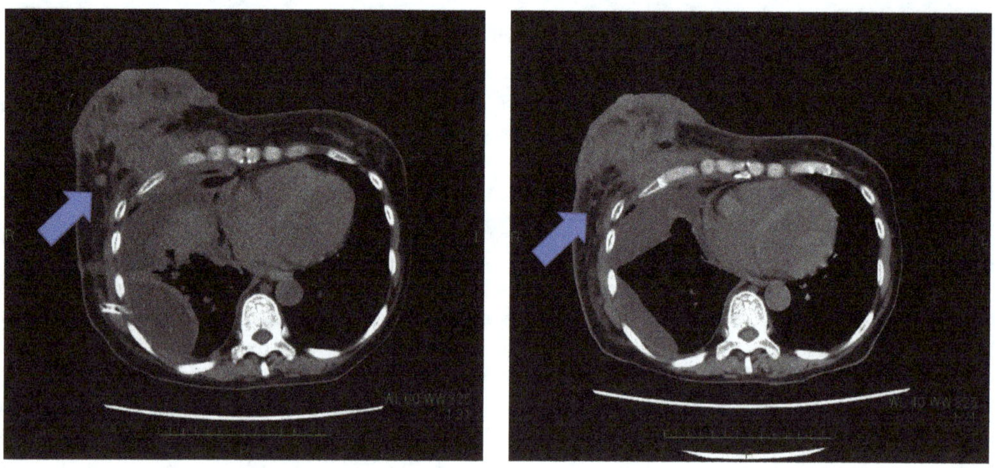

(a) (b)

Figure 3: (a) Breast sections of CT scan before initiation of dabrafenib and trametinib. (b) Same section 2 weeks after treatment initiation. The arrow points to reduced mass and decreased pleural effusion.

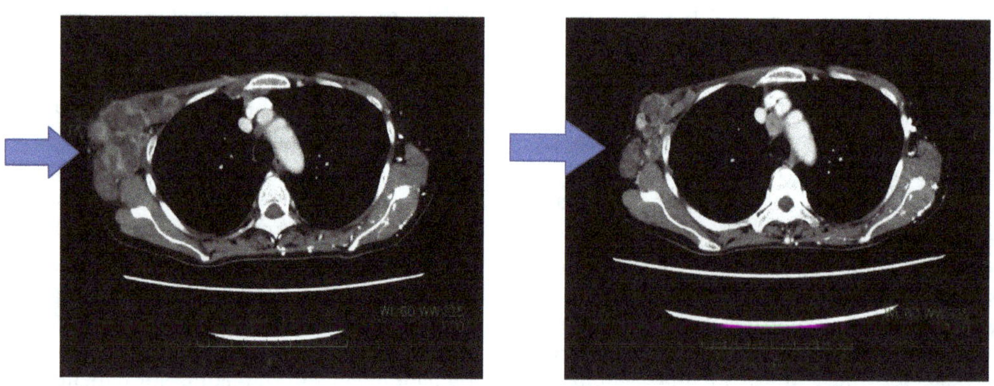

(a) (b)

Figure 4: (a) CT scan section showing right axillary lymph nodes before treatment. (b) CT scan section showing right axillary lymph nodes 6 weeks after treatment initiation. Arrow shows right axillary lymph nodes being decreased after treatment.

Studies on the resistance mechanisms for BRAF and MEK inhibitors have shown secondary RAS mutations, including those of NRAS or KRAS, can contribute to the resistance development by increasing MAPK reactivation [24]. We tried to identify different pre- and posttreatment mutations but could not find any differences using our target sequence panel.

Another report has indicated that cooccurring PI3K-mTOR pathway aberrations in BRAF V600-mutated nonmelanoma tumors are associated with PFS and OS reductions and may predict primary resistance to BRAF-targeted therapy [25]. Our patient had BRAF and PIK3CA mutations at the beginning of treatment; in retrospect, this may explain the reason for the low efficacy of BRAF and MEK inhibition in our patient. Combinations of BRAF, MEK, and PI3K-mTOR pathway inhibitors may be more effective in such patients. A phase I trial of BRAF inhibitor vemurafenib and mTOR inhibitor everolimus for advanced cancer is underway (NCT01596140). More studies are needed for a better understanding of response and resistance to BRAF-targeted therapy in patients with BRAF-mutant breast cancer.

Abbreviations

NGS: Next-generation sequencing
CT: Computed tomography
HER2: Human epidermal growth factor receptor 2
EGFR: Epidermal growth factor receptor
PFS: Progression-free survival
OS: Overall survival
ER: Estrogen receptor
PgR: Progesterone receptors
IHC: Immunohistochemistry
EMA: Epithelial membrane antigen
FEC: Fluorouracil+epirubicin+cyclophosphamide
PD: Progressive disease
MAPK: Mitogen-activated protein kinase.

Ethical Approval

Our institutional ethics committee approved the search through electronic medical records for this paper. The patient also approved and gave consent for the use of her medical records.

Consent

The patient provided a written informed consent for the publication of this case report and all accompanying images.

Authors' Contributions

TS managed this patient in ward and wrote the manuscript. EN decided to perform NGS and managed the patient in the outpatient setting; she also added a substantial contribution by critically proofreading the manuscript. YM and TM are pathologists who made the diagnosis of metaplastic carcinoma and made slides with histopathology pictures. MK, KS, AS, and KY are breast cancer specialists and helped us to choose the medications to prescribe. YF and KT are the department heads and approved all medical decisions. All authors read and approved the final manuscript.

Acknowledgments

The authors would like to thank Enago (https://www.enago.jp) for the English language review.

References

[1] S. R. Lakhani, I. O. Ellis, S. J. Schnitt, P. H. Tan, and M. J. van de Vijver, *WHO Classification of Tumours of the Breast*, IARC Press, Lyon, France, 2012.

[2] C. M. Pezzi, L. Patel-Parekh, K. Cole, J. Franko, V. S. Klimberg, and K. Bland, "Characteristics and treatment of metaplastic breast cancer: analysis of 892 cases from the National Cancer Data Base," *Annals of Surgical Oncology*, vol. 14, no. 1, pp. 166–173, 2007.

[3] E. A. Rakha, P. H. Tan, Z. Varga et al., "Prognostic factors in metaplastic carcinoma of the breast: a multi- institutional study," *British Journal of Cancer*, vol. 112, no. 2, pp. 283–289, 2015.

[4] R. A. Nelson, M. L. Guye, T. Luu, and L. L. Lai, "Survival outcomes of metaplastic breast cancer patients: results from a US population-based analysis," *Annals of Surgical Oncology*, vol. 22, no. 1, pp. 24–31, 2015.

[5] N. Okada, T. Hasebe, M. Iwasaki et al., "Metaplastic carcinoma of the breast," *Human Pathology*, vol. 41, no. 7, pp. 960–970, 2010.

[6] T. Nagao, T. Kinoshita, T. Hojo, H. Tsuda, K. Tamura, and Y. Fujiwara, "The differences in the histological types of breast cancer and the response to neoadjuvant chemotherapy: the relationship between the outcome and the clinicopathological characteristics," *Breast*, vol. 21, no. 3, pp. 289–295, 2012.

[7] H. Davies, G. R. Bignell, C. Cox et al., "Mutations of the BRAF gene in human cancer," *Nature*, vol. 417, no. 6892, pp. 949–954, 2002.

[8] D. B. Solit and N. Rosen, "Resistance to BRAF inhibition in melanomas," *The New England Journal of Medicine*, vol. 364, no. 8, pp. 772–774, 2011.

[9] G. V. Long, D. Stroyakovskiy, H. Gogas et al., "Combined BRAF and MEK inhibition versus BRAF inhibition alone in melanoma," *The New England Journal of Medicine*, vol. 371, no. 20, pp. 1877–1888, 2014.

[10] G. V. Long, D. Stroyakovskiy, H. Gogas et al., "Dabrafenib and trametinib versus dabrafenib and placebo for Val 600 BRAF-mutant melanoma: a multicentre, double-blind, phase 3 randomised controlled trial," *The Lancet*, vol. 386, no. 9992, pp. 444–451, 2015.

[11] C. Robert, B. Karaszewska, J. Schachter et al., "Improved overall survival in melanoma with combined dabrafenib and trametinib," *The New England Journal of Medicine*, vol. 372, no. 1, pp. 30–39, 2015.

[12] Y. Tanabe, H. Ichikawa, T. Kohno et al., "Comprehensive screening of target molecules by next-generation sequencing in patients with malignant solid tumors: guiding entry into phase I clinical trials," *Molecular Cancer*, vol. 15, no. 1, p. 73, 2016.

[13] B. Weigelt, B. Kreike, and J. S. Reis-Filho, "Metaplastic breast carcinomas are basal-like breast cancers: a genomic profiling

analysis," *Breast Cancer Research and Treatment*, vol. 117, no. 2, pp. 273–280, 2009.

[14] A. Prat, J. S. Parker, O. Karginova et al., "Phenotypic and molecular characterization of the claudin-low intrinsic subtype of breast cancer," *Breast Cancer Research*, vol. 12, no. 5, p. R68, 2010.

[15] J. S. Reis-Filho, F. Milanezi, S. Carvalho et al., "Metaplastic breast carcinomas exhibit EGFR, but not HER2, gene amplification and overexpression: immunohistochemical and chromogenic in situ hybridization analysis," *Breast Cancer Research*, vol. 7, no. 6, pp. R1028–R1035, 2005.

[16] J. S. Reis-Filho, C. Pinheiro, M. B. Lambros et al., "EGFR amplification and lack of activating mutations in metaplastic breast carcinomas," *The Journal of Pathology*, vol. 209, no. 4, pp. 445–453, 2006.

[17] The Cancer Genome Atlas Network, "Comprehensive molecular portraits of human breast tumours," *Nature*, vol. 490, no. 7418, pp. 61–70, 2012.

[18] J. S. Ross, S. Badve, K. Wang et al., "Genomic profiling of advanced stage, metaplastic breast carcinoma by next-generation sequencing reveals frequent, targetable genomic abnormalities and potential new treatment options," *Archives of Pathology & Laboratory Medicine*, vol. 139, no. 5, pp. 642–649, 2015.

[19] M. V. Dieci, V. Smutná, V. Scott et al., "Whole exome sequencing of rare aggressive breast cancer histologies," *Breast Cancer Research and Treatment*, vol. 156, no. 1, pp. 21–32, 2016.

[20] J. Albanell, J. A. Elvin, S. M. Ali et al., "BRAF: an emerging target for triple negative breast cancer," *Journal of Clinical Oncology*, vol. 35, Supplement 15, p. 1099, 2017.

[21] J. Albanell, J. A. Elvin, J. Suh et al., "BRAF genomic alterations in breast cancer," *Annals of Oncology*, vol. 27, article vi70, Supplement 6, 2016.

[22] G. S. Falchook, G. V. Long, R. Kurzrock et al., "Dabrafenib in patients with melanoma, untreated brain metastases, and other solid tumours: a phase 1 dose-escalation trial," *The Lancet*, vol. 379, no. 9829, pp. 1893–1901, 2012.

[23] V. Subbiah, R. J. Kreitman, Z. A. Wainberg et al., "Dabrafenib and trametinib treatment in patients with locally advanced or metastatic BRAF V600–mutant anaplastic thyroid cancer," *Journal of Clinical Oncology*, vol. 36, no. 1, pp. 7–13, 2018.

[24] G. V. Long, C. Fung, A. M. Menzies et al., "Increased MAPK reactivation in early resistance to dabrafenib/trametinib combination therapy of BRAF-mutant metastatic melanoma," *Nature Communications*, vol. 5, no. 1, article 5694, 2014.

[25] S. Sen, F. Meric-Bernstam, D. S. Hong, K. R. Hess, and V. Subbiah, "Co-occurring genomic alterations and association with progression-free survival in BRAFV600-mutated non-melanoma tumors," *Journal of the National Cancer Institute*, vol. 109, no. 10, article djx094, 2017.

Undifferentiated Nasopharyngeal Carcinoma Presenting with Shoulder Mass

Cosphiadi Irawan,[1] Rahmat Cahyanur ,[1] and Reyhan Eddy Yunus[2]

[1]*Division of Hematology-Medical Oncology, Department of Internal Medicine, Faculty of Medicine Universitas Indonesia, Dr. Cipto Mangunkusumo General Hospital, Jakarta, Indonesia*
[2]*Department of Radiology, Faculty of Medicine Universitas Indonesia, Dr. Cipto Mangunkusumo General Hospital, Jakarta, Indonesia*

Correspondence should be addressed to Rahmat Cahyanur; rahmat.cahyanur01@ui.ac.id

Academic Editor: Jose I. Mayordomo

Nasopharyngeal cancer (NPC) is the most common cancer among head and neck cancer that usually presented with unilateral neck mass. Unusual symptoms of NPC can lead us to diagnosis misleading and delayed definitive treatment. We present a case of NPC with bone metastasis in the shoulder. A 33-year-old female presented with right shoulder mass caused by undifferentiated carcinoma of unknown primary, based on biopsy of shoulder mass. After four months, she was complaining painless neck swelling, headache, and hearing impairment in the left ear. Bone MRI showed malignant bone tumour in the right humerus. Neck CT scan showed mass in the nasopharyngeal and bilateral lymphadenopathy. Biopsy in nasopharyngeal revealed undifferentiated carcinoma of nasopharyngeal cancer (WHO-3 type A). The patient was diagnosed as NPC stage IVb and thus was treated with palliative chemotherapy. After three cycles of cisplatin docetaxel, patient condition improved.

1. Introduction

Nasopharyngeal cancer (NPC) is the most common head and neck cancer. Southeast Asia including Indonesia is the area with high prevalence of NPC cases. Our hospital, as a national referral hospital, had 878 patients with NPC in 2012-2015. The incidence rate for NPC is estimated 6.2/100000 cases yearly [1].

The most common presenting sign of NPC is unilateral neck mass (approximately 80% cases) [2]. A previous study in Cipto Mangunkusumo General Hospital showed neck lump presented in 58.1% [2]. Suzina and Hamzah also reported in Malaysia that unilateral neck mass was the most common presenting symptom (37.5%) [3]. Lee et al. studied 5020 patients in Hong Kong and showed that neck mass was found in 37.3%. Metastasis deposits were only found in 0.3% cases as the presenting symptoms [4].

This article would like to report a rare clinical presentation of NPC that came to medical facilities due to right shoulder mass. Unusual presenting sign leads to misleading diagnosis and delayed definitive treatment. The case that undifferentiated carcinoma of unknown primary based on biopsy result could be end up in NPC, especially in an endemic area, is important to us.

2. Case Presentation

A 33-year-old female came into the hospital due to right shoulder mass. She felt increasing pain. She reported that the mass grew rapidly. She consulted the orthopaedic, and biopsy was performed. Biopsy result showed undifferentiated carcinoma of unknown primary site. She had been advised to perform further evaluation, but she preferred complementary and alternative medicine for two months.

Two months later, she is complaining painless neck swelling rapidly growing in the left neck. She is also complaining headache and hearing impairment in the left ear. She was referred to the Cipto Mangunkusumo General Hospital for further evaluation, because of facility limitation. Bone MRI of right upper extremities was performed and

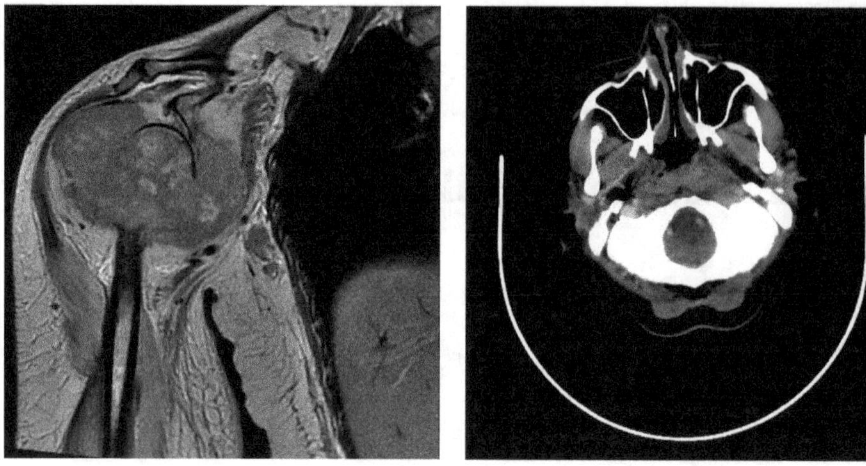

(a) (b)

Figure 1: (a) MRI of right upper extremities showed malignant bone tumour. (b) CT scan of nasopharynx showed mass and bilateral lymphadenopathy.

showed malignant bone tumour in the proximal epimetadiaphysis of the right humerus (Figure 1(a)). Neck CT scan was performed and showed mass in the nasopharyngeal and bilateral lymphadenopathy (Figure 1(b)). Biopsy in nasopharyngeal was performed, and undifferentiated carcinoma of nasopharyngeal cancer (WHO-3 type A) was confirmed from histopathological examination.

In the tumour board meeting, after a review with the previous histopathological data from bone and nasopharynx, this case was concluded as NPC stage T4N3M1 (bone). Palliative treatment was performed with Cisplatin-Docetaxel. After three cycles of chemotherapy, patient condition improved, and pain reduced.

3. Discussion

Metastasis deposit in the bone, described in this case, was uncommon presenting symptoms for NPC cases (0.3% cases). At the moment of shoulder mass being diagnosed, the patient only had mild headache without other symptoms associated with NPC. Wei and Sham classified common symptoms in NPC into four categories: (1) symptoms caused by the presence of tumour mass in the nasopharynx (epistaxis, nasal block, and discharge); (2) symptoms associated with dysfunction of the Eustachian tube symptoms; (3) symptoms associated with the superior enlargement of the tumour (headache, diplopia, facial pain, and numbness); and (4) neck mass [5]. Among the symptoms that had been classified, neck mass is the most common presenting symptom [4]. The patient was first examined in a health facility with limited equipment, located about 800 km from the capital city. The examination that could be performed to determine the diagnosis was only biopsy of shoulder mass, and the result showed undifferentiated carcinoma of unknown primary. As stated before, there was not any ear, nose, and throat (ENT) symptom when undifferentiated carcinoma of unknown primary was diagnosed so examination leading to ENT disease, such as NPC, was not done there.

This case describes undifferentiated carcinoma found in the bone. The literature stated that 20% of the cases of bone metastasis of unknown primary site were undifferentiated carcinoma. Most of the primary site that caused bone metastasis was lung cancer (52-60%), especially among women and young patients. Besides lung cancer, other origins that are commonly possible were renal carcinoma (12%), prostate cancer (10%), and thyroid carcinoma (3%) [6]. The nasopharynx is an uncommon origin site that caused bone metastasis, without the primary being detected clinically. In spite of this, bone metastasis is the most common location of metastasis in nasopharyngeal carcinoma, ranging from 54 to 80%, with the most frequently involved bone metastatic sites were the rib (53.5%), thoracic vertebrae (50.0%), lumbar vertebrae (43.6%), pelvic girdle (42.3%), and lower limb (32.4%) [7].

A histopathological report in this case showed WHO-3 type A. Undifferentiated carcinoma of nasopharynx characteristic has higher incidence of distant metastasis, despite higher local tumour control rate. Undifferentiated carcinoma is common in an endemic area (account 95% cases), including Indonesia. Type A undifferentiated NPC had a 5-year overall survival (30-40%) [8].

In this case, the patient seek out complementary and alternative treatment before going through further examination. It is quite common in Indonesia to seek out traditional treatment. About 31.4% of the population in Indonesia use traditional treatment [9]. In this case, the diagnosis was delayed and so was the medical treatment. NPC itself has a higher rate to be cured if the patients seek medical treatment in an earlier stage. The 5-year overall survival (OS) rates for patients in stages I, II, III, and IV were 90.48%, 76.71%, 76.89%, and 33.87%, respectively ($P = 0.000$) [10]. There will be more cases found untreatable if there is more delay to be diagnosed and proceed with the medical treatment.

This case had been diagnosed as stage IVb based on the AJCC 8th [11]. Palliative intent chemotherapy was planned. Cisplatin and docetaxel were given in this case. After chemotherapy, clinical and CT scan evaluations were done. The neck mass was reduced partially, shoulder mass disappeared, and patient's complain improved [12].

Acknowledgments

This work is supported by Hibah PITTA 2018 funded by DRPM Universitas Indonesia No. 2060/UN2.R3.1/ HKP.05.00/2018.

References

[1] M. Adham, A. N. Kurniawan, A. I. Muhtadi et al., "Nasopharyngeal carcinoma in Indonesia: epidemiology, incidence, signs, and symptoms at presentation," *Chinese Journal of Cancer*, vol. 31, no. 4, pp. 185–196, 2012.

[2] V. F. Jayalie, M. S. Paramitha, J. Jessica et al., "Profile of nasopharyngeal carcinoma in Dr. Cipto Mangunkusumo National Hospital, 2010," *eJournal Kedokteran Indonesia*, vol. 4, no. 3, pp. 156–162, 2016.

[3] S. A. H. Suzina and M. Hamzah, "Clinical presentation of patients with nasopharyngeal carcinoma," *The Medical Journal of Malaysia*, vol. 58, no. 4, pp. 539–545, 2003.

[4] A. W. M. Lee, W. Foo, S. C. Law et al., "Nasopharyngeal carcinoma—presenting symptoms and duration before diagnosis," *Hong Kong Medical Journal*, vol. 3, no. 4, pp. 355–361, 1997.

[5] W. I. Wei and J. S. Sham, "Nasopharyngeal carcinoma," *The Lancet*, vol. 365, no. 9476, pp. 2041–2054, 2005.

[6] A. Piccioli, G. Maccauro, M. S. Spinelli, R. Biagini, and B. Rossi, "Bone metastases of unknown origin: epidemiology and principles of management," *Journal of Orthopaedics and Traumatology*, vol. 16, no. 2, pp. 81–86, 2015.

[7] L. Shen, J. Dong, S. Li et al., "M1 stage subdivision and treatment outcome of patients with bone-only metastasis of nasopharyngeal carcinoma," *The Oncologist*, vol. 20, no. 3, pp. 291–298, 2015.

[8] H. C. Hsu, C. L. Chen, M. M. Hsu, T. C. Lynn, S. M. Tu, and S. C. Huang, "Pathology of nasopharyngeal carcinoma. Proposal of a new histologic classification correlated with prognosis," *Cancer*, vol. 59, no. 5, pp. 945–951, 1987.

[9] Indonesian Ministry of Health, *Laporan Nasional Riskesdas 2018. Report*, Badan Penelitian dan Pengembangan Kesehatan, Jakarta, 2019.

[10] H. Dou, D. Hu, C. Lam, Y. Liu, X. Wang, and W. Zhang, "Retrospective analysis of results of treatment for nasopharyngeal carcinoma in Macao," *Chinese Journal of Cancer Research*, vol. 26, no. 2, pp. 148–158, 2014.

[11] American Joint Committee on Cancer, *8th Edition Implementation Project*, American Joint Committee on Cancer, 2018, October 2018, http://cancerstaging.org/8thEdImplementation/Pages/default.aspx.

[12] A. T. Chan, V. Grégoire, J. L. Lefebvre et al., "Nasopharyngeal cancer: EHNS–ESMO–ESTRO Clinical Practice Guidelines for diagnosis, treatment and follow-up," *Annals of Oncology*, vol. 23, Supplement 7, pp. vii83–vii85, 2012.

23

Salivary Duct Carcinoma: Case Reports and Brief Review of the Literature

Deepti Kantamani, Sai S. Bandaru, Jennifer L. Miatech, and M. Patrick Stagg

Baton Rouge General Medical Center-Bluebonnet, Internal Medicine Residency Program, Baton Rouge, LA, USA 70809-3679

Correspondence should be addressed to Jennifer L. Miatech; jennifer.miatech@brgeneral.org

Academic Editor: Ossama W. Tawfik

Salivary duct carcinoma (SDC) is an uncommon and highly aggressive tumor associated with high morbidity and mortality. According to the World Health Organization, it is an extremely rare malignancy with an estimated incidence of 1-1.2 in 1,000,000 patients. Standard treatment for SDC is wide surgical resection along with lymph node dissection followed by adjuvant radiation therapy. The role of adjuvant chemotherapy is not known. In this report, we present three cases of SDC. A 71-year-old female with T1N0M0 disease was treated with total parotidectomy, ipsilateral neck dissection, and adjuvant radiotherapy without evidence of disease recurrence at 5 months. The second is a 59-year-old female with TXN1M0 disease who was treated with total parotidectomy with ipsilateral level I-IV neck dissection and adjuvant radiotherapy without evidence of disease occurrence at 21 months. The third case is a 79-year-old male with widely metastatic disease, including brain metastases, treated with cranial irradiation, leuprolide, and lapatinib who remains under home hospice care.

1. Introduction

Salivary duct carcinoma (SDC) is a rare, highly aggressive malignancy. The term SDC describes the malignancy that histologically resembles in situ and invasive ductal carcinoma of the breast. The parotid gland is the most commonly involved salivary gland accounting for approximately 80% of tumors, followed by the submandibular gland (8-12%) and minor salivary glands less than 10% [1, 2]. SDC is an extremely rare malignancy with an estimated incidence of 1-1.2 in 1,000,000 patients, with a higher prevalence in men [3]. It is often diagnosed at an advanced stage as it metastasizes early to regional lymph nodes and distant sites. Immunohistochemically, tumor cells are diffusely positive for cytokeratin 7 and androgen receptor stains and may be GATA binding protein 3 positive. HER2/neu positivity occurs in 15-40% of patients with SDC [2]. The mainstay of treatment for SDC is wide surgical resection along with lymph node dissection followed by adjuvant radiation therapy. The role of adjuvant chemotherapy and targeted therapies has limited benefit to date. Overall survival of the metastatic disease is poor, and 60-80% of patients with advanced-stage (T4) die within three years [4].

Adeberg et al. listed 1282 cases of SDC found in the literature between 1987 and 2019 [3]. Most clinical studies of SDC in the literature are institution-based retrospective cohort studies. This malignancy poses a challenge for physicians to provide education and information to the patients regarding the overall prognosis and treatment options given the absence of consensus guidelines. Due to the rarity of this devastating disease, we feel that each case should be reported. We describe three cases of SDC recently encountered in our institution.

2. Case Presentation

2.1. Case I. A 71-year-old African American female with no significant past medical history presented to her primary care physician in September 2020 for progressive swelling in her right parotid region for 3 months associated with a recent onset of dental pain. She denied any previous history of tobacco use or prior radiation exposure. Antibiotics resolved her dental pain without improvement of the right parotid swelling. She was then evaluated by head and neck surgery. Computed tomography (CT) of the head and neck revealed a 1.9 cm heterogeneously enhancing lesion in the anterior, superior superficial parotid gland without any enlarged nodes. She did not have any preoperative facial nerve involvement or lymphadenopathy. She underwent a total parotidectomy with clinically uninvolved margins. The complete facial nerve was dissected free of the neoplasm with gross preservation of function. Postoperatively, she had some weakness in the marginal mandibular branch of the facial nerve, along with weakness in closing her superior palpebral fissure of the right eye. Pathology of resected lesions revealed salivary duct carcinoma that was 1.7 cm in maximum dimension, positive for cytokeratin 7, HER2/neu equivocal 2+, and androgen receptor-positive. The tumor was negative for p40, mucin, estrogen receptor, progesterone receptor, TTF-1, SOX100, mammaglobin, p63, and s-100. HER2/neu was 1+ FISH not amplified. She had no lymphovascular invasion, but perineural invasion was present. Postoperative positron emission tomography (PET) scan before radiation was negative for metastatic disease. The tumor was staged pathologically as T1N0M0 stage I. She received adjuvant radiotherapy incorporating margin positivity with 6600 cGy in 30 fractions to the entire parotid bed and the adjacent nodes with 6000 cGy in 30 fractions. The remainder of her right neck received 5400 cGy in 30 fractions. She completed radiotherapy in January 2021. She developed facial dermatitis and dysgeusia as a result of radiation, but otherwise tolerated therapy. Currently, she is being followed with CT scans every 3 months and is without evidence of disease recurrence to date.

2.2. Case II. A 59-year-old Caucasian female with a past medical history of essential hypertension and a 35 pack-year history of tobacco smoking who first noted a neck mass in December 2018 presented to a head and neck surgeon in May 2019 complaining of a painless left-sided neck mass. She did not have any associated localized or constitutional symptoms. Fine-needle aspiration of the left neck mass in May 2019 returned positive for malignant cells that could not be further classified. PET/CT in June 2019 revealed a 0.9 × 1.0 × 1.2 cm solitary ovoid mass inferior to the left distal portion of the parotid gland. Imaging could not reliably determine if the mass inferior to the parotid gland originated from the parotid gland. The tumor stage was TXN1M0. A core biopsy of the left neck mass on June 20, 2019, showed neoplastic cells but could not be classified further. On July 8, 2019, she underwent an excisional biopsy of the mass by her head and neck surgeon. Intraoperatively, the mass was positioned between the cervical branch and the inferior branch of the marginal mandibular nerve and was firmly adherent to both the nerves. The adherence to the mass necessitated the sacrifice of these nerves. The parotid had no abnormalities on palpation and no clinically positive margins. Several enlarged cervical lymph nodes found on resection were negative for malignancy. Final pathology revealed salivary duct carcinoma involving a single intraparotid or periparotid lymph node with a tumor measuring approximately 9 mm in greatest dimension and is present <1 mm from nearest tissue edge. The tumor cells were positive for GATA-3, BRST-2, cytokeratin 7, and HER2/neu and showed focal scattered positivity for S-100, p63, and p40. Immunohistochemical stains were positive for mammaglobin and androgen receptors. There was no extranodal extension identified. On July 17, 2019, the patient underwent left total parotidectomy and ipsilateral level I-IV neck dissection with excision of sublingual gland and a submandibular gland biopsy. The final pathology showed benign salivary gland tissue in the left parotid, left submandibular gland, and left sublingual gland. All lymph nodes removed from left level I-IV were negative for malignancy. Postoperatively, she developed paresthesia of the left lateral tongue and left lower lip. She completed adjuvant radiotherapy to the postoperative parotid bed and ipsilateral neck with a total dose of 60/57/54 cGy in 30 fractions on October 7, 2019. She developed xerostomia and hypothyroidism as a result of radiation therapy. The patient declined adjuvant platinum-based chemotherapy and targeted therapy. She is followed every 3 months with serial imaging without evidence of disease to date.

2.3. Case III. A 79-year-old Caucasian male presented to his primary care physician for routine follow-up in November 2020. He has a past medical history of insulin-dependent diabetes mellitus, essential hypertension, hyperlipidemia, and coronary artery disease with coronary artery bypass grafting and pacemaker placement. He denied any previous history of tobacco use. On physical examination, a nontender mass on the left side of his neck was easily palpable. Complete review of systems was otherwise negative except for increased forgetfulness. CT scan of the neck revealed a large mass arising from or immediately adjacent to the left parotid gland. Multiple left lung masses representing metastatic disease were also present on this scan. PET scan revealed 2.9 × 3.4 cm hypermetabolic soft tissue mass in the left parotid gland and extensive metastatic disease in the lung, mediastinum, liver, and bones. He underwent an ultrasound-guided biopsy of the left parotid mass and a CT-guided biopsy of a left lung nodule. Pathology revealed salivary duct carcinoma in the parotid and metastatic disease in the lung. Immunohistochemistry was positive for cytokeratin 7, GATA-3, and mammaglobin. HER2/neu and androgen receptors were positive in the lung biopsy. Magnetic resonance imaging (MRI) of the brain contained numerous ring-enhancing lesions, approximately 40-50. He received whole-brain radiation 30 cGy in 10 fractions in December 2020. He tolerated radiation therapy without complication. Following a discussion about goals of care, the patient decided against palliative chemotherapy. He did agree to androgen deprivation therapy with leuprolide. Next-generation sequencing identified no actionable targets except for HER2/neu amplification. He started lapatinib in February 2021. Despite dual therapy with leuprolide and lapatinib, he developed new visual symptoms prompting a repeat MRI of the brain on May 20, 2021, which revealed a mixed response to therapy. The majority of the central nervous system enhancing metastatic lesions decreased in size or resolved compared to the previous MRI on December 8, 2020. However, several new lesions were slightly more prominent than the previous ones. The patient decided to transition to comfort care and has been under home hospice since May 2020.

3. Discussion

Kleinsasser et al. described salivary duct carcinoma (SDC) in 1968 as a salivary malignancy that histologically resembles in situ and invasive ductal carcinoma of the breast [2, 5]. The World Health Organization recognized it as a distinct tumor type in 1991. SDC is rare, accounting for approximately 1 to 3% of all malignant salivary gland tumors [2]. Most tumors arise de novo, although 20% of cases arise secondarily from preexisting benign pleomorphic adenoma (i.e., carcinoma ex pleomorphic adenoma) [6]. The most common presenting symptom is a painless neck mass. Locally advanced disease can involve the facial nerve resulting in facial weakness. According to the case series published by Jaehne et al., which included 50 cases, around 66% present at T3/T4 stage [7, 8]. SDC predominantly affects male patients (66%-75%), presenting with a wide age range from 34 to 83 years and a mean age of diagnosis at 62.5 [8].

SDC is a highly aggressive high-grade salivary malignancy with a tendency for early regional, distant metastasis, and a high-grade recurrence. The most common sites of distant metastasis are the lung, bone, brain, and liver. Perineural invasion, lymphovascular invasion, extracapsular spread, higher N stage, and facial nerve involvement often are considered negative prognostic indicators, although findings are inconsistent. Cheng et al. described that perineural invasion and LVI were frequently present in approximately 57-69% and 61-70% of patients, respectively. Extranodal invasion occurred in 58% of patients [2]. The series published by Jaehne et al. found local disease recurrence in 48% of patients at 17.4 months after initial treatment and distant metastases in 48% after an average of 28 months [8]. The mean survival of patients in this report was 36 to 56 months. The 5-year survival rate for stage I disease was 42%, stage II was 40%, stage III was 30.8%, and stage IV was 23.2% [8]. Patients with parotid gland involvement had a better prognosis than those with submandibular or minor salivary gland involvement.

Currently, no National Comprehensive Cancer Network (NCCN) guidelines for the specific treatment of SDC exist. NCCN guidelines recommend complete surgical excision of tumor for major salivary gland tumors without nodal involvement (N0) with or without neck dissection for high-grade and T3/T4 salivary gland tumors. The recommendation for those with node involvement (N+) is complete surgical resection combined with neck dissection. In addition, they recommend adjuvant radiotherapy for high-risk features like intermediate or high grade, close or positive margins, neural/perineural invasion, lymph node metastasis, lymphatic/vascular invasion, and T3-4 tumors. Postoperative radiotherapy for SDC is an appropriate therapeutic option regardless of stage and margin status [9]. Excellent local control rates can be achieved with extensive (local) surgical treatment and postoperative RT [10]. Smaller trials discuss the activity of chemotherapy regimens including a taxane plus platinum. Randomized clinical trials demonstrating the benefit of cytotoxic chemotherapy are lacking.

SDC treatment is most often with targeted therapy. Androgen receptor expression is seen in over 90% of the cases of SDC, making the tumor a potential target for androgen deprivation therapy [9]. Additionally, HER2 expression occurs in between 15 and 40% of cases [2]. Therapy with trastuzumab for HER2 overexpressing tumors improves overall survival [9]. A case series of 50 tumor samples published by Jaehne et al. showed that the intensity of HER2/-neu expression correlates with the early development of distant metastasis and poor 5-year survival rate. The 2-year, 3-year, and 5-year survival in patients with HER2 1+ were 88.9%, 55.6%, and 11.1% compared to 51.4%, 17.1%, and 0%, respectively, in those with HER2 3+ positivity [8]. Further research regarding androgen deprivation therapy and other targeted therapy is warranted. There are no consensus guidelines in the management of metastatic disease.

We report three cases of SDC. Case 1 is clinically stage 1, T1N0M0 treated with total parotidectomy with ipsilateral neck dissection and adjuvant radiotherapy. She is under close monitoring postradiotherapy and has remained disease-free since January 2021 to date. Case 2 is clinically stage 2, TXN1M0 treated with total parotidectomy with ipsilateral level I-IV neck dissection and adjuvant radiotherapy who remains disease-free since October 2019. Case 3 presented with widely metastatic disease and remains under home hospice care after undergoing cranial irradiation and treatment with leuprolide and lapatinib.

4. Conclusion

The rarity of salivary duct carcinoma and lack of consensus guidelines necessitates the reporting of these cases. We present three cases including staging, therapy, and outcome data to enhance our understanding of this disease and build a more substantial data set for historical controls in future clinical trials. Finally, we hope clinical trials employing robust historical data will soon address the treatment of metastatic SDC, which remains an unmet medical necessity.

Disclosure

All authors have declared that they have no financial relationships at present or within the previous three years with any organizations that might have an interest in the submitted work.

References

[1] A. W. Anwer, M. Faisal, M. Adeel et al., "Clinicopathological behavior and treatment-related outcome of rare salivary duct carcinoma: the Shaukat Khanum Memorial Cancer Hospital experience," *Cureus*, vol. 10, no. 8, article e3139, 2018.

[2] C.-C. Hsu, W.-Y. Li, and P.-Y. Chu, "Salivary duct carcinoma of the supraglottis with a distinct presentation. A case report

and literature review," *Medicine (Baltimore)*, vol. 97, no. 11, article e0095, 2018.

[3] S. Adeberg, P. Windisch, F. Ehret et al., "Intensity modulated radiotherapy (IMRT) with carbon ion boost in the multimodal treatment of salivary duct carcinoma," *Frontiers in Oncology*, vol. 9, p. 1420, 2019.

[4] R. H. W. Simpson, "Salivary Duct Carcinoma: new Developments—Morphological variants including pure in situ high grade Lesions; proposed molecular classification," *Head and Neck Pathology*, vol. 7, no. S1, pp. 48–58, 2013.

[5] O. Kleinsasser, H. J. Klein, and G. Hubner, "Salivary duct carcinoma: a group of salivary gland tumours analogous to mammary duct carcinoma," *Archiv fur klinische und experimentelle Ohren- Nasen*, vol. 192, pp. 100–105, 1968.

[6] M. L. Johnston, S. H. Huang, J. N. Waldron et al., "Salivary duct carcinoma: treatment, outcomes, and patterns of failure," *Head & Neck*, vol. 38, Suppl 1, pp. E820–E826, 2016.

[7] D. Stodulski, B. Mikaszewski, H. Majewska, and J. Kuczkowski, "Parotid salivary duct carcinoma: a single institution's 20-year experience," *European Archives of Oto-Rhino-Laryngology*, vol. 276, no. 7, pp. 2031–2038, 2019.

[8] M. Jaehne, K. Roeser, T. Jaekel, J. D. Schepers, N. Albert, and T. Löning, "Clinical and immunohistologic typing of salivary duct carcinoma: a report of 50 cases," *Cancer*, vol. 103, no. 12, pp. 2526–2533, 2005.

[9] M. Nakaguro, Y. Tada, W. C. Faquin, P. M. Sadow, L. J. Wirth, and T. Nagao, "Salivary duct carcinoma: updates in histology, cytology, molecular biology, and treatment," *Cancer Cytopathology*, vol. 128, no. 10, pp. 693–703, 2020.

[10] A. C. C. Beck, P. J. F. M. Lohuis, A. Al-Mamgani, L. A. Smit, and W. M. C. Klop, "Salivary duct carcinoma: evaluation of treatment and outcome in a tertiary referral institute," *European Archives of Oto-Rhino-Laryngology*, vol. 275, no. 7, pp. 1885–1892, 2018.

24

Breast Cancer Metastasis in a Renal Carcinoma Pulmonary Metastasis: A Rare Example of Tumor-to-Tumor Metastasis

Áurea Lima,[1,2,3] **Isa Peixoto**,[4] **Susana Sarandão**,[5] **Daniel Melo**,[6] **Ângelo Rodrigues**,[7] **and Helena Pereira**[5]

[1]*Medical Oncology Service, Centro Hospitalar de Entre o Douro e Vouga, EPE, Unit of Santa Maria da Feira, R. Dr. Cândido Pinho 5, 4520-211 Santa Maria da Feira, Portugal*
[2]*Molecular Oncology and Viral Pathology Group, Research Center of Portuguese Institute of Oncology of Porto, Portuguese Institute of Oncology of Porto Francisco Gentil, EPE, Rua Dr. António Bernardino de Almeida, 4200-072 Porto, Portugal*
[3]*CESPU, Institute for Research and Advanced Training in Health Sciences and Technologies, Cancer Research Group, R. Central da Gandra, 1317 Gandra, Portugal*
[4]*Medical Oncology Service, Centro Hospitalar Universitário do Porto, EPE, Largo Prof. Abel Salazar 4099-001 Porto, Portugal*
[5]*External Radiotherapy Service, Portuguese Institute of Oncology of Porto Francisco Gentil, EPE, Rua Dr. António Bernardino de Almeida, 4200-072 Porto, Portugal*
[6]*Pathologic Anatomy Service, Centro Hospitalar Universitário de São João, Alameda Prof. Hernâni Monteiro 4200-319 Porto, Portugal*
[7]*Pathologic Anatomy Service, Portuguese Institute of Oncology of Porto Francisco Gentil, EPE, Rua Dr. António Bernardino de Almeida, 4200-072 Porto, Portugal*

Correspondence should be addressed to Áurea Lima; aurealimamd@gmail.com

Academic Editor: Katsuhiro Tanaka

The tumor-to-tumor metastasis phenomenon remains fairly uncommon, with fewer than 100 cases described to present time. Virtually any tumor can be a donor or a recipient neoplasm. Nevertheless, renal carcinomas have been implicated as the most common malignant tumors to harbor metastasis, while lung and breast tumors are the most frequent donors. This article reports an extremely rare case of a breast cancer metastasis in a lung metastasis of clear cell type renal cell carcinoma that met all Campbell and coworkers' tumor-to-tumor metastasis criteria. Additionally, we present the literature case reports of breast cancer metastasis in renal cell carcinomas and try to discuss the mechanisms underlying its occurrence. Since this phenomenon identification will impact the therapeutic strategy and it is not easily detected by image, the anatomopathological study of any and all suspicious lesions is of crucial importance. To the best of our knowledge, this is the first report of a metastasis inside a metastasis.

1. Introduction

Tumor-to-tumor metastasis (TTM) is a term describing the presence of two histologically distinct tumors at one location, each with different morphologic and immunophenotypic features [1]. It is an extremely rare phenomenon in patients with multiple synchronous or metachronous primary malignancies. The most common metastatic donor neoplasms are lung and breast cancers, while meningioma is the most common recipient of metastasis among benign tumors and renal cell carcinoma among malignant tumors [2]. Although the lung is one of the organs most vulnerable to metastases, a lung carcinoma is one of the rarest recipients of TTM [3]. Furthermore, the phenomenon of a metastasis in another metastasis is still a rarer event.

Herein, we report a TTM case of a breast cancer metastasis in a pulmonary metastasis of clear cell type renal cell carcinoma (ccRCC).

This work has been approved by CHEDV's Ethics Committee, according to the Helsinki Declaration of the World Medical Association; also, the patient gave written informed consent to have her case used for this paper.

2. Results

2.1. Patient History and Presentation. We present a 57-year-old woman with a past medical history of stage IV ccRCC (pT3aR0cN0M1) diagnosed in August 2019. During diagnosis and staging evaluation, she was observed to have a 12 mm suspicious lesion on the left kidney and a 20 mm nonsuspicious solid nodule in the right adrenal; the multidisciplinary team (MDT) decided left radical nephrectomy, performed in September 2019, plus clinical and imagological surveillance of the right adrenal nodule. Follow-up exams revealed an increment of 2 mm of the right adrenal nodule without new lesions; MDT decided histological evaluation of the lesion, which revealed a ccRCC metastasis. Since this was a unique metastasis, a right adrenalectomy was performed in February 2020. In March 2020, the patient referred to having a palpable nodule in the left breast. The auxiliary diagnostic tests carried out revealed a stage III invasive ductal carcinoma (IDC) ER 100%, PgR negative, HER2 positive (FISH), and Ki67 > 30%, initially managed with neoadjuvant chemotherapy (CHT) with sequential anthracycline/taxane-based regime combined with dual anti-HER2 blockade (trastuzumab/pertuzumab), followed by surgery (cT3N+/ypT2N1 (3/15)cM0). In November 2020, the follow-up CT scan (Figure 1) showed bilateral pulmonary nodules.

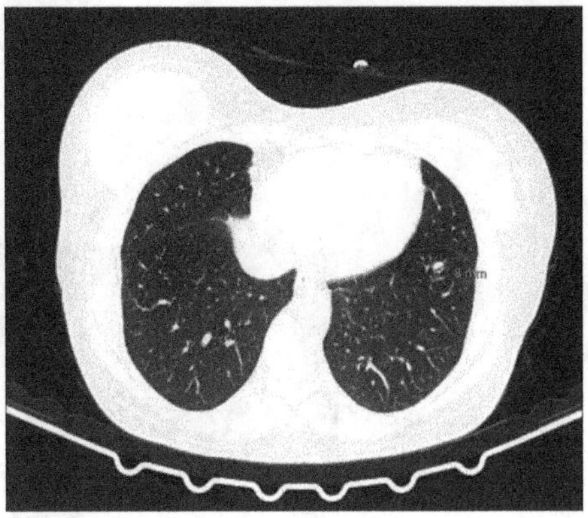

FIGURE 1: Transverse section of a thorax CT scan presenting an 8 mm pulmonary nodule.

2.2. Diagnostic Workup. The patient was asymptomatic, with a Karnofsky performance status (KPS) score of 100. No positive findings were encountered in the anamnesis on physical examination and/or other follow-up exams. PET/CT showed abnormal 18F-FDG uptake in the referred suspected pulmonary nodules, without other hypermetabolic changes that may suggest malignant involvement (Figure 2).

Given the impossibility of performing needle biopsy, the patient was proposed and accepted for surgery. Three pulmonary nodules, located in the left lung (basal, cisural, and upper lobe), were excised. Microscopic examination was performed to all nodules. Cisural and upper lobe nodules corresponded to ccRCC metastasis without additional findings. Microscopic examination (Figures 3 and 4) and immunohistochemical study (Figure 5) of the basal nodule biopsy specimen revealed two distinct neoplasms. The following immunophenotype was observed: CD10+, vimentin+ (heterogenous), MelanA-, inhibin-, CK7-, and ER-, and inside this, another distinct phenotype was observed: CD10-, vimentin-, MelanA-, inhibin-, CK7+ (few cells), ER+, PgR-, GCDFP15-, Cam5.2+, EMA+ (few cells), and CD56-. Therefore, the presented results raised the hypothesis of being a breast cancer metastasis in a lung metastasis of ccRCC.

2.3. Medical Management and Treatment. Concerning the breast cancer, breast MDT proposed the patient, in November 2020, for adjuvant radiotherapy plus hormone therapy with anastrozole and dual anti-HER2 therapy with trastuzumab/pertuzumab (the anatomopathological confirmation of the breast cancer metastasis in the lung metastasis of the ccRCC occurred later in December). As for the ccRCC, urologic MDT proposed the patient, in January 2021, to pazopanib. An overview of patient clinical history and management is given in Figure 6.

3. Discussion

Metastasis from one neoplasm (the donor) to another neoplasm (the recipient) has been described in the literature for many years since Fried published the first documented case of bronchogenic carcinoma metastatic to a meningioma in 1930 [4, 5]. In 1968, Campbell and coworkers proposed the following basic criteria for the diagnosis of TTM: (i) diagnosis of more than one primary tumor; (ii) extravascular metastasis existence; (iii) confirmation that it has not resulted from direct contiguous spread nor from tumor cell embolization; and (iv) in the presence of generalized lymphatic or hematological malignancy, exclusion of those tumors that metastasized to the lymphatic system [1]. During the decades that followed, some authors reported TTM phenomenon, with the donor neoplasm arising from a variety of sites, including the breast. Although the lung is one of the rarest recipients of TTM [3], renal neoplasms, and particularly ccRCC, are the most common tumor metastasis recipient. Additionally, there have been few cases previously reported of metastatic breast cancer within ccRCC (Table 1).

We reported an extremely rare case of breast cancer metastasis in a lung metastasis of ccRCC that met all Campbell and coworkers' TTM criteria.

Although the exact mechanism by which TTM occurs is yet to be understood, two major theories have been described to explain this phenomenon [12–15]. The first one, the

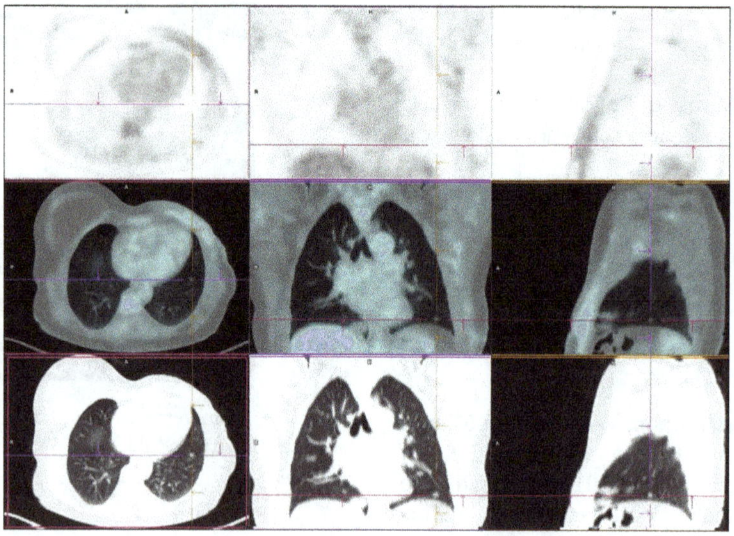

Figure 2: PET/CT images showing an increased metabolic activity in the pulmonary suspected lesion.

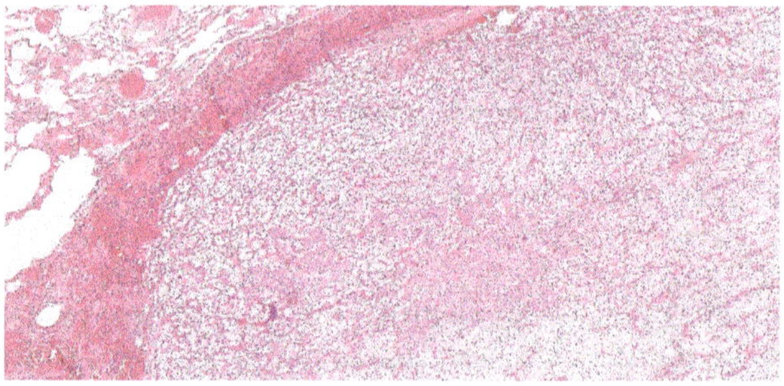

Figure 3: Microscopic examination of the basal nodule biopsy specimen (H&E, 40x). Pulmonary parenchyma (upper left corner) with involvement of epithelial cells with the clear cytoplasm and well-defined cell membrane, interspersed within a highly vascularized stroma, compatible with ccRCC. Inside this, a distinct population cells, arranged in nests, with a more eosinophilic cytoplasm is identified, corresponding to the breast carcinoma.

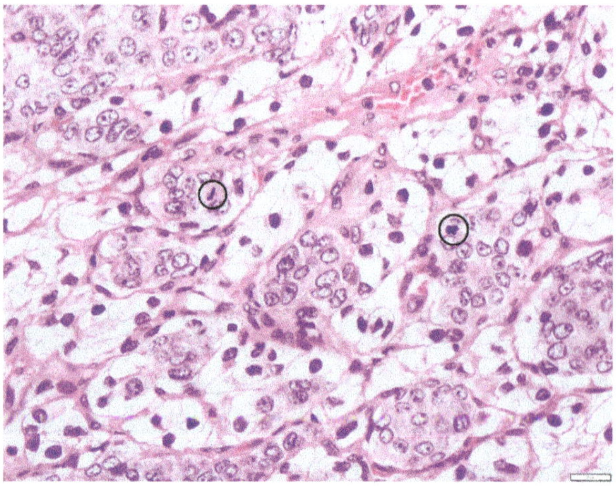

Figure 4: Microscopic examination of the basal nodule biopsy specimen with a high-power field showing the two neoplastic components (H&E, 400x). Note the two mitotic figures on the breast cancer component.

metabolic theory, argues that metastatic tumor cells would preferentially grow in microenvironments with abundant micronutrients, while the second one, the mechanical/anatomic theory, proposes that tumor metastasis is mainly determined by hemodynamic factors of the vascular and lymphatic system, as these factors are most important for successful delivery of metastatic tumor cells. The ccRCC is highly vascularized due to the inactivation of the von Hippel Lindau tumor suppressor gene, which increases hypoxia-inducible factor, leading to increased vascular endothelial growth factor [16]. This, in addition to the fact that kidneys receive approximately 20% of the cardiac output, makes ccRCC a hemodynamically favorable recipient, from a mechanistic perspective [17]. Moreover, and from a metabolic standpoint, ccRCC has increased glycogen and lipid content, which may account for its favorable microenvironment [18]. With this in mind, it is easy to understand why renal cell carcinoma, and in particular ccRCC, is such a frequent recipient of TTM.

Awareness of the TTM phenomenon is important to avoid an incorrect diagnosis and to select the appropriate treatment when unusual malignancies are encountered. In this case, due to their distinct biological behavior, there is not a single effective treatment for both HER2+ breast and ccRC metastatic cancers. Therefore, and since this patient has a good KPS score, both neoplasms were addressed separately. The change of the breast cancer stage led to the alteration of the anti-HER2 treatment strategy, with the initiation of dual blockade, as indicated by Cleopatra trial results for HER2+ metastatic disease [19]. Concerning the ccRCC treatment, our patient was in the International Metastatic Renal Cell Carcinoma Database Consortium (IMRCCDC) favorable risk group. The results of Keynote 426 and of CheckMate 9ER trials support the use of pembrolizumab plus axitinib or nivolumab plus cabozantinib, respectively, as the first-line treatment in metastatic disease for all IMRCCDC risk groups, being the preferred choices in the favorable risk group, but neither of them are reimbursed by the Portuguese

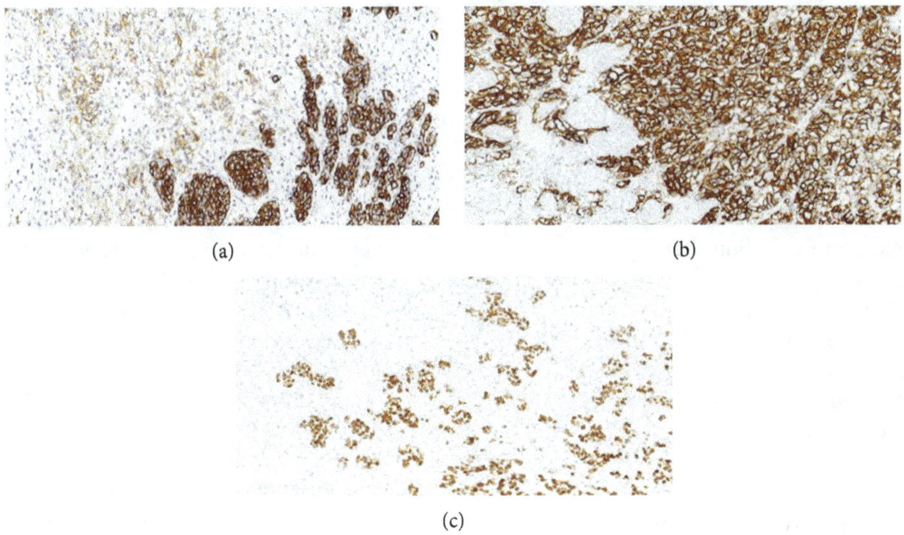

FIGURE 5: Immunohistochemical stains. (a) (Cam5.2, 200x) Both neoplasms are positive for cytokeratins, confirming an epithelial origin of the two neoplastic populations. (b) (CD10, 200x) Strong and diffuse positivity for CD10, characteristic of ccRCC. Highlight the antibody's negativity in the breast carcinoma cell population. (c) (ER, 200x) Strong and nuclear positivity for the antibody directed to ER in breast carcinoma cells. Highlight the antibody's negativity in the ccRCC component.

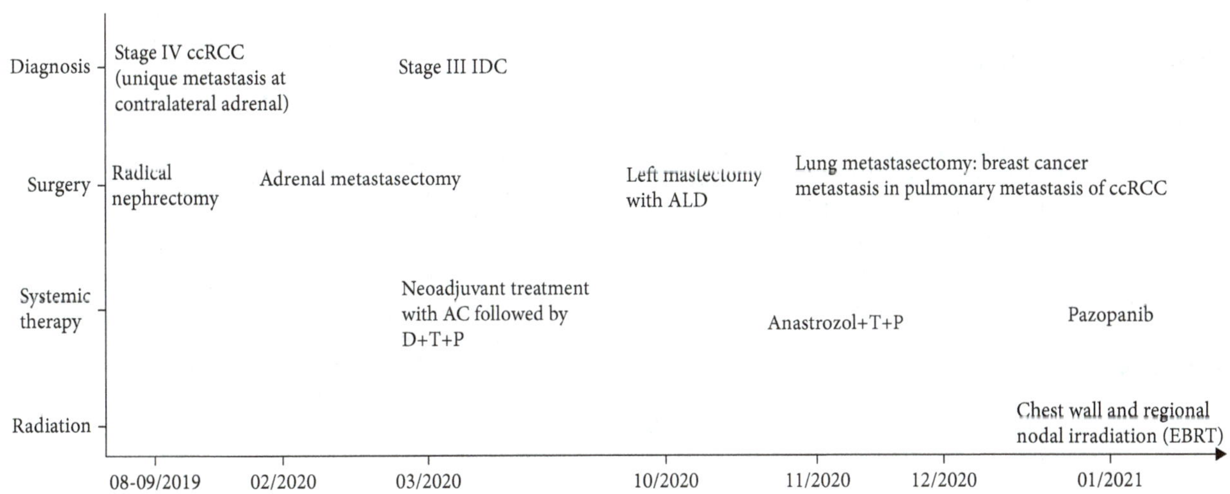

FIGURE 6: Overview of the patient clinical history and management.

TABLE 1: Clinical cases of breast carcinoma to renal cell carcinoma tumor-to-tumor metastasis described in the literature.

Gender	Age (years)	Donor histology	Receipt histology	Location	Reference
Female	79	Invasive ductal carcinoma	Clear cell renal cell carcinoma	Right kidney	[6]
Female	62	Invasive ductal carcinoma	Clear cell renal cell carcinoma	Right kidney	[7]
Female	71	Invasive ductal carcinoma	Clear cell renal cell carcinoma	Right kidney	[8]
Female	74	Invasive ductal carcinoma	Chromophobe renal cell carcinoma	Right kidney	[9]
Female	43	Invasive ductal carcinoma	Clear cell renal cell carcinoma	Left kidney	[10]
Female	57	Invasive lobular carcinoma	Clear cell renal cell carcinoma	Right kidney	[11]

Medicines and Heath Care Products Authority (INFARMED), which justify the option of pazopanib administration for this case therapeutic strategy (noninferior to sunitinib in the COMPARZ trial with better quality of life) [20–22].

We report this case for its rarity. To date, literature reported only six cases of metastasis of breast cancer in renal cell carcinomas. Nevertheless, and to the best of our knowledge, this is the first report of a metastasis inside a metastasis.

Abbreviations

AC:	Doxorubicin and cyclophosphamide
ALD:	Axillary lymph node dissection
ccRCC:	Clear cell type renal cell carcinoma
CHT:	Chemotherapy
CT:	Computed tomography
D:	Docetaxel
EBRT:	External beam radiation therapy
ER:	Estrogen receptor
18F-FDG:	18-F-Fluoro-2-deoxyglucose
FISH:	Fluorescence in situ hybridization
H&E:	Hematoxylin and eosin
HER2:	Human epidermal growth factor receptor 2
IDC:	Invasive ductal carcinoma
IMRCCDC:	International Metastatic Renal Cell Carcinoma Database Consortium
KPS:	Karnofsky performance status
MDT:	Multidisciplinary team
P:	Pertuzumab
PET/CT:	Positron emission computed tomography
PgR:	Progesterone receptor
T:	Trastuzumab
TTM:	Tumor-to-tumor metastasis.

Authors' Contributions

H.P. was responsible for the case management. H.P., A.L., I.P., and S.S. contributed to the case review. D.M. and A.R. conducted the pathological review. A.L. and I.P. were the principal writers of the manuscript. A.L., I.P., S.S., and H.P. edited and provided valuable insight into the preparation of the paper. All authors approved the final paper. Áurea Lima and Isa Peixoto contributed equally to this work.

References

[1] L. V. Campbell Jr., E. Gilbert, C. R. Chamberlain Jr., and A. L. Watne, "Metastases of cancer to cancer," *Cancer*, vol. 22, no. 3, pp. 635–643, 1968.

[2] K. Honma, K. Hara, and T. Sawai, "Tumour-to-tumour metastasis. A report of two unusual autopsy cases," *Virchows Archiv A Pathological Anatomy and Histopathology*, vol. 416, no. 2, pp. 153–157, 1989.

[3] F. Piacentini, G. Rossi, C. Casali, A. Cadioli, E. Barbieri, and V. Guarneri, "Primary pulmonary cancer colliding with metastatic breast carcinoma: hitherto unreported cases of cancer-to-cancer metastasis focusing on clinical implications," *Lung Cancer*, vol. 74, no. 1, pp. 145–148, 2011.

[4] B. M. Fried, "Metastatic inoculation of a meningioma by cancer cells from a bronchiogenic carcinoma," *The American journal of pathology*, vol. 6, 1930.

[5] C. Petraki, ,M. Vaslamatzis, T. Argyrakos et al., "Tumor to tumor metastasis: report of two cases and review of the literature," *International Journal of Surgical Pathology*, vol. 11, no. 2, pp. 127–135, 2003.

[6] I. C. Lakovschek, ,E. Petru, M. J. Pollheimer, M. Ratschek, H. Augustin, and V. Bjelic-Radisic, "A rare case of cancer-to-cancer metastasis: breast cancer to renal cell cancer : case report and review of literature," *Wiener Medizinische Wochenschrift (1946)*, vol. 169, no. 13-14, pp. 350–353, 2019.

[7] M. G. Moller, T. Gribbin, S. Ebrom, G. Padula, and T. L. Fitzgerald, "Breast cancer metastatic to renal cell carcinoma," *Surgery*, vol. 139, no. 4, pp. 577–579, 2006.

[8] M. Urdiales-Viedma, R. J. Luque, F. Valle, and S. Martos-Padilla, "Clear cell renal cell carcinoma metastasized by a breast ductal carcinoma," *Archivos Españoles de Urología*, vol. 69, no. 4, pp. 197–201, 2016.

[9] W. Toro-Zambrano, Á. Gómez-Durán, A. F. Conde-Martin, C. Mayoral-Guisado, A. Ruiz-Guerrero, and A. Rubio-Fernández, "From tumour to tumour: metastasis of invasive ductal breast carcinoma to chromophobe renal cell carcinoma," *Revista Española de Patología*, vol. 50, no. 1, pp. 58–63, 2017.

[10] Z. Huo, Y. Gao, Z. Yu, W. Zuo, and Y. Zhang, "Metastasis of breast cancer to renal cancer: report of a rare case," *International Journal of Clinical and Experimental Pathology*, vol. 8, no. 11, pp. 15417–15421, 2015.

[11] D. Ashman, G. Quiroga-Garza, and D. Lee, "Rare presentation of metastatic lobular breast carcinoma involving clear cell renal cell carcinoma," *Case Reports in Oncological Medicine*, vol. 2020, Article ID 5315178, 5 pages, 2020.

[12] S. Paget, "The distribution of secondary growths in cancer of the breast. 1889," *Cancer Metastasis Reviews*, vol. 8, no. 2, pp. 98–101, 1989.

[13] H. Peinado, H. Zhang, I. R. Matei et al., "Pre-metastatic niches: organ-specific homes for metastases," *Nature Reviews. Cancer*, vol. 17, no. 5, pp. 302–317, 2017.

[14] I. J. Fidler and G. Poste, "The "seed and soil" hypothesis revisited," *The Lancet Oncology*, vol. 9, no. 8, p. 808, 2008.

[15] N. Diseases, "A treatise on tumours. By James Ewing, A.M., M.D., Sc.D., Professor of Pathology at Cornell University Medical College, N.Y.; Pathologist to the Memorial Hospital. Third edition. Royal 8vo. Pp. 1127, with 546 illustrations. 1928. Philadelphia and London: W. B. Saunders Co. Ltd. 63s. net," *British Journal of Surgery*, vol. 16, 2005.

[16] X. Na, G. Wu, C. K. Ryan, S. R. Schoen, P. A. di'santagnese, and E. M. Messing, "Overproduction of vascular endothelial growth factor related to von Hippel-Lindau tumor suppressor gene mutations and hypoxia-inducible factor-1α expression in renal cell carcinomas," *The Journal of Urology*, vol. 170, no. 2, pp. 588–592, 2003.

[17] D. P. Kaufman, H. Basit, and S. J. Knohl, *Physiology, Glomerular Filtration Rate*, StatPearls Publishing, Treasure Island, FL, USA, 2020.

[18] J. H. Pinthus, K. F. Whelan, D. Gallino, J. P. Lu, and N. Rothschild, "Metabolic features of clear-cell renal cell carcinoma: mechanisms and clinical implications," *Canadian Urological Association Journal*, vol. 5, no. 4, pp. 274–282, 2011.

[19] S. M. Swain, J. Baselga, S. B. Kim et al., "Pertuzumab, trastuzumab, and docetaxel in HER2-positive metastatic breast cancer," *The New England Journal of Medicine*, vol. 372, no. 8, pp. 724–734, 2015.

[20] B. I. Rini, E. R. Plimack, V. Stus et al., "Pembrolizumab plus axitinib versus sunitinib for advanced renal-cell carcinoma," *The New England Journal of Medicine*, vol. 380, no. 12, pp. 1116–1127, 2019.

[21] T. K. Choueiri, T. Powles, M. Burotto et al., "Nivolumab plus cabozantinib versus sunitinib for advanced renal-cell carcinoma," *The New England Journal of Medicine*, vol. 384, no. 9, pp. 829–841, 2021.

[22] R. J. Motzer, T. E. Hutson, D. Cella et al., "Pazopanib versus sunitinib in metastatic renal-cell carcinoma," *The New England Journal of Medicine*, vol. 369, no. 8, pp. 722–731, 2013.

25

Bellini Duct Carcinoma Misdiagnosed with Urothelial Papillary Carcinoma

Joey El Khoury,[1,2] Maher Abdessater,[1,2] Rami Halabi,[1,2] Fadi Nasr,[1,3] Johnny Boustany,[1,2] Anthony Kanbar,[1,2] Charbel El Hachem,[1,2] and Raghid El Khoury[1,2]

[1]*Faculty of Medicine and Medical Sciences, Holy Spirit University of Kaslik (USEK), Jounieh, Lebanon*
[2]*Department of Urology, University Hospital Center-Notre Dame des Secours, Byblos, Lebanon*
[3]*Department of Oncology, University Hospital Center-Notre Dame des Secours, Byblos, Lebanon*

Correspondence should be addressed to Maher Abdessater; maher.abdessater@gmail.com

Academic Editor: Raffaele Palmirotta

Background. Collecting (Bellini) duct carcinoma (CDC) or Bellini duct carcinoma (BDC) is a rare subtype of kidney tumors, accounting for less than 3% and known to have the worst prognosis. It is known to have multiple clinical presentations; this is why it can be easily misdiagnosed. The aim of this article is to present a case of CDC that was initially misdiagnosed with urothelial papillary carcinoma (UPC) in a 41-year-old male. *Case Presentation.* Our patient presented with a left flank pain evolving for one month and one episode of gross macroscopic hematuria. Upon presentation, he had left costovertebral angle tenderness. Initial lab tests were normal. Computed tomography revealed a 5 cm solid mass of the left renal pelvis and multiple infracentimetric perihilar lymph nodes. Subsequently, the patient had left nephroureterectomy. Microscopic examination showed the presence of a high-grade urothelial papillary carcinoma of the renal pelvis' lumen. All four of the dissected lymph nodes showed disease metastasis. Three years after establishing the diagnosis, the patient presented again for chronic abdominal pain, with a recent history of weight loss. CT scan showed a left paraaortic mass infiltrating the left psoas muscle over a length of 12 cm. Immunohistochemical profiling of this mass confirmed the diagnosis of Bellini duct carcinoma, rejecting the initial diagnosis of UPC. Therefore, the patient required a cisplatin-gemcitabine-based chemotherapy regimen. *Conclusion.* BDC remains one of the rare aggressive subtypes of RCC, having a multitude of initial clinical presentations and an unfavorable prognosis. In this patient, CDC was masquerading as a transitional cell carcinoma that should always be kept in mind as a possible presentation. Corresponding early imaging and histopathology exams are primordial for a correct diagnosis and thus a better prognosis.

1. Introduction

Collecting duct carcinoma (CDC) is a rare subtype of kidney tumors, accounting for less than 3% and known to have the worst prognosis with its tendency to early metastasis [1]. CDC is also called Bellini duct carcinoma (BDC) because it concerns the distal medullar segment of the collecting duct of Bellini [2]. Commonly, the disease is diagnosed between ages 40 and 71, with a 2 : 1 male to female ratio [1]. African descents are more touched than Caucasians. Unfortunately, given the large spectrum of initial presentation signs and symptoms that mimics other types of renal carcinomas, CDC can be easily misdiagnosed [3]. We hereby report the case of a middle-aged man with misdiagnosed CDC, in order to emphasize the importance of an early and correct diagnosis of this rare disease.

2. Case Presentation

A 41-year-old male, heavy smoker, known to have recurrent urinary stones, presented with left flank pain and one episode of gross hematuria. Upon presentation, he was afebrile and chills were not reported.

Physical examination revealed a soft nontender abdomen with left costovertebral angle tenderness and no palpable lymph nodes.

Blood tests including chemistry (complete blood count, electrolytes, blood urea nitrogen, creatinine blood level, and hepatic enzymes) were normal but urinalysis showed 23 White Blood Cells (WBC) and 38 Red Blood Cells (RBC) per high-power microscopic field in urinary sediment.

Suspicious urinary cytology warranted further investigations. Therefore, computed tomography (CT) urography scan revealed the presence of a 5 cm left renal pelvis mass and multiple infracentimetric perihilar lymph nodes (Figure 1). Subsequently, laparoscopic left nephroureterectomy with perihilar lymph node dissection was performed a few days later.

Gross examination revealed a 3×2.5 cm vegetative tumor of the renal pelvis that infiltrates the adjacent renal parenchyma and the perihilar fat (Figure 2). Microscopic examination showed a high-grade transitional papillary carcinoma of the renal pelvic lumen infiltrating the muscular layer of the renal pelvis, the adjacent renal parenchyma, and the perihilar fat with the presence of multiple tumoral emboli in the adjacent venous structures. The presence of urothelial carcinoma in situ (CIS) was also noted in the mucosa. Four of the six dissected lymph nodes showed disease metastasis.

The patient had adjuvant chemotherapy based on cisplatin-gemcitabine and was on a surveillance protocol (CT and urinary cytology) for two years with no signs of relapse.

After that, he was lost of view for one year and returned back again for periumbilical abdominal pain and a recent history of weight loss. Physical examination and laboratory tests were unremarkable. CT scan showed a left paraaortic mass infiltrating the left psoas muscle over a length of 12 cm (Figure 3). Biopsy of this mass revealed carcinomatous proliferation formed by polygonal cells with eosinophilic and dense cytoplasm containing irregular hyperchromatic nucleus with multiple nucleoli. Occasional clear cells were also seen (Figure 4). These findings required further investigations to confirm the origin of the disease. This is why immunohistochemical profiling was done and showed diffuse and strong positivity of tumoral cells for anti-CK7 and anti-HMWCK while having negative results with CD10 and CD117 stains. Based on these findings, the diagnosis of BDC was maintained, rejecting the initial diagnosis of TCC. The patient was subsequently restarted on a cisplatin-gemcitabine-based chemotherapy regimen.

3. Discussion

Collecting duct carcinoma (CDC) was first described in 1976 by Mancilla-Jimenez et al. [4] as atypical hyperplastic changes of the epithelium adjacent to the collecting ducts. Fleming and Lewi established diagnostic criteria for this special subtype of renal cell carcinoma (RCC) [3] until it was recognized by the World Health Organization (WHO) in 1998 as a new entity [1].

Till 2013, almost 200 cases have been reported in the literature [5] with less than 5 cases reported later [1, 5]. An increased prevalence of BDC was reported in patients with renal failure and nephrolithiasis and on hemodialysis [6], aligning well with our patient's history of recurrent urinary stones.

Symptoms at presentation may resemble RCC in 70% of the cases (gross hematuria, weakness, flank mass or pain, and weight loss). This fact should always be kept in mind since it contributed to our initial misdiagnosis; our patient mostly presented nonspecific symptoms. The rest may be atypical (acute renal failure, metastatic lesions to bones or meninges, and lymphadenopathy) [5–7]. Common metastasis sites include the lungs, bones (as osteoblastic lesions), liver, and adrenal glands [3, 6]. Metastasis or paraneoplastic symptoms are present in 40% of cases at presentation [1]. One asymptomatic case, diagnosed incidentally as a heterogeneous abdominal mass on ultrasonography (US), was described by Kierstan et al. [6].

Laboratory studies are usually normal, though microscopic hematuria and mild anemia were reported in some cases [2, 5, 6]. Alpha-fetoprotein (AFP), cancer embryonal antigen (CEA), and urine cytology might be positive [6] and, in some cases, such as ours, an important clue for a definite diagnosis.

Imaging findings are nonspecific. Computed tomography commonly shows heterogeneous enhancement of a medullary mass with cystic components, poorly defined contour, and extension to the renal pelvis. Infradiaphragmatic thrombus of the inferior vena cava and multiple regional lymphadenopathies were described as signs of locally advanced disease [5]. In addition to the collecting duct mass, our patient showed multiple infracentimetric perihilar lymph nodes, hence considered a locally advanced disease. Heterogeneous masses, irregular borders, variable echoes, and blood flow signals were described on ultrasonography [2, 6]. MRI reveals an isointense image on T1, iso- or hypointense image on T2, and lower enhancement compared to the normal cortex and medulla [4].

The diagnosis is made on pathology, but it can be difficult since it has many common features with other tumors like urothelial papillary carcinoma (our case). However, the latter can be differentiated from CDC by its positive expression of p63, GATA3, and Uroplakin II, while negative for PAX8 [8]. Macroscopically, the tumor looks like a grey to white mass with cyst-like formations resulting from distention of collecting tubules. Invasion of the renal sinus or the cortex, thrombus of the vena cava, enlarged lymph nodes, arterial embolization, and perirenal tissue necrosis are described. Microscopically, the BDC, as seen also in our case, is described as round to polygonal cells with typical knob-like widened portions (cobblestones), acidophilic cytoplasm, and rarely hyperchromatic nuclei arranged in a tubular glandular pattern with multiple atypical mitoses, anaplastic giant cells, chronic interstitial nephritis, areas of hemorrhage, and necrosis [7]. Synchronous carcinoma in situ or dysplastic lesions are typically seen in the adjacent tubules.

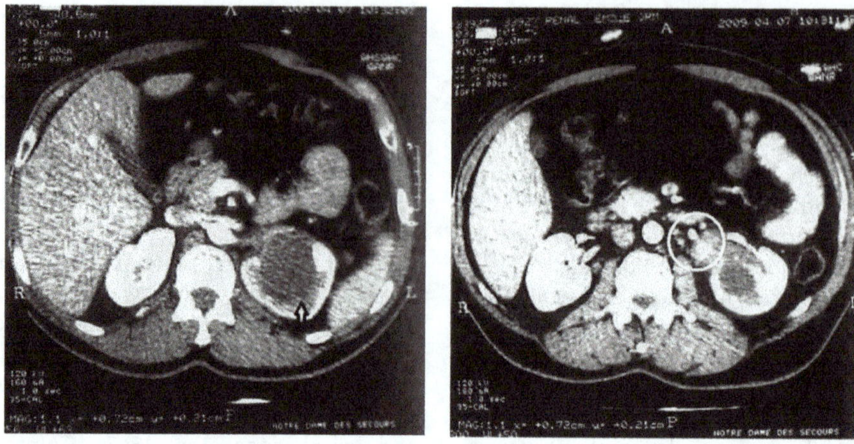

(a) (b)

FIGURE 1: CT scan of the patient showing a 5 cm solid mass of the left renal pelvis (a, arrow) and multiple infracentimetric perihilar lymph nodes (b, circle).

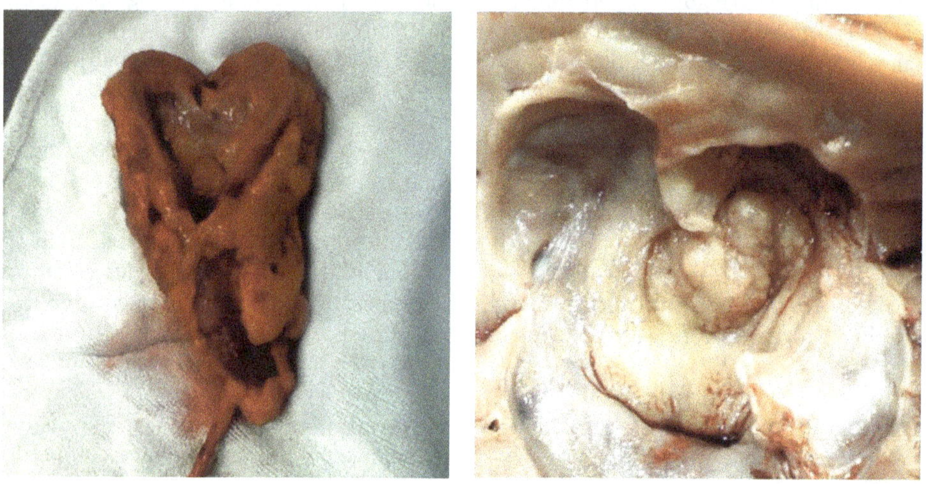

(a) (b)

FIGURE 2: Gross appearance of the left kidney and ureter showing the infiltration of the perihilar fat (a) by a vegetative tumor of the renal pelvis measuring 3×2.5 cm and invading the adjacent renal parenchyma (b).

Immunohistological studies are positive for cytokeratin cocktail, high-molecular weight cytokeratin, pancytokeratin (AE1/AE3) [5, 6], EMA, and Vimentin [2] but negative for CD117 [5]. CD10 and CK7 status is variable [2, 5, 6]. This immunohistological profiling was the tool we used to determine the origin of our paraaortic mass, beyond any reasonable doubt.

Genetically, the disease is associated with deletion of chromosome 1q or loss of chromosomes 1, 6, 8, 11, 18, and 21 without sufficient data on the molecular mechanisms [6].

Detecting the disease at an early stage is the only favorable prognostic factor [2]. In fact, survival in operated patients with low-grade BDC was 5 times more than in those with high-grade disease [2]. The median overall survival is 7.6 months [3], and more than half of the patients die within 2 years form diagnosis [1, 7] due to the dissemination of the disease [7]. Independent factors associated to disease-specific mortality are the following: American Society of Anesthesiologists (ASA) score 3 and 4, tumor size > 7 cm, stage M1, Fuhrman grade 3 and 4 (despite Vancouver conference's suggestion of not assigning a CDC grade, Ciszewski et al. graded patients based on the Fuhrman scale since they examined them before publication of conference recommendations), and lymphovascular invasion [3].

No definitive treatment is established so far [1]. The treatment of choice is radical nephrectomy due to the central location of the disease and the tendency to invade the collecting system [1]. Surgical treatment offers the longest survival if performed when the disease is still localized in the kidney [3]. It was also associated to adjuvant chemotherapy; knowing that both the collecting duct and the urothelial cells originate from divisions of the mesonephric (Wolff) duct, and based on morphologic, antigenic, and cytogenetic similarities between CDC and urothelial carcinoma (UC), the use of similar chemotherapy regimens has been practiced with promising results for future treatment

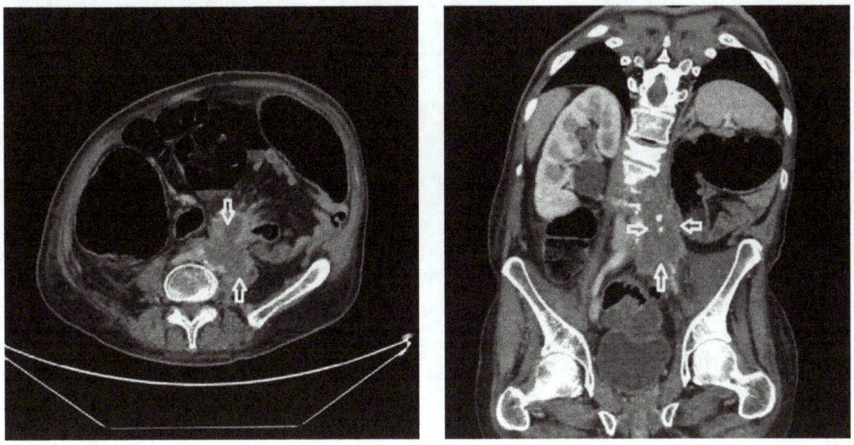

(a) (b)

FIGURE 3: Abdominal CT scan showing a left lateroaortic mass (a) spanning over 12 cm and infiltrating the left psoas and iliac muscles, as well as the left iliac vessels (b).

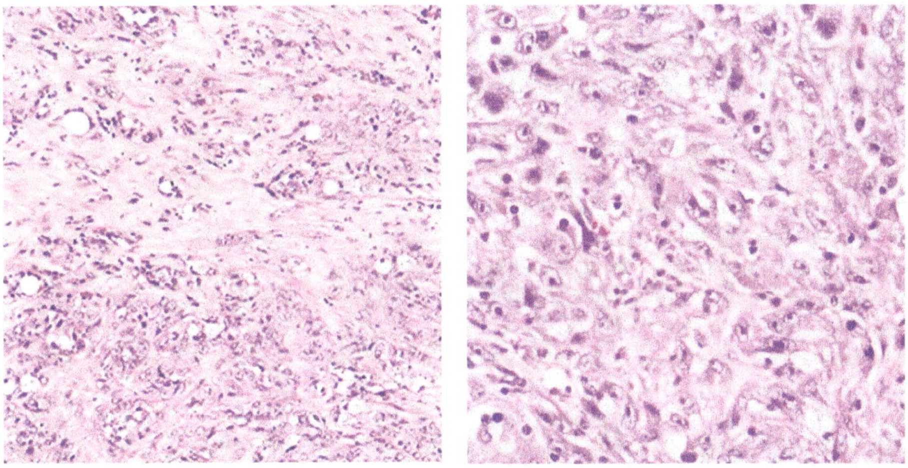

(a) (b)

FIGURE 4: Microscopic appearance of the tumor showing (a) complex, infiltrative, and poorly circumscribed cells with some cords and tubules (×10) and (b) carcinomatous proliferation formed by polygonal cells with eosinophilic and dense cytoplasm and an irregular hyperchromatic nucleus with multiple nucleoli and occasional presence of clear cells (×40).

consideration [9]. Identical to our case, Orsola et al. suggested an association between urothelial carcinoma and CDC and they presented cases where one tumor preceded the other [9]. Our case was considered a diagnostic error more than an evolution of the initial tumor because the previous pathology was not reviewed again. However, the fact that these tumors have the same embryologic origin can highlight the hypothesis that transitional urothelial carcinoma could eventually develop a second type of tumor such as the CDC.

Adjuvant chemotherapy using gemcitabine+cisplatin/-carboplatin made 26% remission rate [1], which was also our informed and optimal treatment of choice, following the radical nephrectomy. Treatment with tyrosine kinase inhibitors (sorafenib, sunitinib, or temsirolimus) is promising in metastatic disease but needs more investigations [5]. Percutaneous biopsy in metastatic disease might be beneficial to guide the management of the advanced disease [3]. Radiotherapy has no place in BDC [6].

Mishra et al. in 2016 treated a locally advanced disease with adjuvant chemotherapy with no disease relapse at 10 months [5]. Li et al. reported the case of a patient with T1aN0M0 disease who rejected chemotherapy when informed of possible side effects but remained disease-free 4 years after surgery [2].

4. Conclusion

BDC remains one of the rare aggressive subtypes of RCC, having a multitude of initial clinical presentations and an unfavorable prognosis. In this patient, CDC was masquerading as a transitional cell carcinoma that should always be kept in mind as a possible presentation. Corresponding early imaging and histopathology exams are primordial for a correct diagnosis and thus a better prognosis.

Consent

Informed consent was obtained from the patient to publish this article.

Acknowledgments

All funding for the publication of this article was funded by the authors' supporting institution.

References

[1] A. A. Salako, T. A. Badmus, I. Ikem et al., "Bellini duct carcinoma of the kidney masquerading as an iliac bone tumour in an adult nigerian," *Pan African Medical Journal*, vol. 27, pp. 1–6, 2017.

[2] Y. Li, L. Jin, J. Liu et al., "Bellini's duct carcinoma: a report of two cases and a review of the literature," *Oncology Letters*, vol. 11, no. 6, pp. 3839–3841, 2016.

[3] S. Ciszewski, A. Jakimów, and B. Smolska-Ciszewska, "Collecting (Bellini) duct carcinoma: a clinical study of a rare tumour and review of the literature," *Canadian Urological Association Journal*, vol. 9, no. 9-10, pp. E589–E593, 2015.

[4] R. Mancilla-Jimenez, R. J. Stanley, and R. A. Blath, "Papillary renal cell carcinoma: a clinical, radiologic, and pathologic study of 34 cases," *Cancer*, vol. 38, no. 6, pp. 2469–2480, 1976.

[5] A. K. Mishra, R. Manikandan, L. N. Dorairajan, J. K. Mittal, and J. S. Rekha, "Bellini duct carcinoma: a rare entity," *Journal of Clinical and Diagnostic Research*, vol. 10, no. 10, pp. 1-2, 2016.

[6] A. Kierstan, M. Sosnowski, R. Minias, and Z. Jabłonowski, "Rare renal tumors - Bellini duct carcinoma," *Central European Journal of Urology*, vol. 63, pp. 190–193, 2010.

[7] M. Sochaj, A. Kierstan, and M. Sosnowski, "C02 Bellini duct carcinoma of the kidney," *European Urology Supplements*, vol. 12, no. 4, article e1110, 2013.

[8] R. Albadine, L. Schultz, P. Illei et al., "PAX8 (+)/p 63 (-) immunostaining pattern in renal collecting duct carcinoma (CDC): a useful immunoprofile in the differential diagnosis of CDC versus urothelial carcinoma of upper urinary tract," *The American Journal of Surgical Pathology*, vol. 34, no. 7, pp. 965–969, 2010.

[9] A. Orsola, I. Trias, C. X. Raventós, I. Español, L. Cecchini, and I. Orsola, "Renal collecting (Bellini) duct carcinoma displays similar characteristics to upper tract urothelial cell carcinoma," *Urology*, vol. 65, no. 1, pp. 49–54, 2005.

26

PD-1 Inhibitor Therapy in a Patient with Preexisting P-ANCA Vasculitis: A Case Report and Review of the Literature

Amanda Ramos,[1] Marcela del Carmen,[2] and Oladapo Yeku[3]

[1]*Division of Gynecologic Oncology, Department of Obstetrics and Gynecology, Hartford Healthcare, Hartford, CT 06102, USA*
[2]*Division of Gynecologic Oncology, Vincent Obstetrics and Gynecology, Harvard Medical School, Boston, MA 02114, USA*
[3]*Gynecologic Cancers Program, Massachusetts General Hospital, Harvard Medical School, Boston, MA 02114, USA*

Correspondence should be addressed to Oladapo Yeku; oyeku@mgh.harvard.edu

Academic Editor: Ossama W. Tawfik

Background. Recurrent endometrial cancer after definitive therapy is a lethal disease. Recently, immune checkpoint inhibitors (ICI) have improved the management of mismatch repair-deficient (MSI-H) endometrial cancer. Autoimmune side effects are known to occur with ICI. As a result, patients with preexisting autoimmune diseases are excluded from studies involving these drugs. This has led to challenges in clinical practice regarding the use of ICI in otherwise eligible patients with underlying autoimmune disease. *Case Presentation.* We present the case of an 81-year-old woman with an underlying autoimmune vasculitis and recurrent, metastatic endometrial adenocarcinoma with microsatellite instability, who was treated with an immune checkpoint inhibitor. This patient received pembrolizumab, an immune checkpoint inhibitor that targets the programmed cell death-1 immune checkpoint. Ultimately, she was treated for 4 months with pembrolizumab and benefited from stable disease during this period. She remained asymptomatic from her underlying autoimmune P-ANCA vasculitis. A review of the scientific literature reveals several cases of the successful use of immune checkpoint inhibitors in patients with autoimmune diseases, including systemic lupus erythematosus, rheumatoid arthritis, and inflammatory bowel disease. *Conclusion.* This is one of the first reports of a patient with an underlying autoimmune vasculitis successfully treated with an immune checkpoint inhibitor without exacerbating her underlying autoimmune condition. Carefully selected patients with underlying autoimmune vasculitis can be safely treated with ICI.

1. Introduction

Recurrent endometrial cancer poses a treatment challenge for both patients and clinicians. Of the approximately 60,000 women who are diagnosed annually with endometrial cancer, about 15% will recur following first-line therapy, the vaginal apex being the most common location for recurrent disease [1, 2].

Immune checkpoint inhibitors (ICI) have revolutionized the treatment of numerous solid tumor malignancies, such as nonsmall cell lung cancer, melanoma, and renal cell carcinoma [3, 4]. Immune checkpoints such as programmed death receptor-1 (PD-1) are transmembrane proteins that are expressed on activated or exhausted cytotoxic T-cells and help prevent against autoimmunity under normal circumstances [5]. When tumor-infiltrating lymphocytes (TILs) recognize an antigen and become activated, PD-1 binds to its natural ligand, programmed death receptor-ligand 1 (PD-L1) expressed on tumor cells, leading to the suppression of cytotoxic T-cell activity. This pathway evolved as a counter-regulatory mechanism to limit inflammation and damage to healthy tissue. Unfortunately, this pathway is also co-opted by tumor cells to evade the immune system [5]. Therapeutic PD-1 blockade inhibits tumor-mediated T-cell suppression but also increases the risk of autoimmunity.

Anti-PD-1 therapy has been evaluated in several solid tumor malignancies. Le et al. [6] reported a 53% objective response rate in patients with mismatch repair-deficient (MSI-H/MMR) endometrial cancer [6]. This led to the FDA approval of pembrolizumab (Keytruda®), an anti-PD-1 ICI, in MSI-H/MMR solid tumors including endometrial cancer. Follow-up studies of pembrolizumab in mismatch repair intact or microsatellite stable (MSS) endometrial cancer reported a 13% objective response rate [7]. For comparison, single-agent cytotoxic chemotherapy has response rates ranging from 4% to 27% in the recurrent setting [8].

Patients with preexisting autoimmune disease have historically been excluded from clinical trials involving ICI. However, as real-world adoption of ICI increases, physicians face the decision of whether or not to use ICI in otherwise suitable patients with underlying autoimmune disease. Unfortunately, there is limited information regarding the safety and efficacy of ICI that can be used to guide treatment decisions in this patient population.

In this report, we present the case of a patient with underlying p-ANCA vasculitis and recurrent mismatch repair-deficient (MSI-H/MMR) endometrial adenocarcinoma treated with pembrolizumab without exacerbation of her underlying autoimmune disease.

2. Case Presentation

The patient is an 83-year-old woman with a history of major depressive disorder, psoriasis, hypertension, and coronary artery disease who presented to our institution in July of 2017 with postmenopausal bleeding. Pelvic ultrasonography performed on September 19, 2017, revealed a diffusely thickened endometrium. An endometrial biopsy revealed grade 1 of 3 endometrioid adenocarcinoma. As a result of these findings, the patient underwent a total laparoscopic hysterectomy, bilateral salpingo-oophorectomy, and lysis of adhesions on August 22, 2017. Intraoperative findings were notable for tumor protruding from the cervical os. On laparoscopic examination, there was no evidence of extrauterine disease. Given the patient's advanced age and extensive adhesive disease, lymph node dissection was omitted.

The final pathology from this procedure was reviewed, revealing a FIGO grade 2 of 3 endometrioid adenocarcinoma of the endometrium measuring 8.4 cm with 18.5 mm of invasion into a 19 mm thick myometrium. Other pathologic findings included lymphovascular space invasion, cervical stromal invasion, and parametrial involvement. Notably, necrotizing arteritis was identified in her adnexa bilaterally in a manner that was substantially more than expected in routine oophorectomy specimens. Immunohistochemistry revealed a loss of MLH1 and PMS2, with further analysis showing MLH1 promoter methylation, consistent with MSI-H/MMR.

One month following her surgery, she was evaluated by her rheumatologist for further workup of the necrotizing arteritis found in her adnexa. Serologic analysis revealed that she was positive for perinuclear antineutrophil cytoplasmic antibody (MPO-ANCA) consistent with p-ANCA vasculitis. Treatment was deferred as she had no other evidence of active vasculitis.

She received adjuvant external beam radiation therapy to the pelvis for a total of 4500 cGy, followed by high dose rate brachytherapy to a total of 700 cGy over three fractions. At the completion of her therapy in December of 2017, she was admitted to the hospital with C. difficile colitis and acute kidney injury with a creatinine of 3.17 mg/dL (reference range; 0.60-1.50 mg/dL). Her creatinine continued to rise despite fluid resuscitation for what was initially considered prerenal azotemia. A repeat CT scan was performed, and this revealed evidence of interstitial lung disease. In the context of her positive p-ANCA titers and history of adnexal vasculitis, the decision was made to treat her for systemic p-ANCA vasculitis. She received solumedrol, rituximab, cyclophosphamide, and plasmapheresis with rapid improvement of her creatinine to baseline prior to discharge. After induction treatment, her steroids were tapered off, and she continued to receive maintenance rituximab.

She was lost to follow-up for several months and returned in August of 2018 for evaluation of vaginal bleeding. Physical examination revealed the presence of a vaginal apex mass that was biopsy-proven to be recurrent endometrial adenocarcinoma. Given her MSI-H/MMR and her inability to tolerate platinum-based cytotoxic chemotherapy due to her poor performance status, the decision was made to start pembrolizumab 200 mg i.v. every three weeks. She underwent three cycles followed by restaging CT scans which showed stable disease (Figure 1(a)). Figure 1(c) displays the patient's creatinine levels (black circle, left *y*-axis) and ANCA (red square, right *y*-axis) plotted over time. Time on pembrolizumab is highlighted in blue. During this treatment period, her renal function was followed closely (Figure 1(c)), and urinalysis was obtained frequently to evaluate for hematuria. She did not develop any signs or symptoms suggestive of a vasculitis flare. Figure 1(b) displays the patient's CA-125 values over the same time period. Despite her stable CA-125 (Figure 1(b)) and radiographically stable disease (Figure 1(a)), the patient gradually became more socially withdrawn, depressed, and decreased her oral intake despite maximal support from her family and treatment by her psychiatrist. The decision was made to stop cancer-directed care and provide comfort measures only. The patient died on December 18, 2018, four months after starting pembrolizumab.

3. Discussion

In this report, we present the case of a patient with underlying p-ANCA vasculitis and recurrent MSI-H endometrial cancer successfully treated with anti-PD-1 immune checkpoint blockade. While this patient did have an underlying autoimmune disorder, the administration of pembrolizumab did not exacerbate her underlying autoimmune condition. Furthermore, she did not experience any immune-related adverse events, and she had stable disease as her best response to treatment. To our knowledge, this is the first report of a patient with underlying p-ANCA vasculitis, and recent treatment with plasmapheresis, prednisone, cyclophosphamide, and rituximab, who was safely treated with pembrolizumab.

Common immune-related adverse events associated with ICI include rash, hypophysitis, hepatitis, hypothyroidism, type-1 diabetes, arthritis, colitis, and pneumonitis [9]. Of these, pneumonitis is the most severe adverse effect seen with

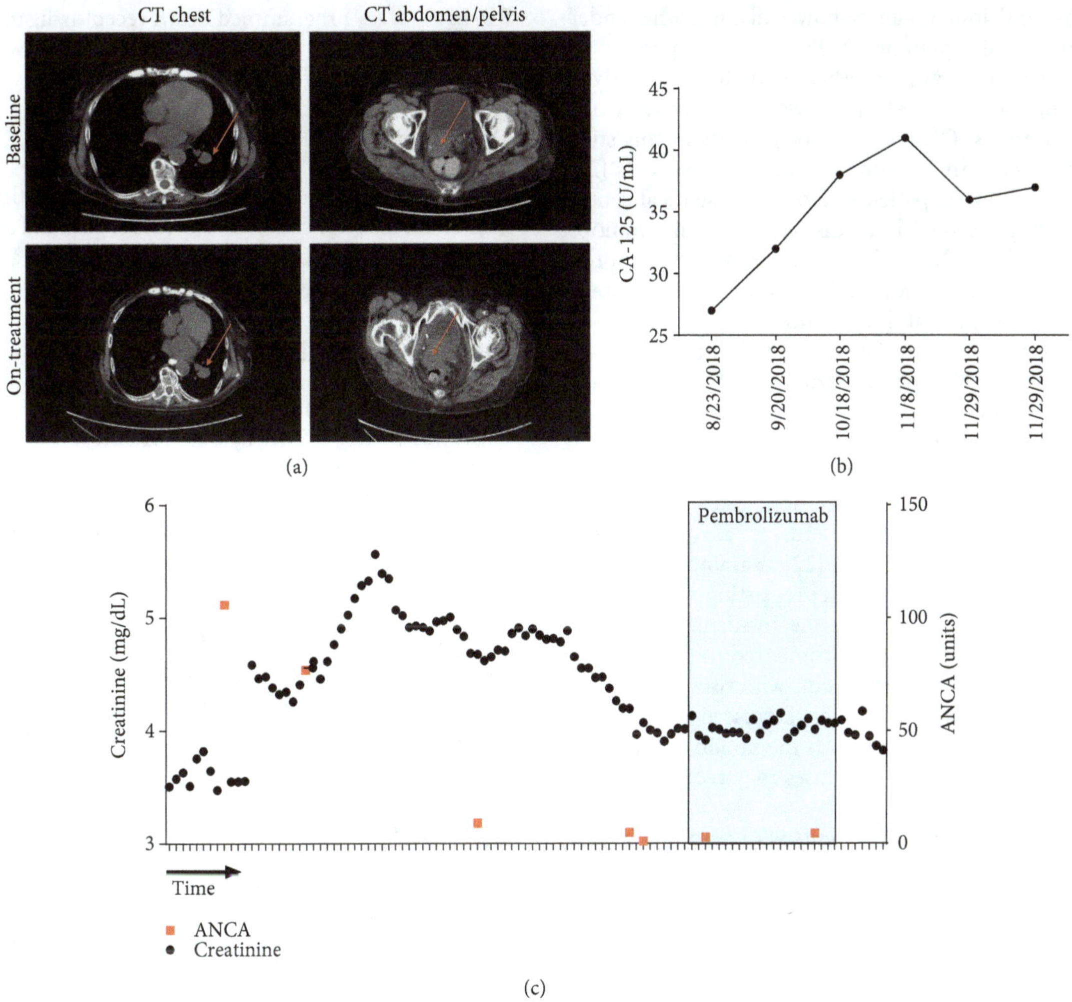

FIGURE 1: Pembrolizumab monotherapy in a patient with underlying p-ANCA vasculitis describes the stability of this patient's malignancy as well as the stability of her underlying autoimmune vasculitis while on pembrolizumab therapy. (a) displays computerized tomography (CT) images at baseline and on-treatment after 3 cycles of pembrolizumab. The size of the vaginal apex mass and lung nodules remained relatively unchanged. Repeat CT scan of the chest, abdomen, and pelvis revealed a pulmonary nodule (1.0 cm), an enlarged perihilar lymph node (1.4 cm), and a right-sided vaginal apex mass (2.8 cm) causing right-sided hydronephrosis (a). (b) CA-125 tumor marker levels are shown. (c) Serum creatinine level over time (black circles, left axis) and ANCA levels (red squares, right axis) are shown. Time on pembrolizumab is highlighted.

PD-1 inhibition [10]. Studies investigating the pathogenesis of immune-mediated toxicities have revealed the presence of T-cell and macrophage infiltration into affected tissues, as well as antibody-dependent complement deposition [11, 12]. There have been at least two documented cases of de novo vasculitis associated with ICI. Cases of giant cell arteritis and polymyalgia rheumatica were documented in 2 case reports after CTLA-4 inhibitor therapy with ipilimumab (Yervoy®) for advanced melanoma [13]. Cases of retinal and uterine vasculitis following ipilimumab and pembrolizumab have also been reported [12–15]. Often, these toxicities result in the discontinuation of therapy.

The antineutrophil cytoplasmic antibody-associated vasculidities are comprised of granulomatosis with polyangiitis, microscopic polyangiitis, and eosinophilic granulomatosis with polyangiitis. These vasculidities are characterized by the presence of autoantibodies directed at neutrophil cytoplasmic constituents such as proteinase-3 and myeloperoxidase [16, 17]. The patient presented in this case study was diagnosed with a myeloperoxidase antineutrophilic cytoplasmic antibody-associated vasculitis (MPO-ANCA), which is a small-vessel vasculitis [18]. PD-1 has been shown to be expressed on B-cells [19]; however, its function in shaping the immune tumor microenvironment has only recently been elucidated [19]. It is theoretically possible that PD-1 inhibition on B-cells could exacerbate an underlying antibody-mediated vasculitis. Patients with preexisting autoimmune conditions such as ANCA-associated vasculitis are excluded from most ICI clinical trials given the concern for increased activation of the immune system and increased risk of inducing or exacerbating autoimmune diseases [20].

Several small retrospective studies have reported exacerbation of underlying autoimmunity by ICI therapy. Johnson et al. [21] reported on 52 patients across 13 medical centers with preexisting autoimmune diseases including rheumatoid arthritis (RA), systemic lupus erythematosus (SLE), scleroderma, and inflammatory bowel disease, who underwent treatment with ipilimumab. Twenty-seven percent (13 patients) experienced an exacerbation of their underlying autoimmune disease. These flares were effectively treated with corticosteroids. Of note, 50% of patients in this study did not experience any immune-related adverse events [21]. In another review of 30 patients across nine medical centers with preexisting autoimmune disease including multiple sclerosis, sarcoidosis, RA, and SLE, treated with ICI, approximately 50% experienced a flare in their underlying disease symptoms [15]. Kehl et al. [20] identified 462 patients with preexisting autoimmune conditions treated with ipilimumab, nivolumab (Opdivo®), pembrolizumab, or atezolizumab (Tecentriq®). In this series, there was no association between immune checkpoint therapy and all-cause hospitalization. However, the authors concluded that patients with preexisting autoimmune disease were more likely to develop immune-related adverse events and, as a result, receive corticosteroids. Yoneshima et al. [22] examined the effects of PD-1 inhibitors on patients with preexisting ANA positive titers. There was no increase in the incidence of adverse events in this patient population compared to patients with negative ANA [22]. However, patients with rising ANA titers on therapy were found to have an increased incidence of grade 3-5 irAEs. This study supports the notion that patients with preexisting autoimmune diseases may receive ICI with close monitoring [22].

There are limited data in patients with preexisting autoimmune vasculitis. A case report by Maul et al. described a patient with preexisting Churg-Strauss disease treated with ICIs [23]. This patient was successfully treated with ipilimumab, followed by the initiation of pembrolizumab monotherapy after the development of colitis secondary to ipilimumab. Since the patient's initial diagnosis of Churg-Strauss, he had been treated with maintenance prednisolone, and this continued while on treatment with ipilimumab [23]. It is possible that, in this case, maintenance prednisolone may have prevented a flare of his underlying condition.

This case report adds to the literature regarding the safety of anti-PD-1 immune checkpoint inhibition in patients with underlying autoimmune disease. This patient with preexisting p-ANCA vasculitis was successfully treated with pembrolizumab (Keytruda®), an anti-PD-1 ICI, without exacerbation of her underlying vasculitis. Additionally, the patient experienced stable disease, an acceptable treatment outcome in elderly patients with incurable cancer, and comorbid medical conditions. Although caution should be taken when treating patients with stable underlying autoimmune disorders with ICIs, flares are not as common as fared, and patients who do develop flares can be readily treated with corticosteroids provided the symptoms are recognized early enough.

Abbreviations

CT: Computerized tomography
ICI: Immune checkpoint inhibitors
TILs: Tumor-infiltrating lymphocytes
PD-1: Programmed death receptor-1
PD-L1: Programmed death receptor-ligand 1
MSI-H/MMR: Mismatch repair-deficient
MSS: Microsatellite stable.

Consent

Written informed consent was obtained from the patient's next of kin for publication of this case report and any accompanying images. A copy of the written consent is available for review by the Editor-in-Chief of this journal.

Authors' Contributions

The collection of data was performed by AR, and the manuscript was written jointly by both AR and OY with the assistance of MD. The figures were created jointly by AR and OY. Informed consent was obtained from the patient's family by AR. All authors read and approved the final manuscript.

Acknowledgments

The authors of this report would like to thank the patient and her family for allowing our team to document her clinical history and sharing her story to help improve the treatment of women and men with preexisting autoimmune conditions and recurrent malignancies.

References

[1] C. L. Creutzberg, W. L. J. van Putten, P. C. M. Koper et al., "Surgery and postoperative radiotherapy versus surgery alone for patients with stage-1 endometrial carcinoma: multicentre randomised trial," *The Lancet*, vol. 355, no. 9213, pp. 1404–1411, 2000.

[2] S. J. Henley, J. W. Miller, N. F. Dowling, V. B. Benard, and L. C. Richardson, "Uterine cancer incidence and mortality — United States, 1999-2016," *MMWR. Morbidity and Mortality Weekly Report*, vol. 67, no. 48, pp. 1333–1338, 2018.

[3] L. Gandhi, D. Rodríguez-Abreu, S. Gadgeel et al., "Pembrolizumab plus chemotherapy in metastatic non-small-cell lung cancer," *The New England Journal of Medicine*, vol. 378, no. 22, pp. 2078–2092, 2018.

[4] M. A. Socinski, R. M. Jotte, F. Cappuzzo et al., "Atezolizumab for first-line treatment of metastatic nonsquamous NSCLC," *The New England Journal of Medicine*, vol. 378, no. 24, pp. 2288–2301, 2018.

[5] A. P. Cogdill, M. C. Andrews, and J. A. Wargo, "Hallmarks of response to immune checkpoint blockade," *British Journal of Cancer*, vol. 117, no. 1, pp. 1–7, 2017.

[6] D. T. Le, J. N. Durham, K. N. Smith et al., "Mismatch repair deficiency predicts response of solid tumors to PD-1 blockade," *Science*, vol. 357, no. 6349, pp. 409–413, 2017.

[7] P. A. Ott, Y. J. Bang, D. Berton-Rigaud et al., "Safety and antitumor activity of pembrolizumab in advanced programmed death ligand 1-positive endometrial cancer: results from the KEYNOTE-028 study," *Journal of Clinical Oncology*, vol. 35, no. 22, pp. 2535–2541, 2017.

[8] K. M. Moxley and D. S. McMeekin, "Endometrial carcinoma: a review of chemotherapy, drug resistance, and the search for new agents," *The Oncologist*, vol. 15, no. 10, pp. 1026–1033, 2010.

[9] I. Puzanov, on behalf of the Society for Immunotherapy of Cancer Toxicity Management Working Group, A. Diab et al., "Managing toxicities associated with immune checkpoint inhibitors: consensus recommendations from the Society for Immunotherapy of Cancer (SITC) Toxicity Management Working Group," *Journal for Immunotherapy of Cancer*, vol. 5, no. 1, p. 95, 2017.

[10] M. Khunger, S. Rakshit, V. Pasupuleti et al., "Incidence of pneumonitis with use of programmed death 1 and programmed death-ligand 1 inhibitors in non-small cell lung cancer: a systematic review and meta-analysis of trials," *Chest*, vol. 152, no. 2, pp. 271–281, 2017.

[11] R. S. Gonzalez, S. N. Salaria, C. D. Bohannon, A. R. Huber, M. M. Feely, and C. Shi, "PD-1 inhibitor gastroenterocolitis: case series and appraisal of 'immunomodulatory gastroenterocolitis'," *Histopathology*, vol. 70, no. 4, pp. 558–567, 2017.

[12] D. R. Minor, S. R. Bunker, and J. Doyle, "Lymphocytic vasculitis of the uterus in a patient with melanoma receiving ipilimumab," *Journal of Clinical Oncology*, vol. 31, no. 20, article e356, 2013.

[13] B. L. Goldstein, L. Gedmintas, and D. J. Todd, "Drug-associated polymyalgia rheumatica/giant cell arteritis occurring in two patients after treatment with ipilimumab, an antagonist of ctla-4," *Arthritis & Rhematology*, vol. 66, no. 3, pp. 768-769, 2014.

[14] J. S. Manusow, L. Khoja, N. Pesin, A. M. Joshua, and E. D. Mandelcorn, "Retinal vasculitis and ocular vitreous metastasis following complete response to PD-1 inhibition in a patient with metastatic cutaneous melanoma," *Journal for Immunotherapy of Cancer*, vol. 2, no. 1, p. 41, 2014.

[15] M. Tocut, R. Brenner, and G. Zandman-Goddard, "Autoimmune phenomena and disease in cancer patients treated with immune checkpoint inhibitors," *Autoimmunity Reviews*, vol. 17, no. 6, pp. 610–616, 2018.

[16] D. B. Johnson, R. J. Sullivan, P. A. Ott et al., "Ipilimumab therapy in patients with advanced melanoma and preexisting autoimmune disorders," *JAMA Oncology*, vol. 2, no. 2, pp. 234–240, 2016.

[17] C. G. Kallenberg, "Pathogenesis and treatment of ANCA-associated vasculitides," *Clinical and Experimental Rheumatology*, vol. 33, 4 Suppl 92, pp. S11–S14, 2015.

[18] E. Suresh, "Diagnostic approach to patients with suspected vasculitis," *Postgraduate Medical Journal*, vol. 82, no. 970, pp. 483–488, 2006.

[19] X. Xiao, X. M. Lao, M. M. Chen et al., "PD-1hi identifies a novel regulatory B-cell population in human hepatoma that promotes disease progression," *Cancer Discovery*, vol. 6, no. 5, pp. 546–559, 2016.

[20] K. L. Kehl, S. Yang, M. M. Awad, N. Palmer, I. S. Kohane, and D. Schrag, "Pre-existing autoimmune disease and the risk of immune-related adverse events among patients receiving checkpoint inhibitors for cancer," *Cancer Immunology, Immunotherapy*, vol. 68, no. 6, pp. 917–926, 2019.

[21] D. B. Johnson and D. Y. Wang, "Immune checkpoint inhibitor therapy in patients with autoimmune disease," *Oncology (Williston Park, N.Y.)*, vol. 32, no. 4, pp. 190–194, 2018.

[22] Y. Yoneshima, K. Tanaka, Y. Shiraishi et al., "Safety and efficacy of PD-1 inhibitors in non-small cell lung cancer patients positive for antinuclear antibodies," *Lung Cancer*, vol. 130, pp. 5–9, 2019.

[23] L. V. Maul, M. Weichenthal, K. C. Kahler, and A. Hauschild, "Successful anti-PD-1 antibody treatment in a metastatic melanoma patient with known severe autoimmune disease," *Journal of Immunotherapy*, vol. 39, no. 4, pp. 188–190, 2016.

27

Primary Leiomyosarcoma of the Gallbladder

Anwar Chammout,[1] Mike Ghabally,[2] Christina Masri,[2] Nour Tantak,[2] Fadi Ward,[2] and Ghefar Omar[3]

[1]*Department of Oncology, University of Aleppo, Faculty of Medicine, Aleppo, Syria*
[2]*University of Aleppo, Faculty of Medicine, Aleppo, Syria*
[3]*Department of Pathology, University of Aleppo, Faculty of Medicine, Aleppo, Syria*

Correspondence should be addressed to Mike Ghabally; mike.ghabally@gmail.com

Academic Editor: Constantine Gennatas

Leiomyosarcoma (LMS) of the gallbladder is an extremely rare entity. Most reported cases were mistakenly diagnosed preoperatively as cholecystitis with or without cholelithiasis. We believe that our article demonstrates the 5th case of gallbladder LMS that was suspected preoperatively to be malignant rather than cholecystitis, which fortunately led to radical resection of the tumor instead of simple cholecystectomy. However, the definitive diagnosis relies exclusively on histological and immunohistochemical techniques. We present a case of a 62-year-old Caucasian female complaining of signs and symptoms suggestive for cholecystitis. On ultrasonography, the gallbladder appeared enlarged and filled with a necrotic mass; thus, the presence of adenocarcinoma was suspected. Multislice Computerized Tomography (MSCT) demonstrated no distant metastasis. An extensive radical cholecystectomy was performed, and histological techniques confirmed a leiomyosarcoma diagnosis. In addition, adjuvant chemotherapy of doxorubicin and ifosfamide was administrated. The patient was on follow-up for 2 years and is doing well till date. The discrimination of gallbladder sarcoma preoperatively remains a clinical and radiological challenge. Although radical resection of the tumor remains the mainstay of the treatment, we believe that adjuvant chemotherapy should be administrated in such cases. However, further studies are required in this field.

1. Introduction

Primary sarcoma of the gallbladder is an extremely rare diagnosis, and one of its common subtypes is leiomyosarcoma (LMS).

This neoplasm was first reported in 1879, while the first detailed description was made by Landsteiner in 1904 [1]. Most reported cases of LMS are made with a primitive diagnosis of cholecystitis with or without cholelithiasis in female patients in their sixth decade [2, 3].

Our search through the medical literature revealed only 22 other case of LMS. Therefore, we believe that our case is the 23rd in this series. This neoplasm is rarely diagnosed preoperatively. The accurate diagnosis is only established with histological and immunohistochemical techniques after cholecystectomy [2, 4].

2. Case Presentation

A 62-year-old Caucasian woman was admitted to the hospital complaining of abdominal pain in the right upper quadrant that started a month ago. The pain was severe, nonradiating, and colic. It was exacerbated by eating fatty meals and was responded to heavy analgesics. She also suffered from nausea, bilious vomiting, constipation, fever reaching 39°C that lasted for 10 days, chills, anorexia, and fatigue. There was no history of weight loss, pallor, jaundice, smoking, or alcohol consumption. Formerly, she was in good health as she did not report any previous illnesses or surgeries and her family history was unremarkable.

On examination, Murphy's sign was positive and there was tenderness over the gallbladder area with a firm palpable mass.

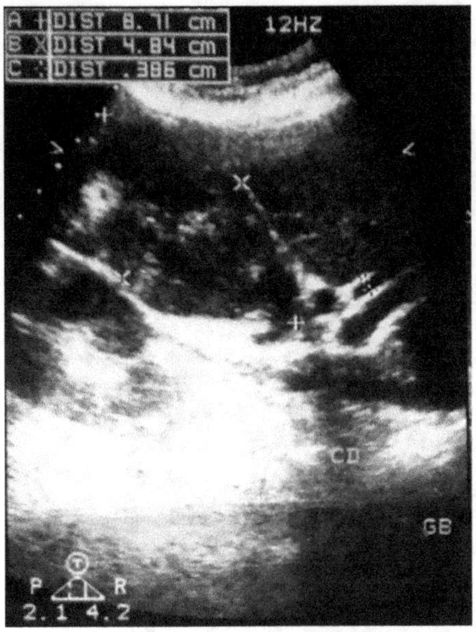

FIGURE 1: Transabdominal ultrasonography.

Laboratory workup showed a normal hemogram and liver function tests. On abdominal ultrasonography, the gallbladder measured 8.7 × 4.8 cm and was filled with necrotized mass and all edges of the gallbladder were clear except for the bottom (Figure 1). Therefore, the presence of a gallbladder adenocarcinoma was suspected. Spleen, pancreas, kidney, and liver were normal. MSCT demonstrated the same findings, and there was no metastasis.

As a result, a provisional diagnosis of gallbladder adenocarcinoma was made and extensive cholecystectomy that involved cholecystectomy, main bile duct resection, and regional lymph node dissection was performed. Intraoperative findings showed no liver metastasis, ascites, peritoneal, or omental deposits. Porta was free, and there was no colonic or duodenal infiltration and no enlarged pericholedochal, paraaortic, or aortocaval lymph nodes.

On microscopy, the tumor consisted of diffuse proliferation of pleomorphic spindle to oval tumor cells with marked variation in size and shape and the presence of many abnormal mitoses and large hyperchromatic nuclei (Figure 2). Furthermore, the gallbladder epithelium mucosa was congested and ulcerated with a mild degree of lymphocytic infiltration.

Immunohistochemical investigations were strongly positive for smooth muscle actin (SMA) and desmin and negative for CK, CD117, and CD34 (Figure 2). Therefore, we put the conclusive diagnosis as primary leiomyosarcoma of the gallbladder. However, we could not perform any further immunohistochemical markers.

Although there is no sufficient evidence regarding the effectiveness of adjuvant chemotherapy with or without radiotherapy, our patient received 6 cycles of adjuvant chemotherapy as the following regimen: (doxorubicin (day 1: 60 mg/m^2)+ifosfamide (days 1-3: 2000 μg/m^2); repeated monthly for 6 cycles). No serious adverse effect or toxicity has occurred. However, radiotherapy is not available in our city. The patient was on follow-up for 2 years; there was no clinical or radiological evidence of recurrence or relapse as observational MSCT scans were clear for any local invasion or distal metastasis, and the patient is doing well till date.

3. Discussion

Sarcoma of the gallbladder is an extremely rare entity that was reported less than 200 times in the medical literature [5]. Older cases agreed that LMS was the most common subtype of Primary Gallbladder Sarcoma (PGBS). On the other hand, recent series revealed that LMS is not as common as previously reported with MFH (malignant fibrous histiocytoma) being the most common subtype [6, 7].

Most of the patients in the reported cases are females (ratio 5 : 1) and mainly in their 6th and 7th decades of life [4–6, 8].

In our search among almost 200 reported PGBSs, there were only 6 cases that were suspected to be malignant preoperatively. Only 4 had the definitive diagnosis of LMS. Thus, our case represents the 5th case in this series [4, 6, 7]. However, the definitive diagnosis relies exclusively on histological and immunohistochemical techniques [8, 9].

Patients with GB sarcoma suffer from nonspecific symptoms that can be divided into two categories [7, 10]. The first category includes symptoms of gallbladder cholelithiasis, including right upper quadrant pain, nausea, vomiting, jaundice, and fever. The second category includes symptoms related to the malignant nature of the disease such as weight loss, fatigue, and anorexia [6–8, 10].

LMS coexists with cholelithiasis in 82% of cases. Therefore, it was related as a primitive factor, although the casual relationship remains circumstantial and unclear [2].

Radiological findings on CT scan and ultrasonography may include a dilated gallbladder, an irregular thickening of the wall, and a necrotizing mass protruding into the lumen [1, 5]. The larger size of the gallbladder, the presence of necrosis, and the polypoidal shape of the tumor should increase the preoperative suspicion of malignancy [6]. It is noteworthy that the diagnosis of such cases and the identification of histopathological subtypes depend on the extent of expertise of the radiologist and pathologist.

The differential diagnosis of a solid polypoidal gallbladder mass is wide and includes adenomas, adenocarcinomas, and neoplastic polyps such as cholesterol polyps, inflammatory polyps, and adenomatous hyperplasia [3, 5]. The definitive diagnosis relies on both morphological features on H&E staining and immunostains [8, 9].

The extensive differential diagnosis of spindle cell tumors of the gallbladder includes leiomyosarcoma, rhabdomyosarcoma, fibrosarcoma, neurosarcoma, epithelioid angiosarcoma, gastrointestinal stromal tumors (GIST), carcinosarcoma, and primary or metastatic undifferentiated carcinoma [1, 3, 5, 7].

Immunohistochemical techniques are the best way to differentiate between sarcomas. The spindle cells in LMS are arranged in a fascicular pattern and have eosinophilic cytoplasm with round to oval nuclei [8]. As previously mentioned, the high positivity for SMA in our case favored the smooth muscle origin of the tumor [1, 10]. In addition,

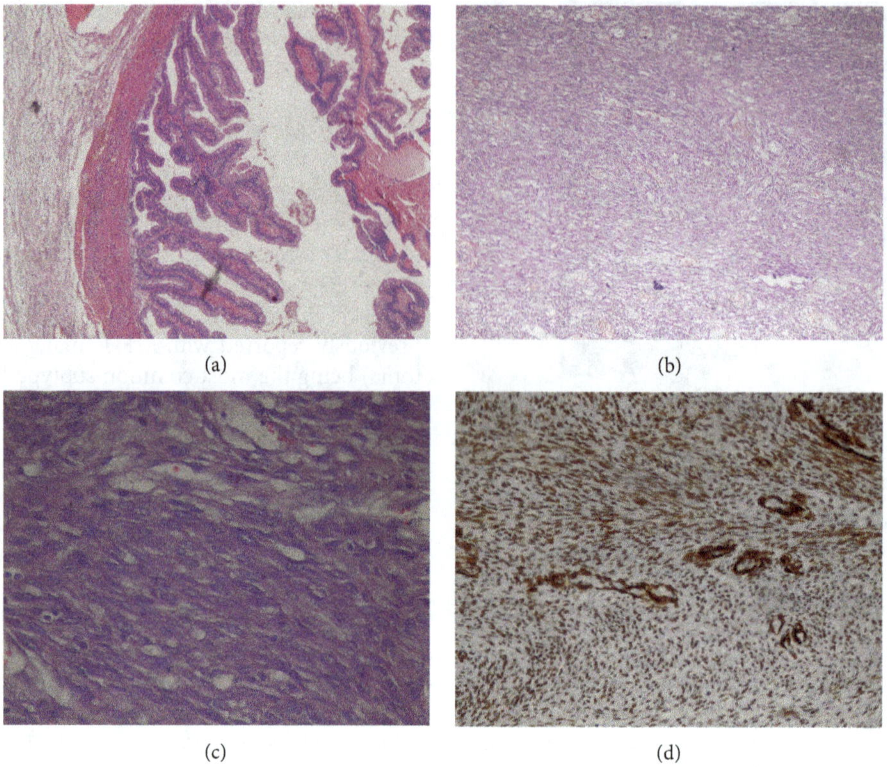

Figure 2: Pathohistochemical profile. (a) Ligand: normal gallbladder mucosa. (b, c) H&E stain shows proliferation of spindle cells arranged in interlacing bundles, pronounced nuclear atypia, pleomorphism, and many atypical mitotic figures (×200 and ×400, respectively). (d) SMA stain: the neoplastic cells show a strong cytoplasmic staining reaction (×200).

desmin was positive. However, immunostains were negative for CK, CD34, and CD117.

LMS of the gallbladder has a very poor prognosis with a 5-year survival rate less than 5% [2, 5, 8, 9]. This is due to the highly malignant nature, rapid progression, and early metastasis [5, 10]. Almost 75% of all patients have liver involvement at the time of diagnosis [2, 7–9]. However, our patient did not have any liver invasion or distal metastasis.

The treatment of choice remains radical cholecystectomy, and in advanced cases, regional lymph node dissection should be performed [2, 5, 8]. Adjuvant chemotherapy with or without radiotherapy has prolonged the overall survival rate in many reported cases of LMS [2, 3, 5, 9]. In our case, the patient underwent and extended radical cholecystectomy with 6 cycles of adjuvant chemotherapy (doxorubicin and ifosfamide) and was on follow-up for 2 years without any clinical or radiological evidence of relapse.

4. Conclusion

LMS of the gallbladder is rare and hard to be differentiated from other malignant subtypes. In most cases, it is falsely diagnosed as cholelithiasis and cholecystitis.

Although radical resection of the tumor remains the mainstay of the treatment, we believe that adjuvant chemotherapy should be administrated in such cases. However, further studies are required in this field.

Abbreviations

CK: Cytokeratin
GB: Gallbladder
GIST: Gastrointestinal stromal tumors
H&E: Hematoxylin and eosin
LMS: Leiomyosarcoma
MFH: Malignant fibrous histiocytoma
MSCT: Multislice Computerized Tomography.
PGBS: Primary Gallbladder Sarcoma
SMA: Smooth muscle actin.

Consent

Informed written consent was obtained from the patient for publication of this report and any accompanying images.

Authors' Contributions

AC was the patient's physician, and he contributed in the following: acquisition of the data, critical revision of the final article, and final approval of the revision to be published. MG, CM, NT, and FW have contributed equally in the following: acquisition of the data, analysis and interpretation of the data, review of the literature, drafting the article, and analysis and interpretation of the imaging findings. GO has contributed to the immunohistochemical parts of the drafting. All authors issued final approval for the version to be submitted.

Acknowledgments

The authors wish to express their thanks to Maryana Sabbagh for her grammatical review.

References

[1] K. Landsteiner, "Ueber das Sarkom der Gallenblase," *Wein Klin Wochenschr*, vol. 17, pp. 163–165, 1904.

[2] C. Fotiadis, A. Gugulakis, L. Nakopoulou, and M. Sechas, "Primary leiomyosarcoma of the gallbladder: case report and review of the literature," *HPB Surgery*, vol. 2, Article ID 79294, 4 pages, 1990.

[3] A. Savlania, A. Behera, K. Vaiphei et al., "Primary leiomyosarcoma of gallbladder: a rare diagnosis," *Case Reports in Gastrointestinal Medicine*, vol. 2012, Article ID 287012, 3 pages, 2012.

[4] J. C. U. Coelho, A. Wallbach, G. Kasting, and R. R. Moreira, "Ultrasonic diagnosis of primary sarcoma of the gallbladder," *Journal of Clinical Ultrasound*, vol. 12, no. 3, pp. 168–170, 1984.

[5] A. L. Im, Y. H. Lee, K. H. Yoon, S. W. Lim, D. E. Park, and K. H. Choi, "Ultrasound and CT findings of primary leiomyosarcoma in the gallbladder: a case report," *Journal of the Korean Society of Radiology*, vol. 70, no. 2, pp. 133–136, 2014.

[6] W. I. Al-Daraji, H. R. Makhlouf, M. Miettinen et al., "Primary gallbladder Sarcoma," *The American Journal of Surgical Pathology*, vol. 33, no. 6, pp. 826–834, 2009.

[7] E. A. Husain, R. J. Prescott, S. A. Haider et al., "Gallbladder sarcoma: a clinicopathological study of seven cases from the UK and Austria with emphasis on morphological subtypes," *Digestive Diseases and Sciences*, vol. 54, no. 2, pp. 395–400, 2009.

[8] A. García-Marín, L. Bernardos-García, J. Martín-Gil, D. Serralta-de-Colsa, and F. Turégano-Fuentes, "Primary leiomyosarcoma of the gallbladder," *Revista Española de Enfermedades Digestivas*, vol. 102, no. 1, pp. 8–67, 2010.

[9] E. Y. Park, H.-I. Seo, S. P. Yun, S. Kim, J. Y. Kim, and K. T. Han, "Primary leiomyosarcoma of gallbladder," *Journal of the Korean Surgical Society*, vol. 83, no. 6, pp. 403–407, 2012.

[10] D. A. Zeig, M. A. Memon, D. R. Kennedy, S. A. Woodward, and R. J. Fitzgibbons Jr, "Leiomyosarcoma of the gallbladder: a case report and Review of the literature," *Acta Oncologica*, vol. 37, no. 2, pp. 212–214, 2009.

Rare Abdominal Wall Metastasis following Curative Resection of Gastric Cancer: What can be Learned from the use of Percutaneous Catheters?

Arthur A. Parsee,[1] Kerry L. Thomas,[1] Masoumeh Ghayouri,[2] Rutika Mehta,[3] Kujtim Latifi,[4] Jennifer Sweeney,[1] Daniel Jeong,[1] and Abraham Ahmed[1]

[1]*Department of Radiology, Moffitt Cancer Center, Tampa, Florida, USA*
[2]*Department of Pathology, Moffitt Cancer Center, Tampa, Florida, USA*
[3]*Department of Gastrointestinal Oncology, Moffitt Cancer Center, Tampa, Florida, USA*
[4]*Department of Radiation Oncology, Moffitt Cancer Center, Tampa, Florida, USA*

Correspondence should be addressed to Arthur A. Parsee; arthur.parsee@moffitt.org

Academic Editor: Jose I. Mayordomo

In cancer care, tissue seeding after curative resections is a known potential complication, despite precautions taken during surgical treatment. We present an uncommon case of an abdominal wall metastasis along the tract of a surgical drain following gastrectomy for gastric adenocarcinoma. To our knowledge, this is the first case of such an occurrence in the setting of a negative staging peritoneal lavage. Aside from the rarity of such a recurrence, this instance highlights an opportunity to reevaluate best practices with regard to the extent of coverage of postoperative salvage radiotherapy. The oncologic patient provides many challenges and may require multiple catheters for drainage and at times infusion of nutrition or therapeutic agents. These foreign bodies should be scrutinized both clinically and radiographically, as they may create vulnerabilities in keeping malignant diseases contained and controlled. We provide a review of the literature with reasonable treatment options for the benefit of future patients.

1. Introduction

Cancer treatment is multidisciplinary and comprehensive with the ultimate goal of tumor eradication to maximize survival and minimize morbidity. Complications must be handled expediently to mitigate morbidity and improve prognosis. Metastatic seeding following resection is a rare but significant occurrence warranting further therapy. Spread patterns of gastric cancer rely primarily on histology, with generic adenocarcinoma mostly involving the liver (48%), followed by the peritoneum (32%) and lung (15%), and least often to the bone (12%) [1]. The signet ring subtype of adenocarcinoma has a predilection for the peritoneum, with a lesser burden in the liver and lungs. The second consideration is tumor location, with cases divided into the cardia and noncardia categories, with the latter also demonstrating a tendency for peritoneal carcinomatosis [1]. This case highlights the presentation and timing with subsequent treatment of an abdominal wall metastasis following total gastrectomy.

2. Case Presentation

A 62 year-old female with no significant past medical history was found to have a normocytic anemia (Hgb 8.6) on routine bloodwork. The primary care provider's workup included upper endoscopy (Figure 1) which revealed a mass 40 cm from the incisors, arising from the gastric cardia, with extension to the gastroesophageal junction. Endoscopic biopsy returned invasive moderately-differentiated gastric adenocarcinoma. Risk factors include smoking (19 pack-years; quit more than 10 years ago) and occasional alcohol consumption of 2-3 drinks per week. No complaints of dysphagia, weight loss, or change in bowel habits. Intermittent gastroesophageal

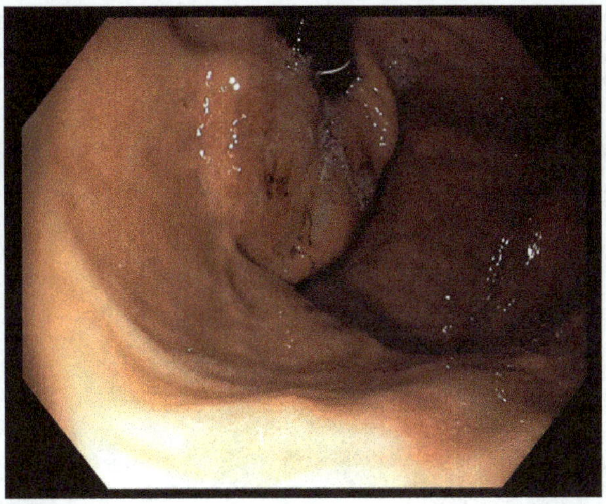

FIGURE 1: EGD photograph—an ulcerated mass 40 cm from incisors is shown, with stigmata of recent bleeding involving the gastric cardia, extending to the gastroesophageal junction.

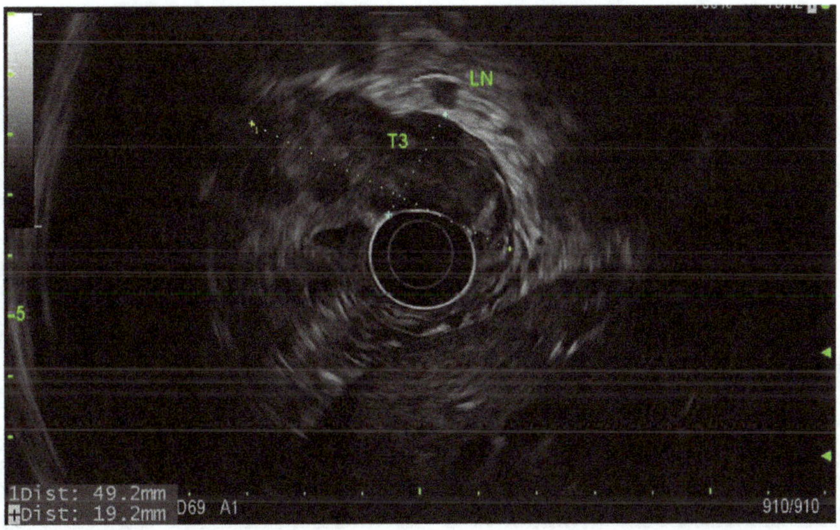

FIGURE 2: EUS—a hypoechoic mass involving two-thirds of the gastric circumference measured 4.8 × 1.9 cm, with serosal invasion and two malignant-appearing lymph nodes (one shown in field-of-view) in the paracardial region (level 16), T3N1MX by endosonographic criteria.

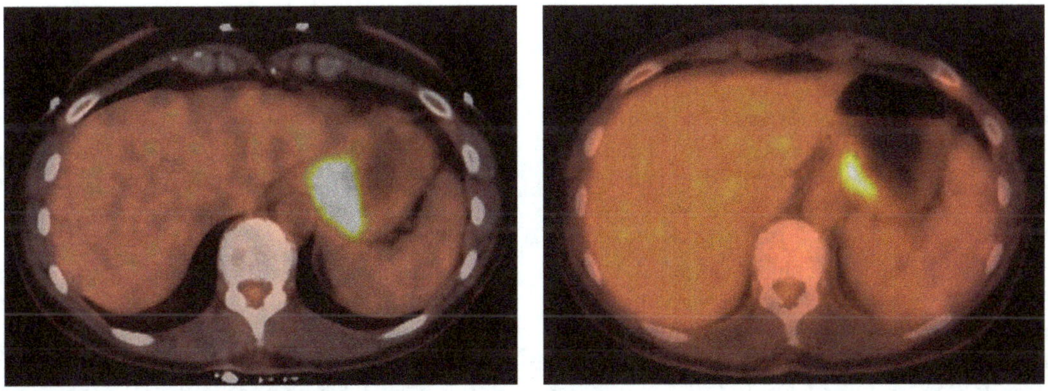

(a) (b)

FIGURE 3: Initial axial fused PET/CT image (a) showing robust hypermetabolism of the gastric cardia (max SUV 10.4) with subsequent axial fused PET/CT image (b.) following neoadjuvant therapy with reduced size and uptake (SUV 4.3), consistent with 60% reduction in FDG concentration.

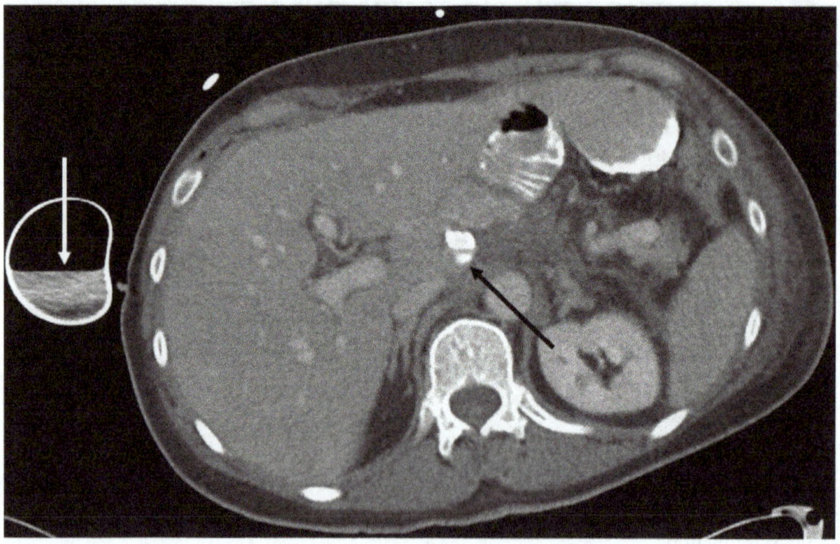

FIGURE 4: Axial postcontrast CT performed in the postoperative period showed leaked contrast concentrated at the tip of the surgical drain (black arrow). Contrast level is also present within Jackson-Pratt drain reservoir (white arrow).

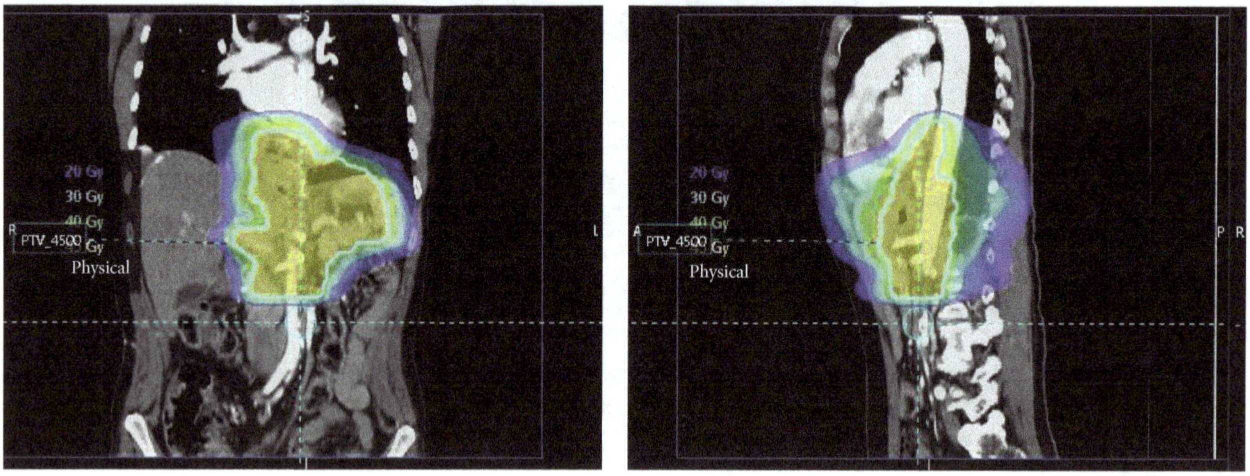

(a) (b)

FIGURE 5: Coronal (a) and sagittal (b) overlays with isodense lines of planned external beam radiotherapy (XRT) with coverage of the surgical bed.

reflux disease (GERD) was treated with pantoprazole. No personal or family history of cancer was noted.

Staging endoscopic ultrasound (Figure 2) demonstrated a well-circumscribed hypoechoic mass measuring up to 4.8 cm with sonographic evidence of serosal invasion. Two malignant-appearing lymph nodes were identified in the paracardial region (level 16) 5 mm from the tumor, lending to staging of T3N1MX. Initial 18-fluoro-deoxyglucose (^{18}FDG) positron-emission tomography/computed tomography (PET/CT) showed concentrated uptake within only the gastric mass, with a standardized uptake value (SUV) of 10.4, but no evidence of distant metastasis. Initial carcinoembryonic antigen (CEA) level was 5.6 ng/mL (normal is less than 5.2).

Diagnostic laparoscopy showed no peritoneal disease, and lavage washings were negative for malignant cells. A multidisciplinary approach concluded the best path towards lessening disease burden prior to a curative resection for a Siewert III gastroesophageal junction cancer [2]. Neoadjuvant chemotherapy was initiated, and it consisted of 6 cycles of 5-fluorouracil, leucovorin, oxaliplatin, and docetaxel (FLOT) with docetaxel being excluded from the last round. A restaging PET/CT (Figure 3) showed reduction in both tumor bulk and FDG avidity by approximately 60%, with CEA level decreased to 2.3 (initially 5.6).

Following standard preoperative cardiac clearance, the patient underwent a robotic-assisted total gastrectomy and D2 lymphadenectomy. En bloc resection included 4 cm of the distal esophagus as well as total omentectomy. Just prior to this, a small lymph node in the splenic hilum was sent for frozen section, which was negative for malignancy. Before construction of the esophagojejunostomy, frozen sections of the resection margins returned, which were also clear of any tumor. A Jackson-Pratt (JP) drain was placed behind

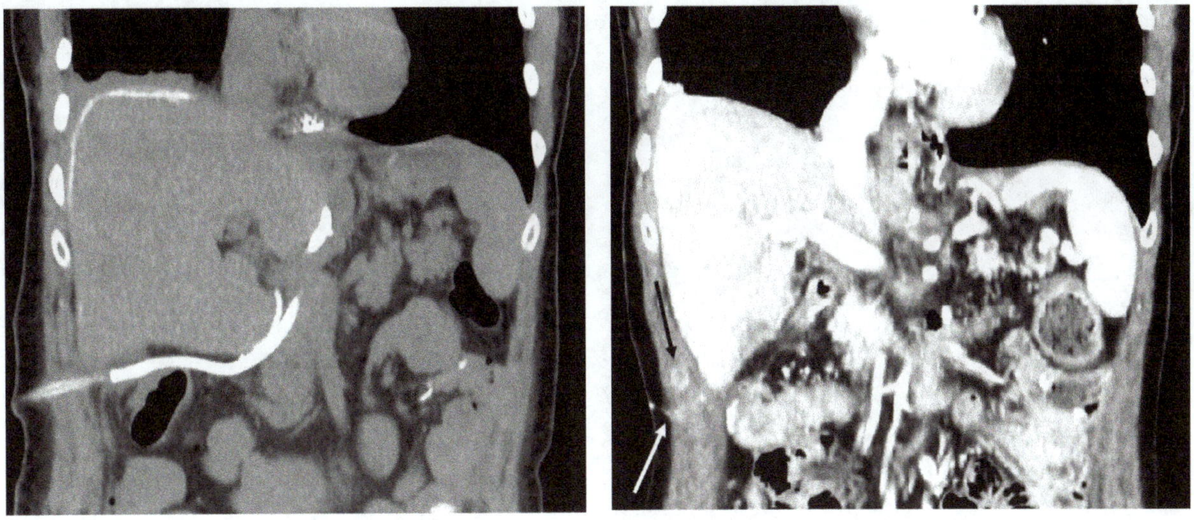

(a) (b)

FIGURE 6: Coronal noncontrast (a) and postcontrast (b) CT reconstructions demonstrating a new vascular nodule (black arrow) in close proximity to the drain tract with the residual barium demarcating tract (white arrow).

the anastomosis. Endoscopic testing was negative for any leaks. A feeding jejunostomy was also placed.

Postoperative recovery was initially as expected, with routine fluoroscopic interrogation of the anastomosis showing no leak with either water-soluble or barium contrast and with normal esophageal motility. On day 4, an episode of fever, tachycardia, and hypertension occurred. Antipyretic and empiric antibiotics were started, and a CT was performed for further investigation (Figure 4). This revealed a small collection of extraluminal contrast near the tip of the surgical drain and a concentration of contrast within the drain's reservoir, both suggesting a small previously occult anastomotic leak. Endoscopy confirmed a small ulceration at the anastomosis, 35 cm from the incisors, which was effectively covered by a 7.0 × 2.3 cm EndoMAXX stent (Merit Medical, South Jordan UT, USA) traversing 31 to 38 cm from the incisors. On day 9, a repeat CT showed a new subphrenic collection as well as more leaked contrast within Morison's pouch. A CT-guided drain was placed to effectively evacuate the subphrenic collection. The remainder of the postoperative course was relatively uneventful, with the jejunostomy removed once the patient was tolerating a soft mechanical diet.

Surgical pathology showed both lymphovascular and perineural invasion, with tumor within 1 mm of the omental margin. Only 2 of 27 nodes were positive, without treatment effect of the primary tumor present, yielding a final stage of ypT4aN1. A regimen of salvage chemoradiation was initiated, which included capectabine, as well as 1.8 Gy fractions divided over 25 sessions, for a total dose of 45 Gy focused on the surgical bed (Figure 5).

Two months later, a near-tripling in CEA (6.4 from 2.3) was concurrent with a new CT finding of a 1.1 cm hypervascular lesion embedded within the right abdominal wall subcutaneous fat (Figure 6) in close proximity to the previous JP surgical drain. This was palpable on the physical exam. An ultrasound was performed (Figure 7) to facilitate targeted

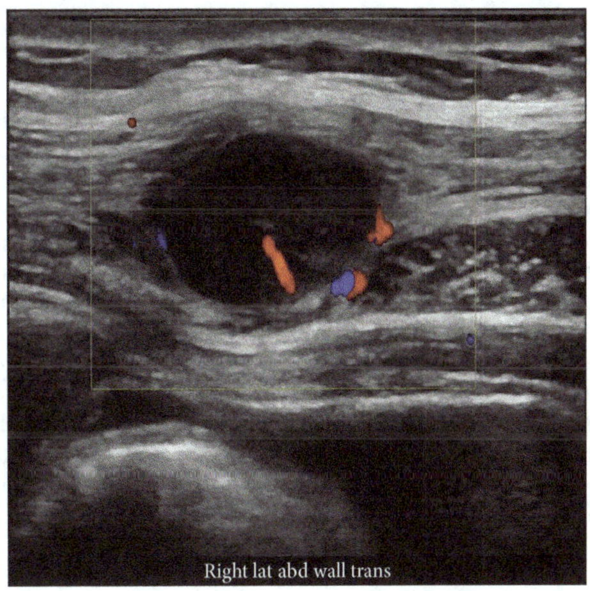

FIGURE 7: Doppler ultrasound confirming the subcutaneous nodule with internal vascularity and distortion of associated subcutaneous tissue planes, performed concurrent with image-guided biopsy.

biopsy. Pathology from core biopsy (Figure 8) showed an identical histological pattern as the original gastric adenocarcinoma. Immunohistochemical analysis was performed in hopes of eliciting additional treatment options. This revealed 3+ expression of the HER2/neu receptor. HER2 testing was not performed on the original endoscopic biopsy or the gastrectomy specimen. A regimen was undertaken consisting of four cycles of calcium folinate, 5-fluorouracil, oxaliplatin, and leucovorin (FOLFOX) as well as Herceptin (trastuzumab). After treatment, the nodule was no longer palpable and had resolved on imaging. The patient is now on maintenance Herceptin alone and is disease free.

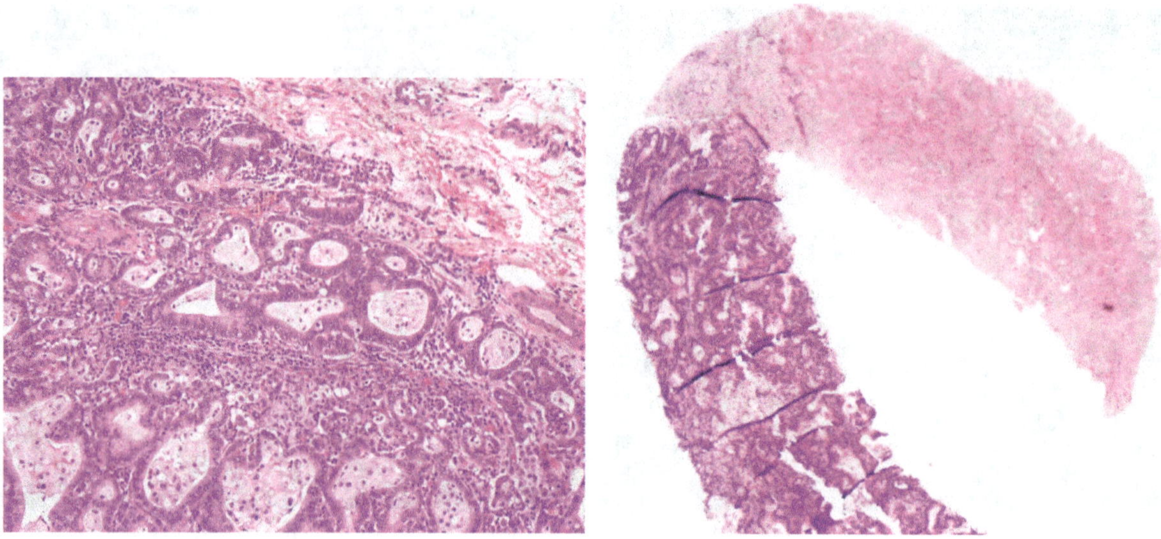

(a) (b)

FIGURE 8: Hematoxylin and eosin-stained histology slides of primary gastric adenocarcinoma at 4x magnification, moderately-differentiated with solid nests and glandular architecture (a). Identical pattern found after biopsy of the abdominal wall mass (b) at 1x magnification.

3. Discussion

Gastric cancer specifically is known to spread primarily via the peritoneum; the two primary paths being stomata-like orifices along the omentum and transvessel migration facilitated by hypoxic-induced factor-1α [3]. Esophagectomy studies have suggested a mechanical disruption of lymphatic channels as being another method for the spread [4]. These studies suggest that the peritoneal fluid at some point becomes contaminated with viable tumor cells, which can be confirmed with lavage of both the peritoneal cavity and surgical wounds. In cases of en bloc resection, a study found that wound washings were positive in 13% of instances, with drained fluid being positive in 9%, in a pool of 184 patients [5]. Studies of upper gastrointestinal cancers with anastomotic leaks are sparse; however, analogous reviews of colorectal cancers did not find that leaks had a significant impact on survival, tract or peritoneal seeding, or local recurrence [6, 7].

Peritoneal lavage has been established as an adjunct in staging, albeit of debated utility [8, 9]. A patient series with exclusive gastrointestinal malignancies found that staging lavage was only helpful in 1.3% of cases in providing useful prognostic information [10]. The most consistent risk factor to consider is the size of the primary tumor at initial staging [11]. The precise moment of seeding may be difficult to determine, as various interventions create a multitude of seeding vulnerabilities. Percutaneous biopsies, whether core or fine needle, provide one possibility of dissemination [12]. Enterostomy tubes for either drainage or feeding deliver yet another path for tumor propagation [13]. The most corroborated risk is transhepatic drainage for malignant biliary obstructions [14–16]. The prevalence of catheter tract seeding is somewhat disputed, with two reviews displaying rates ranging from as low as 6% to as high as 22% [17, 18]. In addition, soft tissue spread is not unique to GI malignancies; for example, an intracranial glioma has been reported to disperse into the peritoneum via a ventricular shunt [19]. Furthermore, seeding is not specific to the peritoneum or abdomen. Malignant effusions spreading from the pleura to the chest wall have been reported to be as high as 22% [20].

As it has been established that tract seeding can arise with a variety of tissue types and through variable media, it is reasonable to undertake protective measures to prevent tract seeding. While surgical literature has described the importance of resecting open biopsy tracts, this appears to be specific to sarcomas and not necessarily applicable to needle biopsies [21]. An argument has been made to justify prophylactic radiation to chest tube sites in the setting of mesothelioma, in the form of a single-dose 10 Gy fraction [22]. While there are several treatment options that may be applied to GI malignancies, it is generally acknowledged that isolated tract metastases, once removed or resolved, generally do not recur [23] as currently holds true in this case.

This report serves as both an example and warning that gastrointestinal cancers with anastomotic leaks can seed catheter tracts, even with a negative staging lavage of the peritoneum. Any catheter site must be scrutinized, as it will extend beyond the irradiated field. Tumor markers and imaging are helpful in diagnosing abdominal wall metastases.

Informed consent was obtained and a copy is available upon request. The case was anonymized, with the exemption from IRB approval.

References

[1] M. Riihimäki, A. Hemminki, K. Sundquist, J. Sundquist, and K. Hemminki, "Metastatic spread in patients with gastric cancer," *Oncotarget*, vol. 7, no. 32, pp. 52307–52316, 2016.

[2] R. BHAvon, H. J. Stein, and J. R. Siewert, "Surgical management of esophagogastric junction tumors," *World Journal of Gastroenterology*, vol. 12, no. 41, pp. 6608–6613, 2006.

[3] F. Sun, M. Feng, and W. Guan, "Mechanisms of peritoneal dissemination in gastric cancer (review)," *Oncology Letters*, vol. 93, no. 4, pp. 243–248, 2017.

[4] T. Nishimaki, T. Suzuki, and K. Hatakeyama, "Implantation metastasis of esophageal carcinoma to the surgical wound after radical esophagectomy," *Surgery*, vol. 119, no. 3, p. 359, 1996.

[5] J. C. Fisher, A. S. Ketcham, R. B. Hume, and R. A. Malmgren, "Significance of cancer cells in operative wounds," *American Journal of Surgery*, vol. 114, no. 4, pp. 514–519, 1967.

[6] F. Jörgren, R. Johansson, L. Damber, and G. Lindmark, "Anastomotic leakage after surgery for rectal cancer: a risk factor for local recurrence, distant metastasis and reduced cancer-specific survival?," *Colorectal Disease*, vol. 13, no. 3, pp. 272–283, 2011.

[7] T. Sueda, M. Tei, Y. Yoshikawa et al., "Prognostic impact of postoperative intra-abdominal infections after elective colorectal cancer resection on survival and local recurrence: a propensity score-matched analysis," *International Journal of Colorectal Disease*, vol. 35, no. 3, pp. 413–422, 2020.

[8] M. Hasbahceci, A. Akcakaya, B. Guler, E. Kunduz, F. U. Malya, and M. Muslumanoglu, "Use of peritoneal washing cytology for the detection of free peritoneal cancer cells before and after ;surgical treatment of gastric adenocarcinoma," *Journal of Cancer Research and Therapeutics*, vol. 14, no. 6, pp. 1225–1229, 2018.

[9] R. K. Freeman and M. A. Wait, "Port site metastasis after laparoscopic staging of esophageal carcinoma," *The Annals of Thoracic Surgery*, vol. 71, pp. 1032–1034, 2001.

[10] E. N. van Dijkum, P. D. Sturm, L. T. De Wit, J. Offerhaus, H. Obertop, and D. J. Gouma, "Cytology of peritoneal lavage performed during staging laparoscopy for gastrointestinal malignancies: is it useful?," *Annals of Surgery*, vol. 228, no. 6, pp. 728–733, 1998.

[11] M. S. Cappell, "Risk factors and risk reduction of malignant seeding of the percutaneous endoscopic Gastrostomy track from pharyngoesophageal malignancy: a review of all 44 known reported cases," *The American Journal of Gastroenterology*, vol. 102, no. 6, pp. 1307–1311, 2007.

[12] K. Shyamala, H. C. Girish, and S. Murgod, "Risk of tumor cell seeding through biopsy and aspiration cytology," *Journal of International Society of Preventive and Community Dentistry*, vol. 4, no. 1, pp. 5–11, 2014.

[13] N. Y. Hsu, T. Y. Lin, C. T. Hsu, and P. P. Tsai, "Tumor seeding of the jejunostomy site after transhiatal esophagectomy for esophageal carcinoma," *Diseases of the Esophagus*, vol. 12, no. 2, pp. 157–159, 1999.

[14] T. Yamakawa, S. Itoh, K. Hirosawa et al., "Seeding of gallbladder carcinoma along the tract after percutaneous transhepatic choledochoscopy," *American Journal of Gastroenterology*, vol. 78, no. 10, pp. 649–651, 1983.

[15] W. S. Kim, K. H. Barth, and M. Zinner, "Seeding of pancreatic carcinoma along the transhepatic catheter tract," *Radiology*, vol. 143, no. 2, pp. 427-428, 1982.

[16] L. Solin and M. Mohiuddin, "Subcutaneous seeding of pancreatic carcinom along a transhepatic biliary catheter tract," *British Journal of Radiology*, vol. 56, no. 671, pp. 883-884, 2014.

[17] S. Talukder, A. Behera, C. Tandup, and S. Mitra, "Isolated implant metastasis in chest wall due to seeding of transpleurally placed PTBD catheter tract in a case of hilar cholangiocarcinoma," *BMJ Case Reports*, vol. 10, no. 1136, p. 219864, 2017.

[18] L. Wang, N. Lin, F. Xin, Q. Ke, Y. Zeng, and J. Liu, "A systematic review of the comparison of the incidence of seeding metastasis between endoscopic biliary drainage and percutaneous transhepatic biliary drainage for resectable malignant biliary obstruction," *World Journal of Surgical Oncology*, vol. 17, no. 1, pp. 116–119, 2019.

[19] S. Stephens, G. Tollesson, T. Robertson, and R. Campbell, "Diffuse midline glioma metastasis to the peritoneal cavity via ventriculo-peritoneal shunt: case report and review of literature," *Journal of Clinical Neuroscience*, vol. 67, pp. 288–293, 2019.

[20] K. Cattapan, W. Tanomkiat, S. L. Geater, and N. Kiranantawat, "Procedure-related tumour seeding in lung cancer with malignant pleural effusion: radiological features and outcomes," *Journal of Medical Imaging and Radiation Oncology*, vol. 62, no. 5, pp. 619–624, 2018.

[21] I. Barrientos-Ruiz, E. J. Ortiz-Cruz, J. Serrano-Montilla, D. Bernabeu-Taboada, and J. J. Pozo-Kreilinger, "Are biopsy tracts a concern for seeding and local recurrence in sarcomas?," *Clinical Orthopaedics and Related Research®*, vol. 475, no. 2, pp. 511–518, 2017.

[22] H. Carette, J. C. Faivre, J. Salleron et al., "Irradiation préventive en une séance de 10 Gy des sites d'intervention pleurale des patients atteints de mésothéliome pleural malin : étude de cohorte rétrospective monocentrique," *Cancer radiotherapie: journal de la Societe francaise de radiotherapie oncologique*, vol. 21, no. 8, pp. 774–783, 2017.

[23] E. Koffi, V. Moutardier, A. Sauvanet, R. Noun, J. F. Fléjou, and J. Belghiti, "Wound recurrence after resection of hepatocellular carcinoma," *Liver Transplantation and Surgery*, vol. 2, no. 4, pp. 301–303, 1996.

29

Stage IV Small Lymphocytic Lymphoma Presenting with Unilateral Vision Loss

Christopher Le, Adam Jacob, Devarajan Iyengar, John Dedousis, and Antonios Tsompanidis

Department of Graduate Medical Education, CarePoint Health Bayonne Medical Center, 29 E. 29th Street, Bayonne, NJ 07002, USA

Correspondence should be addressed to Christopher Le; topherle@gmail.com

Academic Editor: Jeanine M. Buchanich

Small lymphocytic lymphoma (SLL) is a manifestation of chronic lymphocytic leukemia (CLL) in which malignant B-cell lymphocytes accumulate in the lymph nodes or bone marrow. In this report, we describe the medical course of a patient diagnosed with stage IV small cell lymphocytic lymphoma, who presented to the emergency room with acute neurologic manifestations of SLL.

1. Introduction

SLL is a form of non-Hodgkin lymphoma that involves malignant proliferation of B-cells in lymph nodes and other lymphoid tissues. SLL is often categorized along with CLL because they share many of the same clinical features but differ in the site of B-cell proliferation. CLL/SLL is the most common form of leukemia in the United States, making up about 25-30% of all diagnosed leukemia cases [1]. These leukemia cases have a stronger disposition for males compared to female, with the ratio of cases about 1.5 : 1 [1], most often diagnosed in the elderly population > 60 years old. The incidence of SLL is very low in patient categorized with CLL, as about 10% of patient have only nodal involvement.

Most patients present asymptomatically, with leukocytosis found incidentally on routine blood analysis. The patient may show symptoms of anemia, thrombocytopenia, chronic infections, hepatosplenomegaly, or lymphadenopathy at presentation, but these are much less common than the asymptomatic patient. More rarely, patients present with classic B-symptoms including fever, unexplained weight loss, or night sweats. Because SLL is an uncommon, indolent disease, patients are often asymptomatic for years and may eventually present due to complications of metastases.

2. Case Presentation

The patient is a 71-year-old Hispanic male with a past medical history of hypertension, COPD, and prostate cancer in remission post-radiation presented to the emergency department in May 2017 with a one-month history of neck swelling, sore throat, and ear pain. CT scan of the neck soft tissue showed multiple enlarged cervical lymph nodes in the submandibular, submental, posterior cervical, and jugulodigastric regions extending into the supraclavicular area (Figure 1). On the exam, the patient had left posterolateral oral pharyngeal soft tissue enlargement and possible left palatine tonsil involvement. Unfortunately, he left against medical advice before any further evaluation could be performed.

In November 2017, the patient returned to the emergency department with a 2-day history of headache, neck pain, painless vision loss in the right eye, and enlarging cervical and inguinal lymphadenopathy. Significant findings on examinations were complete right eye blindness and bilateral nontender lymphadenopathy in the cervical, supraclavicular, and axillary regions. On fundoscopic examination of the right eye, no retinal hemorrhages were appreciated. However, there was concern for optic nerve swelling and possible increased intraocular pressure.

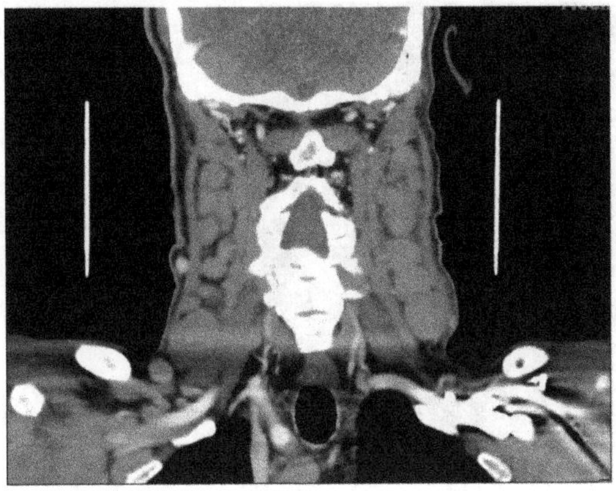

Figure 1: CT of the soft tissue in the neck showing diffuse cervical lymphadenopathy.

Lab work was significant for leukocytosis of 47,600/μL with 86% lymphocytes (10% atypical lymphocytes), hemoglobin of 8.3 g/dL, platelet count of 46,000/μL, and LDH of 4067 U/L. Due to the high leukocytosis and acute vision loss, there was concern for a retinopathy secondary to hyperviscosity syndrome. However, serum viscosity was 1.1 cP (range: 1.1-1.8 cP). Furthermore, CTA of the head and neck and carotid ultrasound were unremarkable showing no significant stenoses, which ruled out hyperviscosity syndrome and any vascular etiology for his vision loss. MRI of the brain showed no evidence of acute infarction or any enhancing mass lesion, which ruled out any acute etiology within the brain as the cause of his vision loss. CT of the chest, abdominal, and pelvis showed extensive mediastinal and retroperitoneal lymphadenopathy with splenomegaly (Figure 2). MRI of the brain and orbits showed a minimal focal area of enhancement within the right optic nerve inside of the optic canal (Figure 3).

Peripheral blood smear showed normocytic, hypochromic red blood cells, lymphocytosis comprised of small and large lymphocytes with few atypical lymphocytes, and thrombocytopenia without clumping. Biopsy was obtained from a paraaortic lymph node instead of the enlarged cervical lymph nodes to differentiate prostate cancer metastasis from a primary malignancy such as leukemia or lymphoma, as prostate cancer is unlikely to metastasize in cervical lymph nodes. The biopsy was consistent with B-cell chronic lymphocytic leukemia. Flow cytometry was positive for CD38 and ZAP-70. Bone marrow biopsy showed chronic lymphocytic leukemia greater than 90% of the cellularity with near total displacement by small lymphocytic infiltrate. Fluorescence in situ hybridization was positive for trisomy 12 and deletion of TP53 on chromosome 17 at p13. Immunohistochemical analysis of a paraaortic lymph node was positive for CD20, PAX5, CD5, CD23, BCL2, and CD43, but negative for Cyclin D1 and p53.

The patient was diagnosed with extensive stage IV small cell lymphocytic lymphoma with infiltration of the right posterior optic nerve. The patient was started on a regimen of rituximab and bendamustine. However, there was a concern that chemotherapy would not adequately penetrate the blood brain barrier to decrease the size of the intracranial lesion. Thus, palliative local radiation was initiated. Through radiation treatments directed at the lesion on his optic nerve, the patient slowly regained vision in his right eye.

3. Discussion

Chronic lymphocytic leukemia (CLL) is caused by the dysregulated growth and differentiation of malignant white blood cells in the bone marrow. These malignant white blood cells present in the blood often infiltrate other organs, such as the liver, spleen, and skin. Small lymphocytic leukemia (SLL) is a variant of CLL, in which most of the malignant white blood cells are present in lymph nodes. A previous study done in 2016 showed that any significant central nervous system involvement of CLL/SLL was an extremely rare consequence, with about 80% of the CNS symptoms occurring due to other causes [2]. CNS involvement in CLL/SLL is often undiagnosed or does not show any clinical signs or symptoms, but patients with CNS involvement have a median survival time of 12 months after diagnosis [3]. Studies have shown that CNS involvement in the progression of CLL/SLL occur in untreated patients while correlation with stage, duration, gender, age, WBC count, or immunologic phenotype has not been shown [4].

While the mechanism of spread into the CNS is not well understood to this point, several cases have been presented that postulate possible sites of entry into the CNS. The dura can act as a barrier to prevent direct invasion into the deeper layers of the CNS. However, spread into the CNS may come as a result of hematogenous or lymphomatous spread that perforates dural vessels and nerves into the arachnoid space [5]. Some studies have linked integrin CD49d, the α chain of the $\alpha 4\beta 1$, with migration of malignant cells across vascular endothelium, showing clinical relevance to disease progression. In addition, extensive bone marrow infiltration has been linked to high CD49d expression [6].

The differential diagnosis for this patient, who presented with sudden onset right eye vision loss, is broad. Important diagnoses to consider include optic neuropathy, optic neuritis, autoimmune disorders, inflammatory pseudotumors, and other compressive neuropathies, including optic nerve glioma, optic nerve meningioma, optic nerve or orbital metastases, inherited disorder, and toxic, nutritional, or metabolic optic neuropathies [7]. Urgent ophthalmology consult may be necessary in order to influence the differential, ordering of subsequent testing, and prevention of further progression of the disease. If there is high clinical suspicion of CLL/SLL involvement in the optic nerve, immediate orbital radiation and induction chemotherapy may be necessary to preserve vision. MRI of the brain and orbit should be done as soon as possible to narrow down the differential, visualize any possible compressive lesions, and determine location of the disease [8].

Optic nerve biopsy can also be considered; however, this carries the risk of permanent vision loss and results may vary due to small biopsy collection in order to preserve vision [9]. In a study performed by Levin et al., 14 of 15 patients that underwent optic nerve biopsy were able to get a definitive

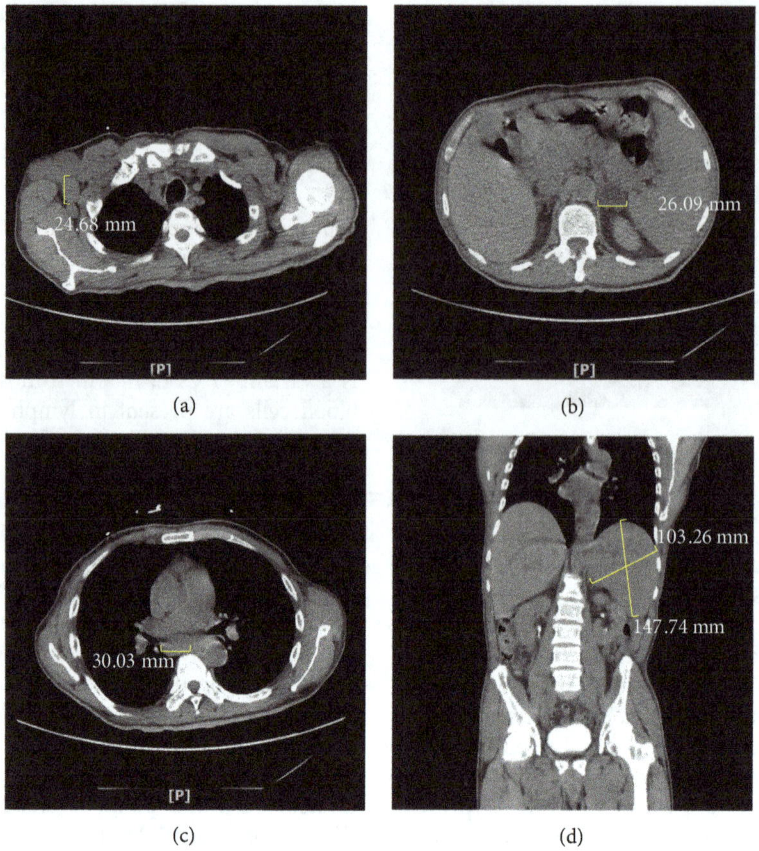

FIGURE 2: CT of the chest, abdomen, and pelvis. (a) Axillary lymphadenopathy. (b) Retroperitoneal lymphadenopathy. (c) Paraaortic lymphadenopathy. (d) Splenomegaly.

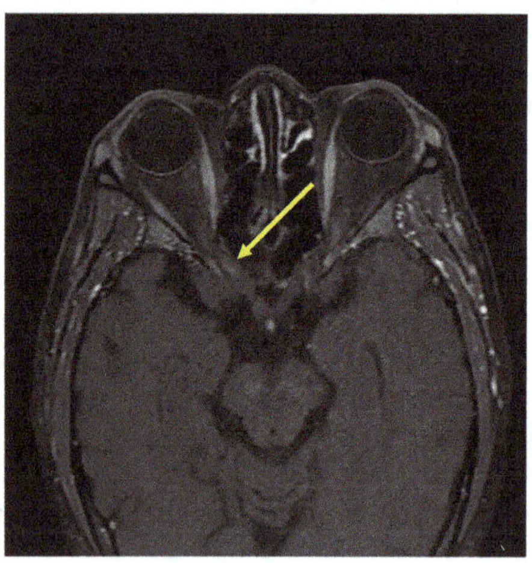

FIGURE 3: MRI of the brain and orbits with contrast showing lymphoma infiltration in the right optic nerve.

diagnosis. Of those patients, 4 who had an unaffected fellow eye were prevented from further vision loss, and 6 patients with tumors had the etiology of their vision loss confirmed [10]. Kim et al. presented two cases in which patients with B-cell non-Hodgkin lymphoma had optic nerve involvement and underwent optic nerve biopsy. Results of one biopsy showed mononuclear cells invading the fibrovascular pial septa surrounding bundles of necrotic fibers. The other showed the fibrovascular septa of the optic nerve infiltrated by lymphocytes and histiocytes [5]. Optic nerve biopsy results were also presented in a case by Myers et al. in a patient with recurrent vision loss and a history of T lymphoblastic lymphoma in remission. The biopsy showed lymphoblastic infiltration with atypical lymphoid cells with morphology like the original disease [8].

Standard treatment for early, stable CLL disease is observation monitoring. For initial management of CLL in advanced and active disease, ibrutinib (NCCN Category 1) or venetoclax plus obinutuzumab (NCCN Category 2A) are preferred treatment options regardless of del(17p)/TP53 mutation status. Other alternative first-line therapy options include chlorambucil plus anti-CD20 antibody (NCCN Category 2A; ESMO Grade A, Level 1) or bendamustine plus anti-CD20 monoclonal antibody (ESMO Grade B, Level 1). Our patient was placed on rituximab and bendamustine as it was thought to be better tolerated in an older patient than ibrutinib due to its toxicities with his multiple comorbidities and poor prognosis. For patients with SLL, regional radiation is often used. Lymphomas are among the group of tumors that are exquisitely sensitive to radiation therapy. In a study done by Johannsson et al., patients with disseminated CLL and indolent non-Hodgkin lymphoma (iNHL) were treated with low-dose radiotherapy (4 Gy in 2 fractions) for palliative treatment. Patients with CLL had an overall response rate of 71% (29% complete response, 42% partial response) with a median duration of response of about 22 months and no significant side effects. The study concluded that low-dose radiotherapy is a highly effective palliative treatment for masses in patients with disseminated CLL and iNHL [11]. In a study done by Pacelli et al., rare orbital tumors treated with radiotherapy had subjective and objective improvement of visual and ocular symptoms without evidence of disease progression [12].

Our case showed the rapid progression of the disease within the span of 6 months from the first clinically reported symptoms. The patient experienced severe neurologic symptoms, including complete right-sided, painless vision loss and right-sided headache and neck pain. The patient had a history of lymphadenopathy without a diagnosis of CLL/SLL, further complicating the case. While the clinical manifestations of this type of leukemia can be variable, CNS involvement provides a particularly unfavorable prognosis. However, the role of CNS involvement in SLL should be studied further to better understand disease progression.

4. Conclusion

SLL is an indolent form of lymphoma and patients often experience asymptomatic lymphadenopathy with no other symptoms. While cytopenias and bone marrow failure are common, neurologic manifestations of SLL are very rare but should be included in the differential of patients with sudden onset neurological symptoms and progressive lymphadenopathy.

Consent

Informed consent was obtained from the patient's sister as he is now deceased.

Acknowledgments

All funding for the publication of this article was funded by the author's supporting institution, CarePoint Health Bayonne Medical Center.

References

[1] R. L. Siegel, K. D. Miller, and A. Jemal, "Cancer statistics, 2018," *CA: a Cancer Journal for Clinicians*, vol. 68, no. 1, pp. 7–30, 2018.

[2] P. Strati, J. H. Uhm, T. J. Kaufmann et al., "Prevalence and characteristics of central nervous system involvement by chronic lymphocytic leukemia," *Haematologica*, vol. 101, no. 4, pp. 458–465, 2016.

[3] A. A. Moazzam, J. Drappatz, R. Y. Kim, and S. Kesari, "Chronic lymphocytic leukemia with central nervous system involvement: report of two cases with a comprehensive literature review," *Journal of Neuro-Oncology*, vol. 106, no. 1, pp. 185–200, 2012.

[4] K. Rakul Nambiar, T. Anoop, and N. Prakash, "CLL with CNS involvement-a diagnostic dilemma," *Acta Scientific Cancer Biology*, vol. 1, no. 1, pp. 17–19, 2017.

[5] J. L. Kim, P. R. Mendoza, A. Rashid, B. Hayek, and H. E. Grossniklaus, "Optic nerve lymphoma: report of two cases and review of the literature," *Survey of Ophthalmology*, vol. 60, no. 2, pp. 153–165, 2015.

[6] C. M. Rojas-Hernandez, J. Nemunaitis, K. D. Marjon, D. Bustamante, Q.-Y. Zhang, and J. M. Gillette, "Chronic lymphocytic leukemia with clinical debut as neurological involvement: a rare phenomenon and the need for better predictive markers," *BMC Hematology*, vol. 17, no. 1, 2017.

[7] G. Ahle, V. Touitou, N. Cassoux et al., "Optic nerve infiltration in primary central nervous system lymphoma," *JAMA Neurology*, vol. 74, no. 11, pp. 1368–1373, 2017.

[8] K. A. Myers, A. Nikolic, K. Romanchuk et al., "Optic neuropathy in the context of leukemia or lymphoma: diagnostic approach to a neuro-oncologic emergency," *Neuro-Oncology Practice*, vol. 4, no. 1, pp. 60–66, 2017.

[9] M. Dayan, J. Elston, and B. McDonald, "Bilateral lymphomatous optic neuropathy diagnosed on optic nerve biopsy," *Archives of Ophthalmology*, vol. 118, no. 10, pp. 1446–1449, 2000.

[10] M. H. Levin, J. J. Ney, S. Venneti et al., "Optic nerve biopsy in the management of progressive optic neuropathy," *Journal of Neuro-Ophthalmology*, vol. 32, no. 4, pp. 313–320, 2012.

[11] J. Jóhannsson, L. Specht, J. Mejer, and B. A. Jensen, "Phase II study of palliative low-dose local radiotherapy in disseminated indolent non-Hodgkin's lymphoma and chronic lymphocytic leukemia," *International Journal of Radiation Oncology • Biology • Physics*, vol. 54, no. 5, pp. 1466–1470, 2002.

[12] R. Pacelli, L. Cella, M. Conson et al., "Fractionated stereotactic radiation therapy for orbital optic nerve sheath meningioma–a single institution experience and a short review of the literature," *Journal of Radiation Research*, vol. 52, no. 1, pp. 82–87, 2011.

30

Primary Eccrine Porocarcinoma of the Breast: A Case Report and Review of Literature

Yi Xin Li[1], **Mihir Gudi**[2], **and Zhiyan Yan**[3]

[1]*Duke-NUS Medical School, Singapore*
[2]*Department of Pathology and Laboratory Medicine, KK Women's and Children's Hospital, Singapore*
[3]*Breast Department, KK Women's and Children's Hospital, Singapore*

Correspondence should be addressed to Zhiyan Yan; yan.zhiyan@singhealth.com.sg

Academic Editor: Katsuhiro Tanaka

Eccrine porocarcinoma (EPC) is a rare cutaneous neoplasm, with less than 500 reported cases worldwide since it was first described in 1963. EPC tends to affect the elderly and most commonly affects the head and neck. The mainstay of EPC treatment is surgery, with lymphadenectomy in the case of nodal involvement or presence of unfavourable characteristics. No evidence exists to guide the use of adjuvant chemotherapy or radiation. EPC is prone to misdiagnosis given its multiple clinical and histopathological mimics, especially in uncommon sites of presentation such as the breast. Herein, we report the case of a 59-year-old woman who presented with a left breast skin lump. The biopsied specimen revealed an infiltrative carcinoma involving the dermis and epidermis with positive IHC staining for P63 and CK5/6 and negative staining for ER, PR, and HER2. The tumour was resected and diagnosed as EPC with atypical features as overlapping characteristics of squamous cell carcinoma (SCC) were detected on histopathological analysis. In our case, a simple mastectomy with broad margins and axillary lymph node dissection with adjuvant radiotherapy to a dose of 60 Gy failed to achieve loco-regional control with nodal recurrence occurring 4 months postsurgery—a testament to the aggressive course of this rare malignancy.

1. Introduction

Eccrine porocarcinoma is a rare, invasive, and highly aggressive cutaneous tumour originating from the intraepidermal eccrine sweat duct (acrosyringium), first described by Pinkus and Mehregan in 1963 [1]. Its exact prevalence is unknown but estimated to constitute 0.005% to 0.01% of all skin cancers [2]. EPC has no predisposition for ethnicity or gender and tends to occur in older people in the sixth to seventh decade of life although there is a wide distribution of presenting ages ranging from 7 months to 97 years [3]. Surgical resection remains the mainstay treatment of choice by general consensus with limited evidence on the benefit of adjuvant radio- or chemotherapy [4]. To our knowledge, only 3 cases of primary EPC in the breast have been reported [4–6]. We present a rare case of primary breast EPC in a 59-year-old woman with lymph node metastasis and discuss the clinical presentation and histopathological findings and review the pertinent literature.

2. Case Report

A 59-year-old woman with a positive family history of breast cancer presented with a superficial left breast lump of 5 months duration without nipple discharge. Her preexisting medical conditions were hypertension, dyslipidemia, and diabetes. Examination revealed a 3×3 cm raised polypoid lesion at the left periareolar region with palpable left axillary lymphadenopathy (Figure 1(a)). Figure 1(b) shows the axillary lymph node dissection specimen.

Bilateral mammography revealed a 3.7 cm circumscribed opacity at the left periareolar region (Figure 2(a)), while ultrasonography showed a $3.3 \times 3.0 \times 0.9$ cm oval hypoechoic mass (Figure 2(b)) with left axilla lymphadenopathy

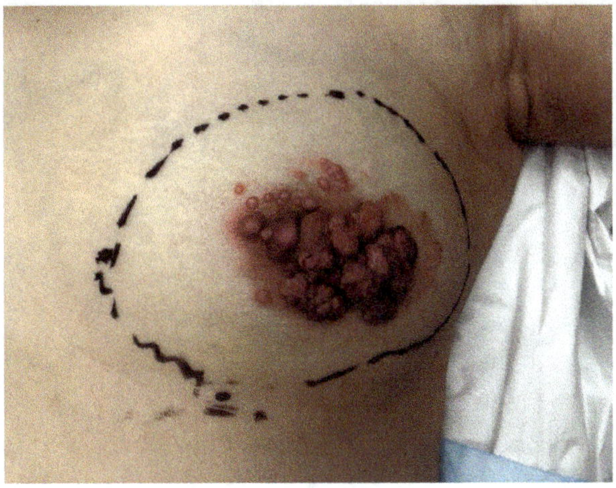

(a)

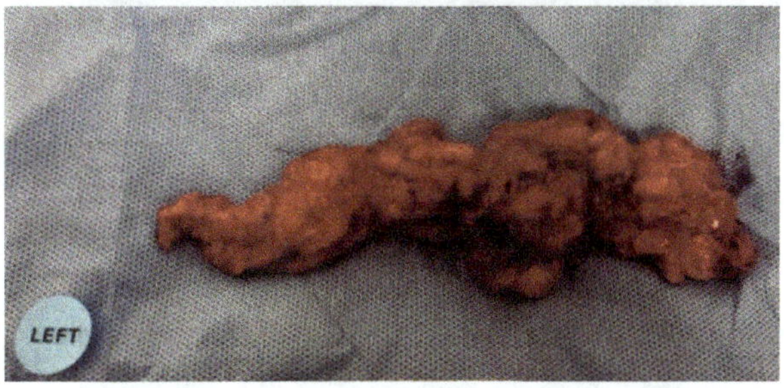

(b)

FIGURE 1: (a) Clinical appearance of the breast lesion. (b) Clinical appearance of the axillary dissection specimen.

(Figure 2(c)). Punch biopsy demonstrated an infiltrative carcinoma involving the dermis and epidermis. Immunohistochemical (IHC) staining was P63 and CK5/6 positive and mammaglobin, estrogen receptor (ER), progesterone receptor (PR), and HER-2 negative. Core biopsy confirmed positive nodal involvement while Computed Tomography (CT) imaging did not detect metastasis. These findings suggested a primary skin cancer instead of breast carcinoma.

Our patient underwent a simple mastectomy with 4 cm gross margins as well as an axillary lymph node dissection up to level II (Figure 1(b)). Macroscopically, the tumour was continuous with the epidermis with subcutis and breast parenchyma invasion; its maximal diameter and thickness were 6 cm and 1.3 cm, respectively. 12 out of 17 lymph nodes were positive for metastasis with extranodal extension present in several involved nodes. The largest nodal metastatic focus measured about 4.5 cm. The surgical margins were tumour-free.

Histologically, the tumour was poorly differentiated, consisting of infiltrative islands (Figure 3(a)) of solid sheets, nests, and cords of rounded to polygonal cells surrounded by desmoplastic stroma. Areas of necrosis (Figure 3(b)) and keratinisation were observed together with nuclear pleomorphism and conspicuous mitoses (Figure 3(c)). Lymphovascular invasion was identified (Figure 3(d)). Ductal and glandular structures were not identified. IHC staining was negative for CK7, CEA, ER (Figure 4(a)), PR, and HER2, focally positive for EMA, P16, and GATA3 (Figure 4(b)), and diffusely positive for CK5/6 (Figure 4(c)) and p63.

The diagnosis of EPC with atypical features of SCC was made, and subsequently, the patient underwent 6 weeks of adjuvant radiotherapy (60 Gy in 30 fractions) to the left axilla and chest wall 2 months postsurgery. The dose and fractionation were extrapolated from treatment guidelines for head and neck SCC given that SCC features were present in this case [7]. However, CT imaging detected nodal recurrence 2 days before the last dose of radiotherapy. The patient rejected reexcision and palliative chemotherapy and is managed supportively at 1-year follow-up.

3. Discussion

EPC is prone to misdiagnosis given its variable presentations. Clinically, EPC can present as ulcerating polypoid, exophytic growths, or verrucous plaques and be misdiagnosed as SCC, Bowen's disease, seborrheic keratosis, or pyogenic granuloma; histopathologically, EPC also has to be distinguished from basal cell carcinoma, hidradenocarcinoma, and most importantly SCC [5].

In our case, additional clinical mimics such as an invasive mammary ductal carcinoma had to be considered as well. However, triple assessment pointed towards a primary skin neoplasm instead of breast carcinoma. Differentials were narrowed to either a sweat gland tumour or squamous cell carcinoma (SCC), its main histologic mimic. On histological analysis, the absence of visible ductal lumina is uncharacteristic of EPC while the remarkably uniform "poroid" appearance of tumour cells is highly unusual for SCC. IHC staining result was equivocal for either diagnosis although negative CK7 and CEA staining is uncommon in EPC [8]. This atypical case demonstrates the utility of identifying additional IHC stains to differentiate EPC from SCC (e.g., S-100, CD117, CK19, and nestin) given their treatment differences which impact prognosis and survival [9, 10]. On the overall, given the tumour's morphology which was more suggestive of EPC instead of SCC, our patient was diagnosed with EPC and the diagnosis is supported by the tumour's highly aggressive nature given its early recurrence despite intensive treatment.

The etiology behind EPC development is unknown. Suggested risk factors include exposure of skin to burns, trauma or radiotherapy, immunosuppression, and prolonged exposure to ultraviolet light which were all absent in our patient [11]. EPC can arise de novo or via malignant transformation of a benign eccrine poroma usually over many years [12]. Reportedly, up to 18% to 50% of EPCs degenerate from initially benign poromas [8]. Unlike poromas which primarily present in regions with high densities of eccrine sweat glands (palmoplantar regions),

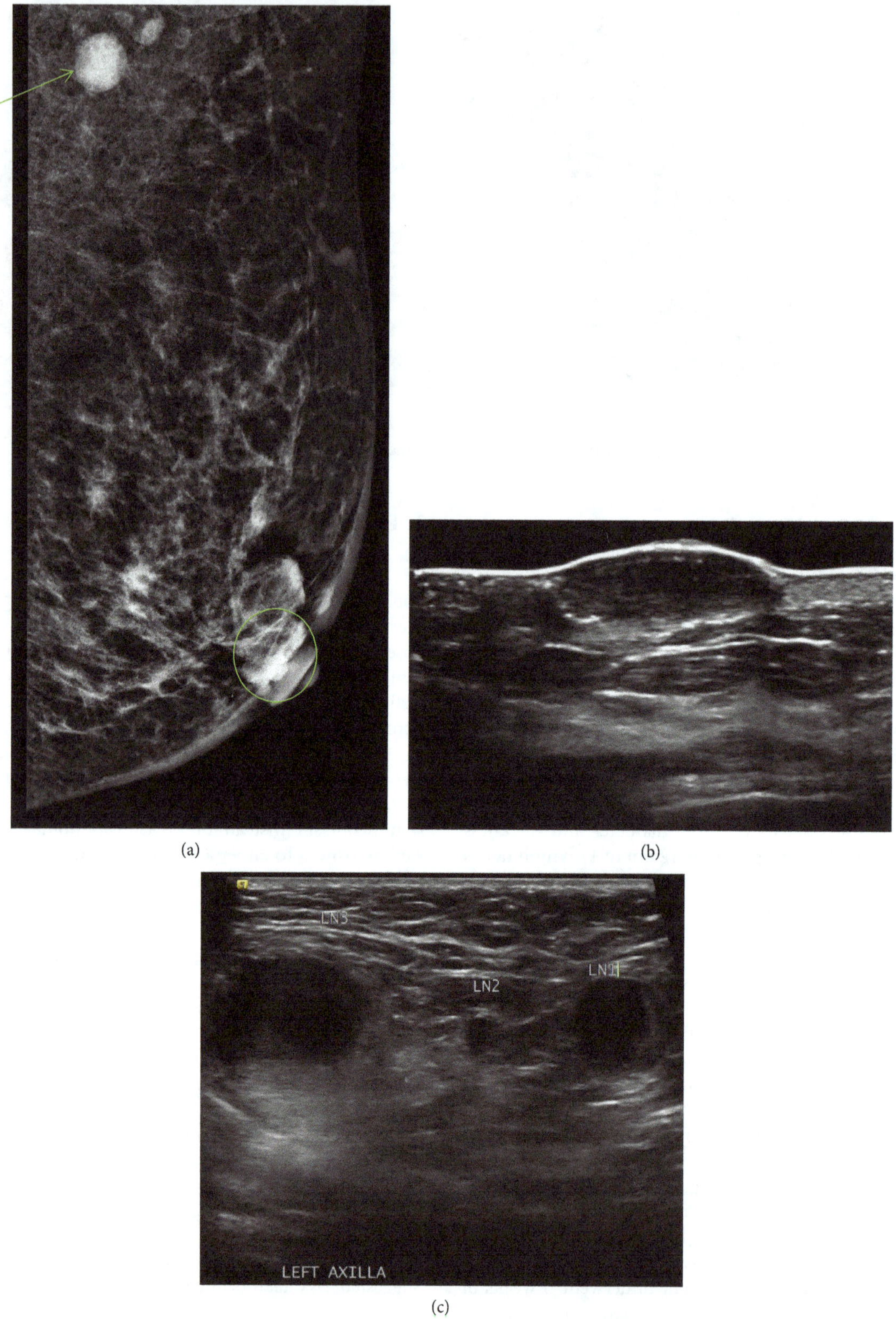

FIGURE 2: (a) Mediolateral oblique mammogram of the left breast showing a circumscribed periareolar opacity (circle) and dense axillary lymph node (arrow). (b) Superficial hypoechoic nodule on left breast sonography. (c) Lymphadenopathy on left axilla sonography.

EPC occurs rarely in these regions and more frequently at the head and neck followed by lower extremities [3]. However, EPC can affect any body part, and to our knowledge, only 3 cases of primary breast EPC have been reported [4–6]. An overview of these patient characteristics and treatment outcomes are summarised in Table 1 which largely correlates with our understanding of EPC presentation and aggressive natural history. The histopathological

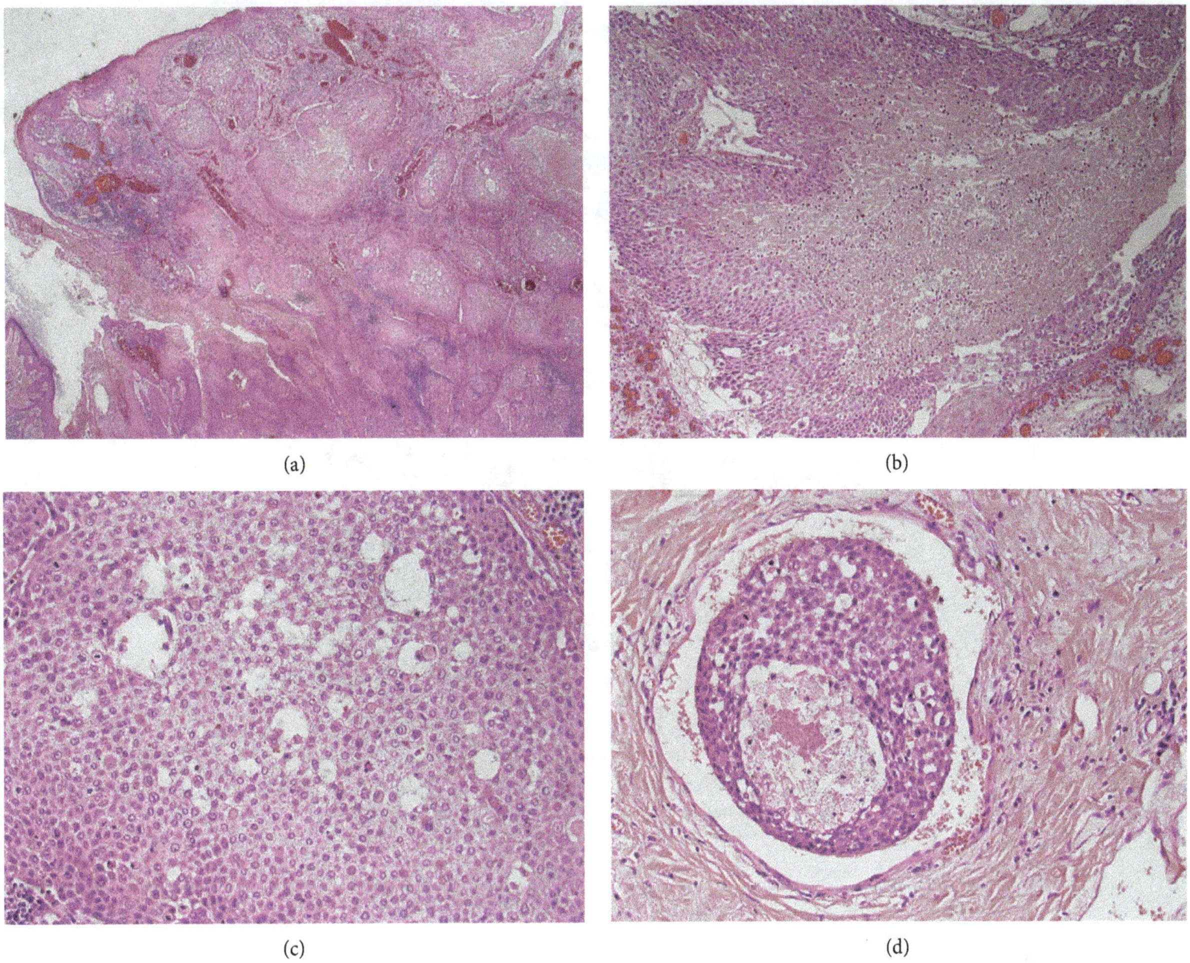

FIGURE 3: Tumour H&E sections: (a) skin-based carcinoma showing islands of infiltrating tumour (×40); (b) focus of central necrosis (×100); (c) cytoplasmic clearing within tumour islands with nuclear pleomorphism (×100); (d) focus of lymphovascular invasion (×200).

and immunohistochemical features in these cases were also typical unlike in our case where diagnosis of EPC was not as straightforward.

There is no standard guideline for EPC treatment. However, the first-line approach by consensus is surgical resection either with Mohs Micrographic Surgery (MMS) or more commonly a Wide Local Resection (WLE) with broad margins (>2 cm), without which prognosis and survival rates are significantly poorer [13]. The curative rate of WLE is reportedly 80% with a 20% probability of local or nodal recurrence despite negative excision margins as realised in our case [13].

The benefit of adjuvant radio and chemotherapy in EPC remains unproven. Le et al. reported that adjuvant radio or chemotherapy did not significantly improve prognosis or overall survival in their meta-analyses of 120 EPC head and neck cases [14]. However, there may be a role for adjuvant radiotherapy in EPC with positive resection margins or presence of poor prognostic features (as "infiltrative" or "pushing" subtypes of EPC, >14 mitoses per high-power field, lymphovascular invasion, and tumoural involvement > 7 mm) as in our case, given the higher risk of recurrence and metastasis [15, 16]. In cases of recurrent and/or metastatic EPC, individual reports have demonstrated the possibility of partial or complete remission with adjuvant chemotherapy such as docetaxel and 5-fluorouracil [6, 17, 18]. Unconventional treatments have also been utilised in recurrent and/or metastatic EPC such as immunotherapy (interferon alpha, interleukin 2, and pembrolizumab), isotretinoin, electrochemotherapy, intralesional photodynamic therapy, CyberKnife radiosurgery, and hormonal treatment (tamoxifen) in the case of positive ER/PR receptors with variable success [19–25].

Recent research may shed light on the high rates of recurrence in EPC even with adjuvant treatment—Taghizadeh-Hesary et al. highlighted the importance of mitochondria's role in cancer metabolism such as mediating efflux pump expression and scavenging reactive oxygen species (ROS) which confers resistance to chemo- and radiotherapy [26]. A stronger functional mitochondrial status may explain why some cancers such as EPC are highly recurrent and resilient. Further research into antimitochondrial therapy may thus have potential in improving treatment outcomes for these cancers.

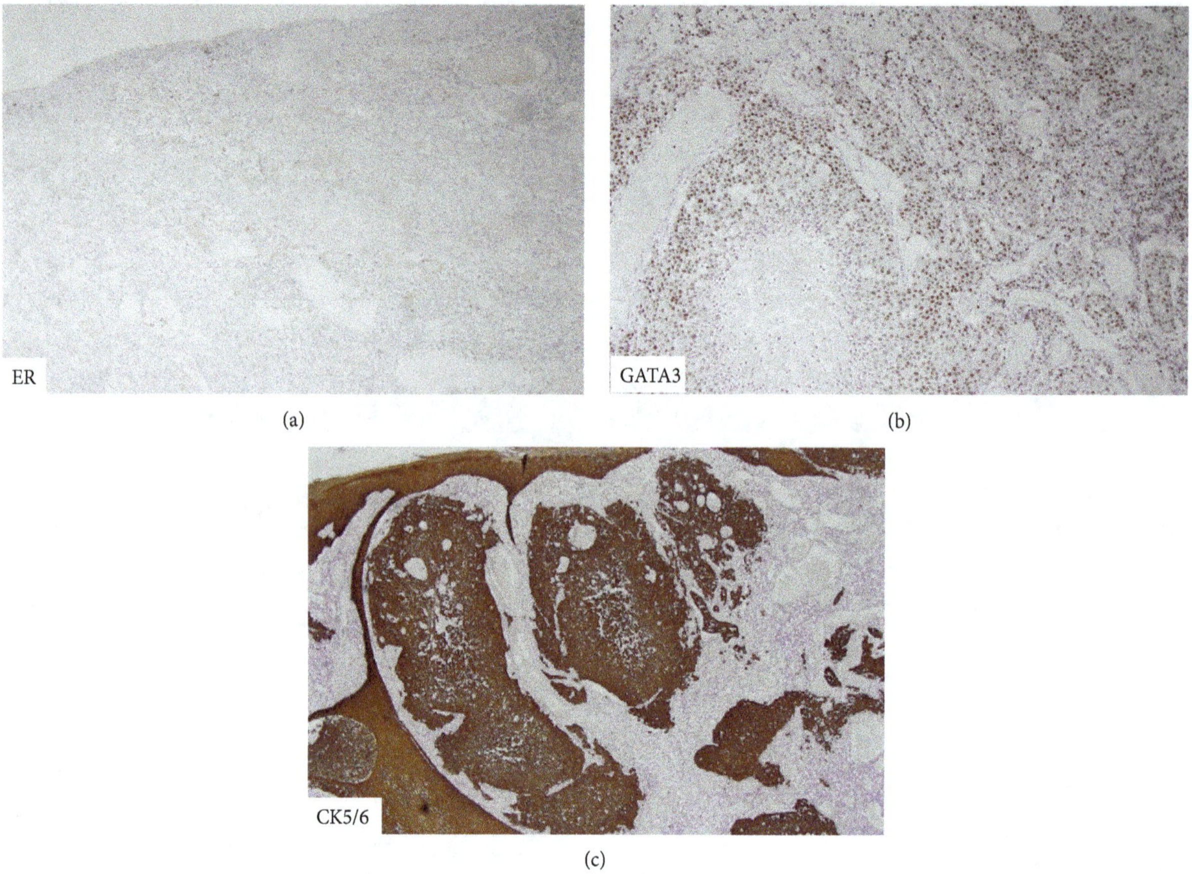

Figure 4: Immunohistochemistry analysis results: (a) ER (-); (b) GATA 3 (+); (c) CK5/6 (+).

Table 1: General characteristics, EPC histopathological and immunohistochemical features, treatment modalities, and outcomes in terms of response or survival.

Age/sex	Site and largest dimension (mm)	Lymph node/ distant metastasis	Histopathological and IHC features of EPC	Treatment received	Treatment outcome	First author and year
92/F	Right breast, 60 mm	+	n.a.	Surgery (mastectomy)	Palliative care, adjuvant therapy rejected	Bonito (2020)
74/F	Right breast, 45 mm (first recurrence)	—	Infiltrative subtype with squamous differentiation and lymphovascular invasion Negative postop margins IHC positive for p63, CK5, and EMA and negative for ER and PR	Surgery (WLE) followed by reexcision (WLE) and adjuvant RT (66 Gy)	Overall survival of 3.3 years; first recurrence 22.5 months after initial resection and patient died 17.5 months after reexcision and adjuvant RT	Morten (2018)
54/M	n.a.	+	Unknown subtype IHC positive for AE1/AE3 and CEA and negative for S-100 and CK5/6	Surgery (WLE) followed by chemotherapy (cisplatin, 5-fluorouracil, and docetaxel) and reexcision (WLE)	Local recurrence and metastasis 1 year postop; complete remission achieved after docetaxel chemotherapy	Aaribi (2013)

M: male; F: female; n.a.: not available.

4. Conclusion

EPC is a rare and aggressive skin neoplasm with a high risk of misdiagnosis due to multiple clinical and histopathological mimics. It has a high propensity for dermal lymphatic invasion which leads to frequent nodal involvement and distant metastasis with a high risk of recurrence. A multidisciplinary approach towards diagnosis and early intervention with frequent follow-up surveillance is therefore essential in pursuit of complete remission.

References

[1] M. Gabrielle, M. A. S. Baker, and M. P. Hoang, "Vulvar adnexal lesions: a 32-year, single-institution review from Massachusetts General Hospital," *Archives of Pathology & Laboratory Medicine*, vol. 137, no. 9, pp. 1237–1246, 2013.

[2] H. Pinkus and A. H. Mehregan, "Epidermotropic eccrine carcinoma," *Archives of Dermatology*, vol. 88, no. 5, pp. 597–606, 1963.

[3] A. M. Salih, F. H. Kakamad, H. O. Baba et al., "Porocarcinoma; presentation and management, a meta-analysis of 453 cases," *Annals of Medicine and Surgery*, vol. 20, pp. 74–79, 2017.

[4] A. Correa Bonito, R. Á. de la Hoz, C. Marín Campos, B. Doblado Cardellach, and P. E. Martín, "Porocarcinoma Located in the Breast: A Case Report," *Cirugía Española*, vol. 98, no. 9, pp. 561–563, 2020.

[5] C. Monten, J. Berwouts, L. Veldeman, D. Creytens, and G. Braems, "A case of eccrine porocarcinoma, located in the breast : the pitfalls reviewed," *Medical Case Reports*, vol. 4, no. 3, 2018.

[6] I. Aaribi, A. Mohtaram, M. Ben Ameur el Youbi et al., "Successful management of metastatic eccrine porocarcinoma," *Case Reports in Oncological Medicine*, vol. 2013, 3 pages, 2013.

[7] National Comprehensive Cancer Network, "Squamous cell skin cancer (Version 1.2022)," April 2022, https://www.nccn.org/professionals/physician_gls/pdf/squamous.pdf.

[8] A. Nazemi, S. Higgins, R. Swift, G. In, K. Miller, and A. Wysong, "Eccrine porocarcinoma: new insights and a systematic review of the literature," *Dermatologic Surgery*, vol. 44, no. 10, pp. 1247–1261, 2018.

[9] K. Goto, T. Takai, T. Fukumoto et al., "CD117 (KIT) is a useful immunohistochemical marker for differentiating porocarcinoma from squamous cell carcinoma," *Journal of Cutaneous Pathology*, vol. 43, no. 3, pp. 219–226, 2016.

[10] M. Mahalingam, J. E. Richards, M. A. Selim, A. Muzikansky, and M. P. Hoang, "An immunohistochemical comparison of cytokeratin 7, cytokeratin 15, cytokeratin 19, CAM 5.2, carcinoembryonic antigen, and nestin in differentiating porocarcinoma from squamous cell carcinoma," *Human Pathology*, vol. 43, no. 8, pp. 1265–1272, 2012.

[11] A. M. Salih, F. H. Kakamad, R. A. Essa et al., "Porocarcinoma: a systematic review of literature with a single case report," *International Journal of Surgery Case Reports*, vol. 30, pp. 13–16, 2017.

[12] R. Fernández-Ferreira, G. Alvarado-Luna, D. Motola-Kuba, I. Mackinney-Novelo, E. E. Cervera-Ceballos, and R. Segura-Rivera, "Intergluteal cleft eccrine porocarcinoma with metastasis to inguinal region and lung: case report and review of the literature," *Case Reports in Oncology*, vol. 13, no. 3, pp. 1463–1473, 2021.

[13] S. S. Song, W. Wu Lee, M. S. Hamman, and S. I. Jiang, "Mohs micrographic surgery for eccrine porocarcinoma: an update and review of the literature," *Dermatologic Surgery*, vol. 41, no. 3, pp. 301–306, 2015.

[14] N. S. Le, S. Janik, D. T. Liu et al., "Eccrine porocarcinoma of the head and neck: meta-analysis of 120 cases," *Head & Neck*, vol. 42, no. 9, pp. 2644–2659, 2020.

[15] A. Robson, J. Greene, N. Ansari et al., "Eccrine porocarcinoma (malignant eccrine poroma)," *The American Journal of Surgical Pathology*, vol. 25, no. 6, pp. 710–720, 2001.

[16] B. Fionda, A. Di Stefani, V. Lancellotta et al., "The role of postoperative radiotherapy in eccrine porocarcinoma: a multidisciplinary systematic review," *European Review for Medical and Pharmacological Sciences*, vol. 26, no. 5, pp. 1695–1700, 2022.

[17] E. de Bree, E. Volalakis, D. Tsetis et al., "Treatment of advanced malignant eccrine poroma with locoregional chemotherapy," *The British Journal of Dermatology*, vol. 152, no. 5, pp. 1051–1055, 2005.

[18] T. A. Plunkett, A. M. Hanby, D. W. Miles, and R. D. Rubens, "Metastatic eccrine porocarcinoma: response to docetaxel (Taxotere) chemotherapy," *Annals of Oncology*, vol. 12, no. 3, pp. 411–414, 2001.

[19] R. Dummer, J. C. Becker, B. Boser, A. A. Hartmann, and G. Burg, "Successful therapy of metastatic eccrine poroma using perilesional interferon alfa and interleukin 2," *Archives of Dermatology*, vol. 128, no. 8, pp. 1127-1128, 1992.

[20] K. A. Lee, M. Cioni, A. Robson, and V. Bataille, "Metastatic porocarcinoma achieving complete radiological and clinical response with pembrolizumab," *BML Case Reports*, vol. 12, no. 9, article e228917, 2019.

[21] M. Friedland, A. Bajracharya, and Z. Arlin, "Malignant eccrine poroma and isotretinoin," *Annals of Internal Medicine*, vol. 100, no. 4, p. 614, 1984.

[22] L. Borgognoni, L. Pescitelli, C. Urso et al., "A rare case of anal porocarcinoma treated by electrochemotherapy," *Future Oncology*, vol. 10, no. 15, pp. 2429–2434, 2014.

[23] D. Torchia, A. Amorosi, and P. Cappugi, "Intralesional photodynamic therapy for eccrine porocarcinoma," *Dermatologic Surgery*, vol. 41, no. 7, pp. 853-854, 2015.

[24] T. Fujimura, A. Hashimoto, S. Furudate, Y. Kambayashi, T. Haga, and S. Aiba, "Successful treatment of eccrine porocarcinoma metastasized to a cervical lymph node with CyberKnife radiosurgery," *Case Reports in Dermatology*, vol. 6, no. 2, pp. 159–163, 2014.

[25] U. Schröder, V. Dries, J. P. Klussmann, C. Wittekindt, and H. E. Eckel, "Successful adjuvant tamoxifen therapy for estrogen receptor-positive metastasizing sweat gland adenocarcinoma: need for a clinical trial?," *The Annals of Otology, Rhinology, and Laryngology*, vol. 113, no. 3, pp. 242–244, 2004.

[26] F. Taghizadeh-Hesary, H. Akbari, and M. Bahadori, "Anti-mitochondrial therapy: a potential therapeutic approach in oncology," 2022, Preprints.org.

31

A South African Breast Implant-Associated Anaplastic Large Cell Lymphoma: Clinical Presentation and Six-Year Follow-Up

Alexandra Grubnik,[1] Yastira Ramdas,[1,2] Barend Van der Bergh,[1] Simon Nayler,[1,3,4] Carol-Ann Benn,[1,5] and Bernardo L. Rapoport[1,2,6]

[1]*Netcare Breast Care Centre of Excellence, Milpark Hospital, 9 Guild Road Parktown, South Africa*
[2]*Department of Immunology, Faculty of Health Sciences, University of Pretoria, Corner Doctor Savage Road and Bophelo Road, Pretoria 0002, South Africa*
[3]*Drs Gritzman & Thatcher Inc. Laboratories, 4 Main Street, Bordeaux, Randburg, Johannesburg 2194, South Africa*
[4]*University of the Witwatersrand, Donald Gordon Medical Centre, 21 Eton Road, Parktown Johannesburg, 2193, South Africa*
[5]*Helen Joseph Hospital Breast Care Clinic, Department of Surgery, Faculty of Health Sciences, University of the Witwatersrand, 1 Perth Road, Auckland Park, Johannesburg, 2092 Gauteng, South Africa*
[6]*The Medical Oncology Centre of Rosebank, 129 Oxford Road, Johannesburg 2196, South Africa*

Correspondence should be addressed to Bernardo L. Rapoport; bernardo.rapoport@up.ac.za

Academic Editor: Katsuhiro Tanaka

Breast augmentation is the most common surgical procedure for women globally, with 1,795,551 cases performed in 2019. Breast implant-associated anaplastic large cell lymphoma (BIA-ALCL) is highly uncommon, with 733 reported cases as of January 2020. In South Africa, there are less than 4000 breast augmentation surgeries annually. This case presents the first case report documentation of a South African woman diagnosed with BIA-ALCL. The patient was a 61-year-old woman who consulted the Breast Care Centre of Excellence in Johannesburg in 2015. She had a prior history of bilateral augmentation mammoplasty with subsequent implant exchange. The patient presented with periprosthetic fluid with a mass-like enhancement on the left breast. Aspiration of the mass-like fluid was positive for CD45, CD30, and CD68 and negative for CD20 and ALK-1, indicative of BIA-ALCL. Surgical treatment included bilateral explantation, complete capsulectomies, and bilateral mastopexy. Macroscopic examination of the left breast capsulectomy demonstrated fibrous connective tissue. The histological examination of the tumor showed extensive areas of broad coagulative necrosis with foamy histiocytes. Immunohistochemistry examination of this tumor showed CD3-, CD20-, and ALK-1-negative and CD30- and CD68-positive stains. PCR analysis for T-cell clonality showed monoclonal T-cell expansion. These findings confirm the presence of BIA-ALCL. The patient recovered well after surgery and did not require adjuvant therapy. A patient with a confirmed diagnosis of BIA-ALCL was successfully treated with explantation and complete capsulectomy. She was followed up regularly for six years, and the patient remains well and in remission.

1. Background

Breast augmentation remains the most common procedure globally, with 1,795,551 performed in 2019 [1]. An estimated 10 million women have implants globally [2]. In South Africa, 3297 breast augmentation cases with silicone implants were recorded in 2016 [2]. Breast implant-associated anaplastic large cell lymphoma (BIA-ALCL), a subtype of T-cell non-Hodgkin's lymphoma, is associated with textured surface breast implants [3, 4]. The cause of BIA-ALCL remains unknown, although several theories, including biofilm, viral, shedding of particles, and genetic predisposition, have been proposed [5–9].

BIA-ALCL is a novel malignant entity. It was first described in 1997 and reported by the Food and Drug Administration (FDA) in 2011 [10–11]. In 2016, the World

Health Organization (WHO) categorized it as a unique disease [10]. NCCN diagnosis and treatment guidelines were published in 2016 and updated in 2019 [11].

As of January 2020, 733 cases of BIA-ALCL were reported to the FDA, including 36 deaths [10]. The incidence and risk of BIA-ALCL have risen considerably from early reports of 1 per million to current estimates of between 1/2,832 and 1/30000, and in specific cohorts, an incidence of as high as 1/355 was reported [10, 12, 13]. The disease incidence mainly depends on the "population" (implant type and characteristics) examined and increased awareness of the disease [14]. To our knowledge, this is the first peer-reviewed case report of a patient with BIA-ALCL in South Africa and the African continent.

2. Case Presentation

A 61-year-old woman initially had a bilateral breast augmentation with Nagor-textured silicone implants in 1994. She had bilateral implant exchange with Allergan, smooth implants in subpectoral pockets, and mastopexy in 2007. She presented to the Breast Care Centre of Excellence in Johannesburg in 2015 with initial swelling of the left breast. Mammography, ultrasound, and MRI revealed a periprosthetic fluid collection and mass-like enhancement on the left breast at the 4 o'clock region showing sustained peripheral enhancement (Figure 1). Family history: the father died of colon cancer. Fluid was aspirated, and cytologic smears on a tissue block were analyzed by hematoxylin-eosin stain and immunohistochemistry. The tumor cells were positive for CD45, CD3, and CD30. Additionally, CD68 was positive in a population of reactive background histiocytes. The tumor was negative for ALK-1, and CD20 was indicative of BIA-ALCL. Preoperative positron emission topography (PET) demonstrated level 1 lymph nodes on the left. The patient was discussed at a multidisciplinary team (MDT) meeting at the Breast Care Centre of Excellence. The patient underwent "en bloc" capsulectomy, which includes removing the implant, capsule, and eventual mass surrounded by a margin of healthy tissue. Surgery and recovery were uneventful. Macroscopic examination of the right breast capsulectomy tissue confirmed a fibrotic capsule showing typical pseudosynovial metaplasia. The left breast capsulectomy revealed similar fibrous connective tissue with the tumor biopsy showing extensive areas of broad coagulative necrosis with foamy histiocytes (Figure 2).

The tumor infiltrated the superficial aspect of the capsule only. The ink margins were clear. Immunohistochemistry examination of this tumor showed CD3-, CD20-, and ALK-1-negative and CD3-, CD30-, and CD68-positive stains. PCR analysis for T-cell clonality showed monoclonal T-cell expansion (Figures 3(a)–3(e)) [15]. DNA was extracted from the submitted sample using QIAGEN® QIA amp DNA FFPE tissue kit. Clonality was performed by the IdentiClone™ TCRB+TCRG T-clonality Assay. The PCR product was electrophoresed with the Bio Rad® system. The PCR showed monoclonal bands (Figure 4). The following abnormalities were detected: **A**-Vβ+Jβ1+Jβ2 regions TCRB; **B**-VB+Jβ2 regions TCRB; **C**-Dβ+Jβ1+Jβ2 regions TCRB; **A**-Vδ1-8, Vδ10, + multiple Jδ regions TCRG; and **B**-Vδ9, Vδ11+multiple Jδ regions TCRG.

These abnormalities were detected on the gel electrophoresis according to the Euroclonality/Biomed-2 guidelines for interpretation and reporting Ig/TCR clonality in suspected lymphoproliferation [16].

Histological examination of a gland removed below the low age of the pectoralis minor muscle (level 1 axillary lymph node) showed a reactive lymph node without evidence of lymphoma involvement.

Following surgery, the patient noted reduced swelling and pain. A six-week follow-up examination revealed no inflammation, reduced pain levels, and no evidence of recurrence. No axillary or supraclavicular pathological lymphadenopathy was seen.

Follow-up visits consisted of physical examination, full blood counts, serum chemistry tests, ultrasound of the breast, chest roentgenograms, and ultrasound of the abdomen and pelvis or computerized body tomography. The patient was followed up at a six-month interval for five years. Currently, the patient is followed up yearly, and she remains in remission at year six.

3. Discussion

BIA-ALCL was first reported in 1997 [17]. The risk of BIA-ALCL increases yearly, with breast augmentation being the most common surgery performed annually for women. Still, there are global discrepancies between surgeon preferences, costs, and various implant technologies [14].

The reported incidence of BIA-ALCL is increasing. This may be due to increased disease awareness. BIA-ALCL is exclusively associated with textured implants, with no confirmed cases in patients with only smooth devices to date [11, 15, 18, 19]. Like our patient, patients with smooth implants at the time of BIA-ALCL diagnosis were found to have a mixed implant history with the previous textured devices. In 2019, the FDA recommended a global voluntary recall of Allergan Biocell textured implants, following findings of increased BIA-ALCL risk with these devices [15]. Shortly following this announcement, several regulatory boards, including France and Canada, have banned macrotextured implants, thus significantly increasing public awareness of BIA-ALCL. Another possible reason is underestimating the actual incidence in published studies with a short median follow of 2-4 years. BIA-ALCL usually occurs after a median of 6-13 years [11, 13].

Breast non-Hodgkin's lymphoma (NHL) is primarily B-cell in origin (95%). T-cell lymphomas of the breast have 3 different subtypes, including anaplastic lymphoma kinase- (ALK-) negative ALCL, ALK-positive ALCL, and cutaneous ALCL [20].

Epidemiologically, non-Hodgkin's lymphomas associated with the breast account for less than 2% of extranodal NHL and less than 1% of NHL, with most presenting as diffuse B-cell, marginal zone lymphoma and follicular lymphoma [21]. BIA-ALCL is a rare subtype of T-cell lymphoma pathologically associated with CD30-positive, ALK-negative ALCL. The risk of women with implants

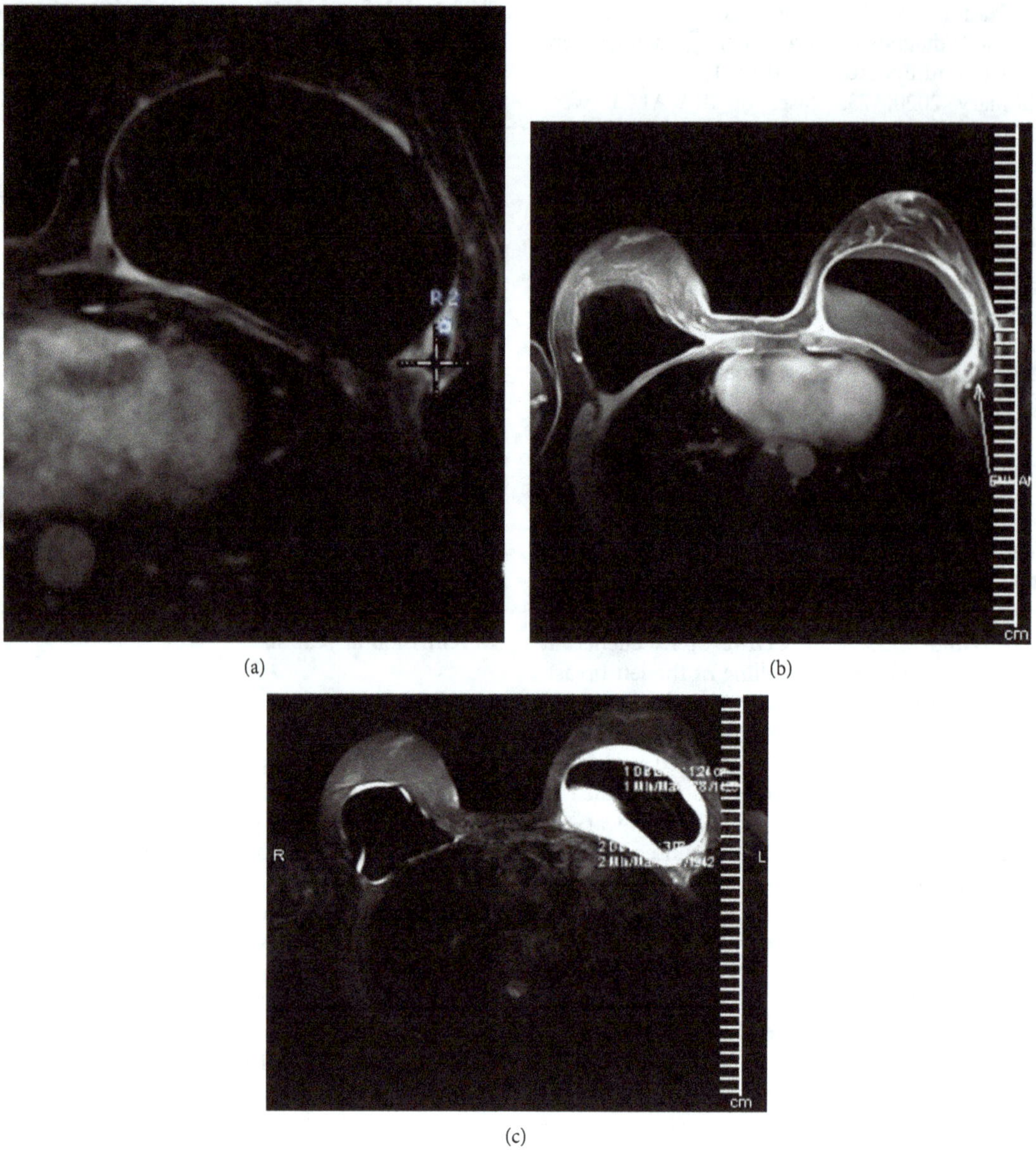

Figure 1: (a–c) MRI images of periprosthetic fluid and mass.

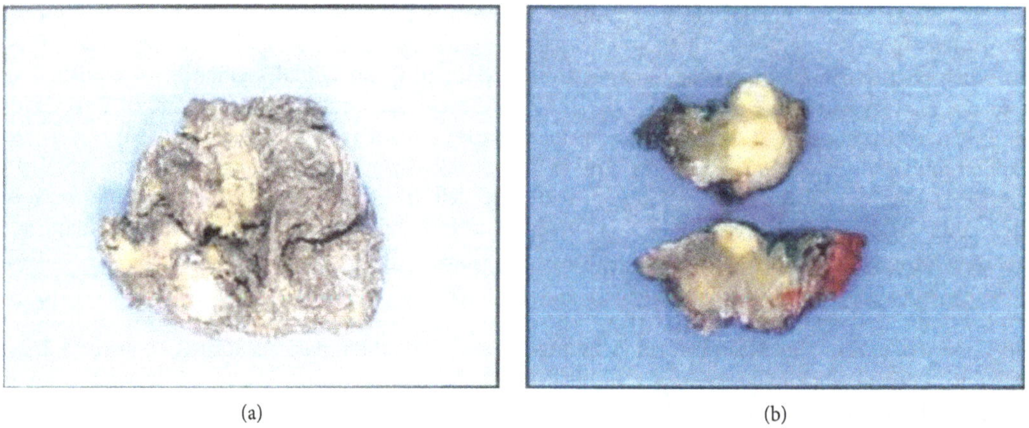

Figure 2: Macroscopy examination: (a) right breast capsulectomy with a mass of 47 g and (b) left breast capsulectomy and implant 294 g.

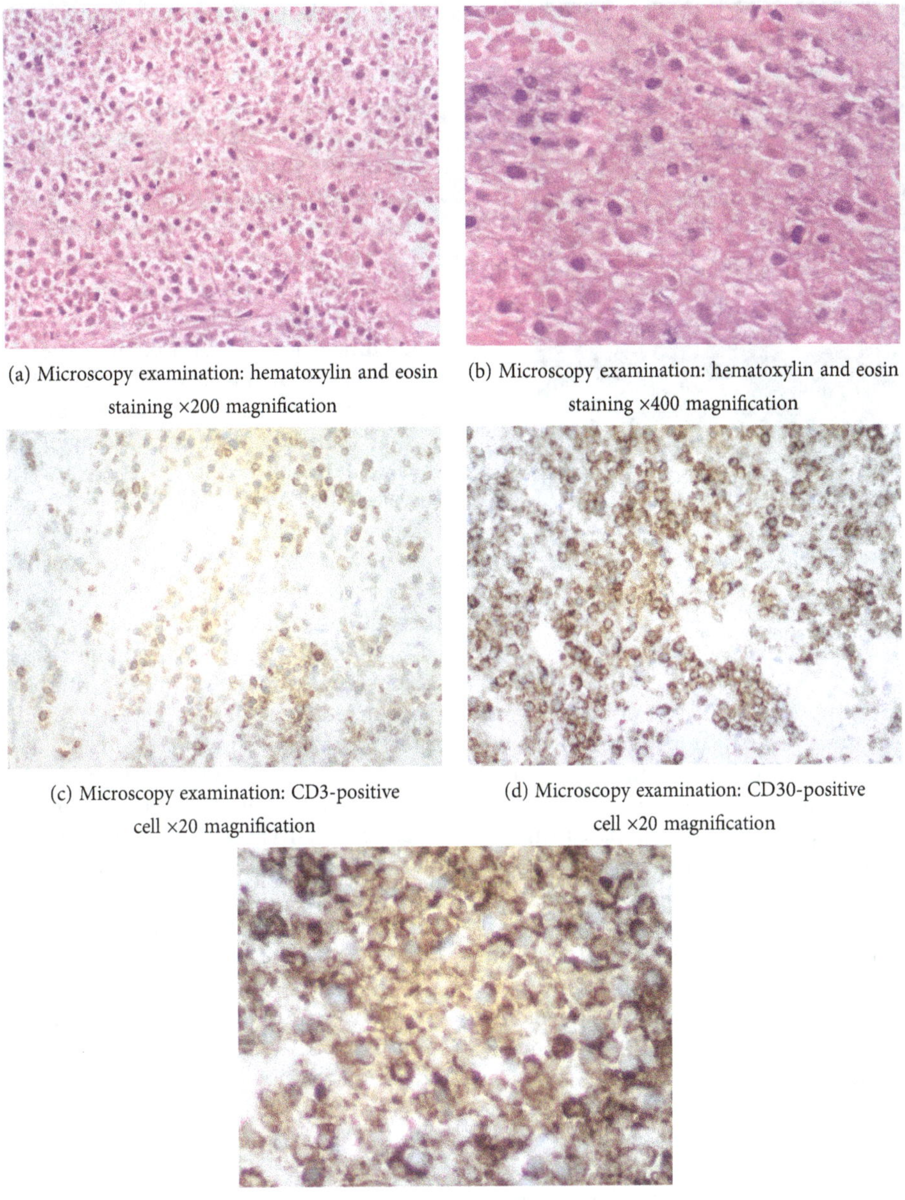

(a) Microscopy examination: hematoxylin and eosin staining ×200 magnification

(b) Microscopy examination: hematoxylin and eosin staining ×400 magnification

(c) Microscopy examination: CD3-positive cell ×20 magnification

(d) Microscopy examination: CD30-positive cell ×20 magnification

(e) Microscopic examination: CD30-positive cell ×400 magnification

FIGURE 3: (a–e) Microscopic examination.

contracting BIA-ALCL is relatively low, and it was only recently classified as a unique disease [22]. A recent European study by the Committee on Device Safety and Development (CDSD) reported 420 cases in Europe, with an overall prevalence of 1:13,745 cases in the 28 member states of the European Union (EU-28). Countries where specific measures have been implemented to tackle BIA-ALCL account for 61% of the EU-28 population and actively reported 382 cases with an overall prevalence of 1:9121 [23]. The disease is treated primarily surgically and is associated with a good prognosis with an overall survival rate of 93-94% at three years and 89-91% at five years [24–26].

The pathogenesis of BIA-ALCL remains unknown; however, chronic inflammation and abnormal immune response may be associated with this disease. The cause for such a response may be bacterial biofilm. Hu et al. found Ralstonia pickettii in more than half of diseased capsules [5]. Kadin et al. demonstrated that BIA-ALCL cells might be derived from lymphocytes with Th1/Th17 polarization in capsular tissues and surrounding seromas, suggesting a chronic bacterial antigen stimulation of the liposaccharide coat of Gram-negative bacteria and a persistent T-cell proliferation might support BIA-ALCL initiation and disease progression [27]. Another theory suggests that the immune response is caused by silicone particles shed from the surface of textured implants [8]. In a separate report, Kadin et al. showed that the BIA-ALCL microenvironment is characterized by high levels of interleukin-13 and IgE, suggesting that the immune response underlying BIA-ALCL has the profile of chronic allergic reaction [28]. Di Napoli et al. reported novel insights

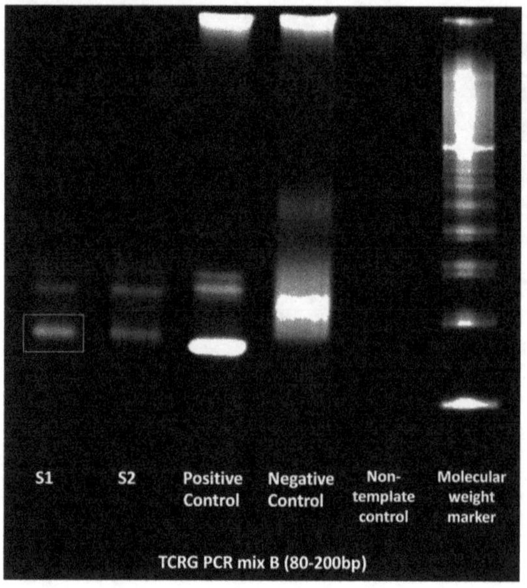

Figure 4: Gel electrophoresis showing clonal band for T-cell receptor gamma. The tumor is shown in the S1 band.

on the pathogenesis of BIA-ALCL [7]. By performing gene expression profiling, the investigators compared the transcriptional profiles of BIA-ALCL with those of normal T-cells and other peripheral T-cell lymphomas. Compared to normal CD4+ T-cells, BIA-ALCL was associated with an upregulation of genes involved in cell motility processes, including chemokine receptor 6 (CCR6), MET, hepatocyte growth factor (HGF), and chemokine (C-X-C motif) ligand 14 (CXCL14) [7]. Several reports suggest activation of the JAK-STAT3 pathway in 13-26% of BIA-ALCL cases [9].

BIA-ALCL typically presents with late seroma in 60-90% of cases [16]. It may also present with a solid mass in the capsule adjacent to the breast implant in 8-24% of cases and, less commonly, with lymphadenopathy (4-12%) or local and systemic symptoms like skin rash and fevers (<5%) [11, 21, 26]. The majority of cases present at an average of 8-10 years after implantation [29]. Patients with suspected BIA-ALCL typically present with unilateral breast swelling. An ultrasound should be performed, and if fluid is present, fine needle aspiration of a minimum of 50 ml of fluid should be undertaken [11]. Fluid is sent for cytology, CD30 immunochemistry, and flow cytometry [11, 29]. A core needle biopsy is recommended if a solid mass is present [11]. A positron emission tomography scan (PET CT scan) is performed for staging before surgery to avoid distortion for 2-3 months afterward [11].

Once the diagnosis is made, the patient should be managed by a multidisciplinary team comprising oncologists, pathologists, radiation oncologists, surgeons, and plastic surgeons. Staging investigations include serum chemistry, serum lactate dehydrogenase, C-reactive protein, $\beta 2$ microglobulin, bone marrow examination (aspiration, biopsy, and flow cytometry), and PET CT scan [11]. However, there are limitations to the current diagnosis methods mentioned owing to patients that underwent aspiration of the effusion or patients undergoing implant and capsule removal, which can affect the CD30 immunochemistry [30]. A recent report by Di Napoli et al. outlines biomarkers that might help to differentiate between BIA-ALCL from all types of benign late seromas. It has been reported that benign effusions may also have an oligo-/monoclonal expansion of CD30+ cells, challenging the diagnosis of BIA-ALCL [31]. Di Napoli et al. applied a multiplexed immuno-based assay to BI-ALCL seromas. The researchers found that BI-ALCL is characterized by a Th2-type cytokine milieu associated with significantly high levels of IL-10, IL-13, and eotaxin, which discriminate BIA-ALCL from all types of reactive seroma. Additionally, the authors found that a cutoff value of IL10/IL-6 ratio of 0.104 is associated with a specificity of 100% and a sensitivity of 83% in distinguishing effusions due to BIA-ALCL [31].

Treatment guidelines for the management of BIA-ALCL are well established [11]. There is a consensus reached between the surgical and oncology communities. In most cases, complete surgical excision of the lymphomatous tumor mass and the breast implant with en block capsulectomy is recommended. Complete surgical excision prolongs overall survival and event-free survival [26]. Additionally, if BIA-ALCL with positive lymph nodes is present, adjuvant chemotherapy may be required, with brentuximab vedontin considered the preferred first line [32]. If residual disease is present, radiotherapy is advised [11, 33]. The prognosis is favorable; a study of 87 diagnosed BIA-ALCL patients reported an overall survival of 94% and 91% at three and five years, respectively, with event-free survival recorded at 49% at five years [26]. Similar results are noted in smaller study groups, and a longer-term follow-up of 60 patients reported a median OS of 12 years, OS at three and five years measured at 97% and 92%, respectively [34].

Of interest is the fact that this manuscript is the first peer-reviewed documented case of BIA-ALCL reported in South Africa, confirmed after an extensive PubMed and literature review of cases prior to 2021.

4. Conclusion

This case describes the successful surgical treatment and six-year long-term follow-up of a BIA-ALCL South African patient.

Ethical Approval

Ethical approval was not required for this study by local and national guidelines.

Consent

Written informed consent was obtained from the patient to publish this case report and any accompanying images.

Authors' Contributions

All authors contributed equally to the conceptualization of the manuscript. AG, YR, BVDR, CB, and BLR provided clinical input. SN provided pathology input. YR, AG, BVDB, and BLR provided editorial oversight. All authors provided a critical appraisal of the manuscript and approved its submission.

Acknowledgments

Professor BL Rapoport is supported by the Cancer Association of South Africa (CANSA) and the National Research Foundation (NRF) of South Africa.

References

[1] International Society of Aesthetic Plastic Surgery, "International Survey on Aesthetic/Cosmetic Procedures Performed in 2019," 2020, https://www.isaps.org/wp-content/uploads/2020/12/Global-Survey-2019.pdf.

[2] International Society of Aesthetic Plastic Surgery, "International Study on Aesthetic/Cosmetic Procedures Performed in 2016," 2017, https://www.isaps.org/wp-content/uploads/2017/10/GlobalStatistics2016-1.pdf.

[3] A. Skelly and L. Guo, "Breast implant-associated anaplastic large cell lymphoma: a clinical update," *Annals of Plastic Surgery*, vol. 86, 3S Supplement 2, pp. S154–S158, 2021.

[4] M. W. Clemens, R. C. DeCoster, B. Fairchild, A. A. Bessonov, and F. Santanelli di Pompeo, "Finding consensus after two decades of breast implant-associated anaplastic large cell lymphoma," *Seminars in Plastic Surgery*, vol. 33, no. 4, pp. 270–278, 2019.

[5] H. Hu, K. Johani, A. Almatroudi et al., "Bacterial biofilm infection detected in breast implant-associated anaplastic large-cell lymphoma," *Plastic and Reconstructive Surgery*, vol. 137, no. 6, pp. 1659–1669, 2016.

[6] V. Tabanelli, C. Corsini, S. Fiori et al., "Recurrent PDL1 expression and PDL1 (CD274) copy number alterations in breast implant-associated anaplastic large cell lymphomas," *Human Pathology*, vol. 90, pp. 60–69, 2019.

[7] A. Di Napoli, L. De Cecco, P. P. Piccaluga et al., "Transcriptional analysis distinguishes breast implant-associated anaplastic large cell lymphoma from other peripheral T-cell lymphomas," *Modern Pathology*, vol. 32, no. 2, pp. 216–230, 2019.

[8] N. J. Hallab, L. Samelko, and D. Hammond, "The inflammatory effects of breast implant particulate shedding: comparison with orthopedic implants," *Aesthetic Surgery Journal*, vol. 39, Supplement 1, pp. S36–S48, 2019.

[9] P. Rastogi, E. Riordan, D. Moon, and A. K. Deva, "Theories of etiopathogenesis of breast implant-associated anaplastic large cell lymphoma," *Plastic and Reconstructive Surgery*, vol. 143, no. 3S, pp. 23S–29S, 2019.

[10] D. A. Arber, A. Orazi, R. Hasserjian et al., "The 2016 revision to the World Health Organization classification of myeloid neoplasms and acute leukemia," *Blood*, vol. 127, no. 20, pp. 2391–2405, 2016.

[11] M. W. Clemens, E. D. Jacobsen, and S. M. Horwitz, "2019 NCCN consensus guidelines on the diagnosis and treatment of breast implant-associated anaplastic large cell lymphoma (BIA-ALCL)," *Aesthetic Surgery Journal*, vol. 39, Supplement 1, pp. S3–S13, 2019.

[12] D. J. Collett, H. Rakhorst, P. Lennox, M. Magnusson, R. Cooter, and A. K. Deva, "Current risk estimate of breast implant-associated anaplastic large cell lymphoma in textured breast implants," *Plastic and Reconstructive Surgery*, vol. 143, no. 3S, pp. 30S–40S, 2019.

[13] P. G. Cordeiro, P. Ghione, A. Ni et al., "Risk of breast implant associated anaplastic large cell lymphoma (BIA-ALCL) in a cohort of 3546 women prospectively followed long term after reconstruction with textured breast implants," *Journal of Plastic, Reconstructive & Aesthetic Surgery*, vol. 73, no. 5, pp. 841–846, 2020.

[14] P. I. Heidekrueger, S. Sinno, D. A. Hidalgo, M. Colombo, and P. N. Broer, "Current trends in breast augmentation: an international analysis," *Aesthetic Surgery Journal*, vol. 38, no. 2, pp. 133–148, 2018.

[15] "Medical device reports of breast implant-associated anaplastic large cell lymphoma," 2021, https://www.fda.gov/medical-devices/breast-implants/medical-device-reports-breast-implant-associated-anaplastic-large-cell-lymphoma.

[16] A. W. Langerak, P. J. Groenen, M. Brüggemann et al., "Euro Clonality/BIOMED-2 guidelines for interpretation and reporting of Ig/TCR clonality testing in suspected lymphoproliferations," *Leukemia*, vol. 26, no. 10, pp. 2159–2171, 2012.

[17] J. A. Keech Jr. and B. J. Creech, "Anaplastic T-cell lymphoma in proximity to a saline-filled breast implant," *Plastic and Reconstructive Surgery*, vol. 100, no. 2, pp. 554-555, 1997.

[18] G. S. Brody, D. Deapen, C. R. Taylor et al., "Anaplastic large cell lymphoma occurring in women with breast implants: analysis of 173 cases," *Plastic and Reconstructive Surgery*, vol. 135, no. 3, pp. 695–705, 2015.

[19] E. L. Doren, R. N. Miranda, J. C. Selber et al., "U.S. epidemiology of breast implant-associated anaplastic large cell lymphoma," *Plastic and Reconstructive Surgery*, vol. 139, no. 5, pp. 1042–1050, 2017.

[20] N. E. K. DePaola and H. Coggins, "Breast implant-associated anaplastic large cell lymphoma: what we know," *Journal of the Advanced Practitioner in Oncology*, vol. 10, no. 1, pp. 54–61, 2019.

[21] C. Y. Cheah, B. A. Campbell, and J. F. Seymour, "Primary breast lymphoma," *Cancer Treatment Reviews*, vol. 40, no. 8, pp. 900–908, 2014.

[22] M. W. Clemens, G. S. Brody, R. C. Mahabir, and R. N. Miranda, "How to diagnose and treat breast implant-associated anaplastic large cell lymphoma," *Plastic and Reconstructive Surgery*, vol. 141, no. 4, pp. 586e–599e, 2018.

[23] F. Santanelli di Pompeo, M. Sorotos, M. W. Clemens, and G. Firmani, "European Association of Plastic Surgeons (EURAPS) committee on device safety and development breast implant-associated anaplastic large cell lymphoma (BIA-ALCL): review of epidemiology and prevalence assessment in Europe," *Aesthetic Surgery Journal*, vol. 41, no. 9, pp. 1014–1025, 2021.

[24] B. Z. Dashevsky, K. M. Gallagher, A. Grabenstetter et al., "Breast implant-associated anaplastic large cell lymphoma: clinical and imaging findings at a large US cancer center," *The Breast Journal*, vol. 25, no. 1, pp. 69–74, 2019.

[25] A. Marra, G. Viale, S. A. Pileri et al., "Breast implant-associated anaplastic large cell lymphoma: a comprehensive review," *Cancer Treatment Reviews*, vol. 84, article 101963, 2020.

[26] M. W. Clemens, L. J. Medeiros, C. E. Butler et al., "Complete Surgical Excision Is Essential for the Management of Patients With Breast Implant-Associated Anaplastic Large-Cell Lymphoma," *Journal of Clinical Oncology*, vol. 34, no. 2, pp. 160–168, 2016.

[27] M. E. Kadin, A. Deva, H. Xu et al., "Biomarkers Provide Clues

to Early Events in the Pathogenesis of Breast Implant-Associated Anaplastic Large Cell Lymphoma," *Aesthetic Surgery Journal*, vol. 36, no. 7, pp. 773–781, 2016.

[28] M. E. Kadin, J. Morgan, H. Xu et al., "IL-13 is produced by tumor cells in breast implant-associated anaplastic large cell lymphoma: implications for pathogenesis," *Human Pathology*, vol. 78, pp. 54–62, 2018.

[29] C. M. McCarthy, N. Loyo-Berríos, A. A. Qureshi et al., "Patient registry and outcomes for breast implants and anaplastic large cell lymphoma etiology and epidemiology (PROFILE): initial report of findings, 2012-2018," *Plast Reconstr Surg*, vol. 143, pp. 65S–73S, 2019.

[30] A. E. Quesada, L. J. Medeiros, M. W. Clemens, M. C. Ferrufino-Schmidt, and S. Pina-Oviedo, "Miranda RN. Breast implant-associated anaplastic large cell lymphoma: a review," *Modern Pathology*, vol. 32, no. 2, pp. 166–188, 2019.

[31] A. Di Napoli, D. Greco, G. Scafetta et al., "IL-10, IL-13, Eotaxin and IL-10/IL-6 ratio distinguish breast implant-associated anaplastic large-cell lymphoma from all types of benign late seromas," *Cancer Immunology, Immunotherapy*, vol. 70, no. 5, pp. 1379–1392, 2021.

[32] S. Horwitz, O. A. O'Connor, B. Pro et al., "Brentuximab vedotin with chemotherapy for CD30-positive peripheral T-cell lymphoma (ECHELON-2): a global, double-blind, randomised, phase 3 trial," *The Lancet*, vol. 393, no. 10168, pp. 229–240, 2019.

[33] P. Turton, D. El-Sharkawi, I. Lyburn et al., "UK Guidelines on the Diagnosis and Treatment of Breast Implant-Associated Anaplastic Large Cell Lymphoma (BIA-ALCL) on behalf of the Medicines and Healthcare products Regulatory Agency (MHRA) Plastic, Reconstructive and Aesthetic Surgery Expert Advisory Group (PRASEAG)," *Journal of Plastic, Reconstructive & Aesthetic Surgery*, vol. 74, no. 1, pp. 13–29, 2021.

[34] R. N. Miranda, T. N. Aladily, H. M. Prince et al., "Breast implant-associated anaplastic large-cell lymphoma: long-term follow-up of 60 patients," *Journal of Clinical Oncology*, vol. 32, no. 2, pp. 114–120, 2014.

32

Recurrent Solitary Fibrous Tumor in Intradural Extramedullary Space: Case Report and Review of the Literature

Neris Dincer,[1] **Melisa Bagci**,[1] **Metin Figen**,[1] **Adem Yilmaz**,[2] **Ahmet Mesrur Halefoglu**,[3] **Canan Tanik**,[4] **and Esengul Kocak Uzel**[1]

[1]*Department of Radiation Oncology, Şişli Etfal Teaching and Research Hospital, Istanbul, Turkey*
[2]*Department of Neurosurgery, Şişli Etfal Teaching and Research Hospital, Istanbul, Turkey*
[3]*Department of Radiology, Şişli Etfal Teaching and Research Hospital, Istanbul, Turkey*
[4]*Department of Pathology, Şişli Etfal Teaching and Research Hospital, Istanbul, Turkey*

Correspondence should be addressed to Esengul Kocak Uzel; dresengulkocak@gmail.com

Academic Editor: Ossama W. Tawfik

Solitary fibrous tumor/hemangiopericytoma (SFT/HPC) is a rare neoplasm arising from spindle cells and most commonly arising from pleura. Spinal SFT/HPC is a rare entity; hence, it is not on the top of the differential diagnosis list when a clinician faces a spinal lesion. In the review of the literature, there exist less than 50 case reports of intradural extramedullary SFT/HPC. Here, we present a 54-year-old female patient who underwent subtotal surgical excision of an intradural extramedullary spinal mass pathologically reported to be SFT/HPC and had symptomatic recurrence in the 3rd year of follow-up. Surgical intervention was unachievable and the patient was given 45 Gy to the surgical cavity followed by a 5.4 Gy boost to visible tumor with external radiotherapy. Patient reported significant relief of her symptoms. We aim to contribute to the formation of a treatment algorithm for this rare entity.

1. Introduction

Solitary fibrous tumors (SFT) (formerly known as hemangiopericytoma (HPC)) are rare mesenchymal neoplasms originating from spindle cells [1]. Although the majority arise from pleura, 60% of SFTs originate outside the pleura [2], and SFTs are deemed to arise anywhere in the body. CD34 is a sensitive marker though it is not specific, and lately specific markers are identified [3]. Although surgery with negative margins is the mainstay treatment, the role of chemotherapy and radiotherapy is under debate [4]. This report presents a case of intradural extramedullary (IDEM) SFT in the thoracic spine.

2. Case Report

Our patient is a 54-year-old female with a past medical history including asthma and peptic ulcer disease. Her family history is free of malignant diseases. In 2016, patient's chest X-ray examination found a suspicious lesion. Magnetic resonance imaging (MRI) was ordered for further investigation in November 2017 since the patient was complaining of back pain. MRI revealed a spinal lesion 12 × 10 mm in diameter at the level of second thoracic vertebra (T2) (Figures 1(a) and 1(b)). The patient was referred to surgery and one month later underwent total laminectomy at the level of second thoracic vertebra (T2) and subtotal excision of intradural extramedullary lesion with neuromonitoring. The lesion involved nerve roots; complete resection could not be achieved due to perioperative neuromonitor signals. Postoperative neurological examination showed motor strengths as 3/5 for the left thigh, 3/5 for the left knee, 0/5 for the left foot, and 4/5 for the left hand. Patient was started on corticosteroid. Left lower extremity strength improved to 4/5, and the patient was discharged on postoperative day 4. A follow-up physical examination and MRI examination were planned for the patient 45 days after the surgery. Pathology report confirmed a WHO 2016 Grade 1 solitary fibrous tumor positive

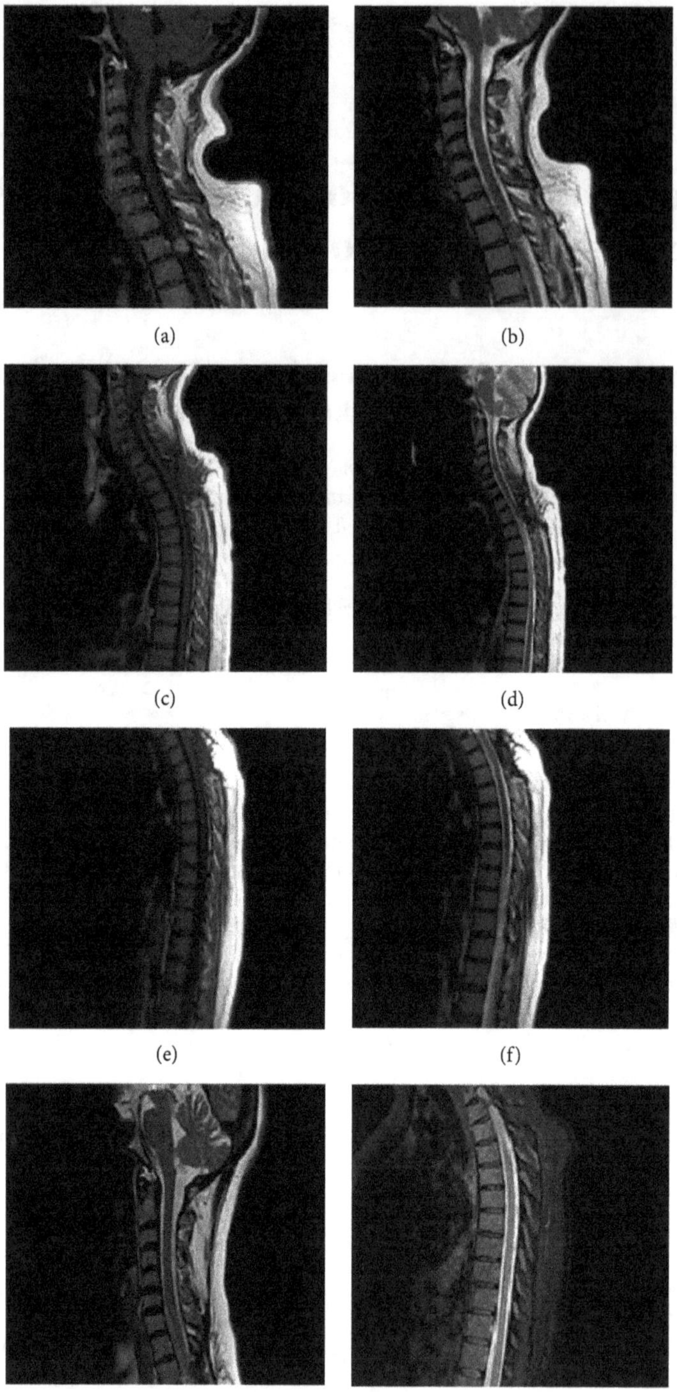

(a) (b) (c) (d) (e) (f) (g) (h)

Figure 1: MRI images on preoperative, 3 months postoperative, 1 year postoperative, and current period. (a, b) (08.12.2017) Preoperative MRI reveals a lesion 12 × 10 mm in diameter, hypointense in both T1-w and T2-w, heterogeneously contrast enhancing with gadolinium. (c, d) (06.03.2018) Postoperative MRI reveals a paracentral mass located in the posterior edge of the spinal canal with minimal contrast enhancement. (e, f) (19.01.2019) Control MRI reveals. (g, h) (18.02.2021): MRI at current presentation reveals a lesion which is moderately hypointense in T1-w and hypointense in T2-w with homogeneous contrast enhancement.

for CD34 and negative for S100, epithelial membrane antigen (EMA), and p53 (Figure 2). Thereafter, the patient underwent routine follow-up. MRI was performed 45 days after the surgery, and it was consistent with a remnant paracentral mass (Figures 1(c) and 1(d)). Control MRI a year after showed regression of the lesion (Figures 1(e) and 1(f)). In June 2020, no intraspinal mass lesion was revealed on MRI. In January 2021, the patient came for routine follow-up with a complaint of bilateral pain in her upper extremities as well as back pain. MRI examination of the

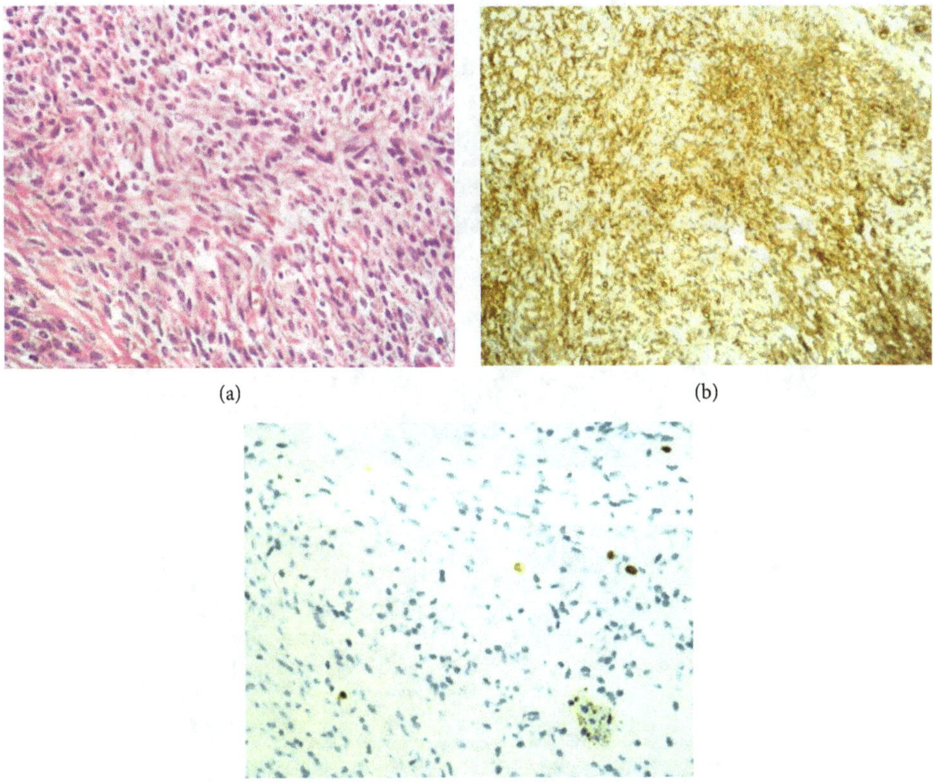

FIGURE 2: Pathology slides. (a) Hematoxylin and eosin staining of z200 magnification reveals spindloid nuclei and thin vascular structures. (b) Diffuse staining with CD34 at ×200 magnification. (c) 1-2% proliferation index with Ki-67 at ×200 magnification.

patient was consistent with an intradural extramedullary lesion 10 × 5 mm in diameter which was compressing the spinal canal in the left paramedian area at the level of T2.

The patient was presented at the multidisciplinary tumor board for treatment options. Given the critical anatomic location and close involvement with nerve roots, the patient was found unsuitable for surgery. Eventually, the board decided on the referral to the radiation oncology clinic. A repeat contrasted thin-slice MRI of cervical and thoracic spine was performed (Figures 1(g) and 1(h)). The report confirmed the recent findings. Patient underwent 1 mm thin slice treatment-planning computer tomography (CT) with intravenous contrast infusion. CT-MRI image fusion was acquired with the preoperative and present MRI for better discrimination of the resection cavity and the boundaries of the present lesion to achieve improved target delineation for treatment planning [5]. Gross tumor volume (GTV) was defined as the postoperative surgical cavity and clinical target volume (CTV) was extended 2 cm above and below the GTV. Planned RT dose was 45 Gray (Gy) in 25 fractions (1.8 Gy/fraction) and a boost of 5.4 Gy in 3 fractions (1.8 Gy/fraction). Organs at risk (OAR) were determined as the spinal cord, lungs, and esophagus in accordance with the atlas of dose constraints in thoracic radiotherapy published by Kong et al. [6]. Maximum point dose constraint to the spinal cord was determined to be 45 Gray (Gy) in accordance with the Quantitative Analyses of Normal Tissue Effects in the Clinic (QUANTEC) model to avoid any radiation-related side effect, namely, myelopathy [7]. Treatment planning was done with conformal three-dimensional (3D), intensity-modified radiation therapy (IMRT), and volumetric modulated arc therapy (VMAT, hereinafter referred to as ARC) approach, respectively (Figure 3). QUANTEC normal tissue tolerances were taken into consideration and the calculations were made accordingly (Table 1) [8]. ARC was the chosen modality with optimal spinal cord protection compared to 3D and tolerable treatment duration for patient comfort and cooperation to stand immobile during the treatment compared to IMRT.

3. Discussion

Primary spinal cord tumors are rare neoplasms that constitute 4.5% of central nervous system (CNS) tumors in adults [9]. Their primary treatment is surgical resection if possible [10], and radiotherapy can ensue if total resection is not achieved [11]. They are classified according to their location as extradural, intradural extramedullary and intramedullary. Extradural tumors are most common followed by intradural extramedullary (IDEM) tumors. Meningioma, schwannoma, and neurofibroma comprise the majority of intradural extramedullary tumors [12]. Solitary fibrous tumors of intradural extramedullary space is a rare entity. They correspond to the

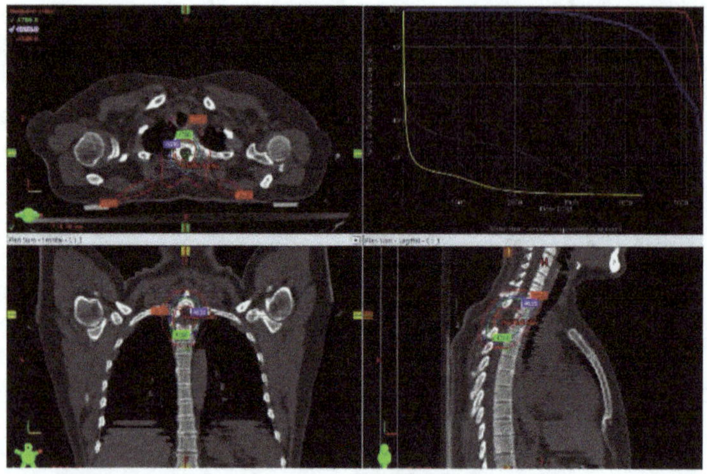

(a)

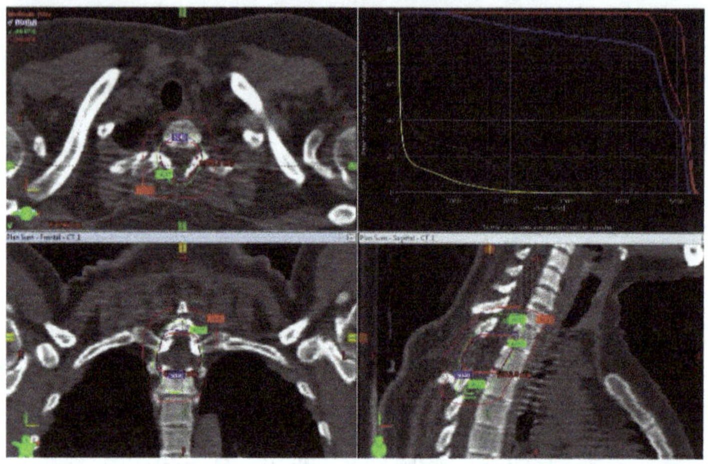

(b)

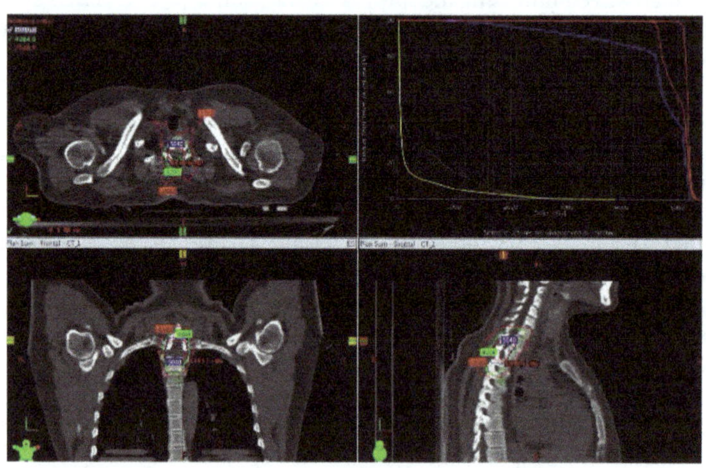

(c)

Figure 3: Plan summations and dose volume histogram (DVH) of 3DCRT, IMRT, and ARC. (a) Plan summations on axial (upper left), frontal (lower left), and sagittal (lower right) views and DVH graph (upper right) of conformal three-dimensional plan. Outer red line of plan summations represents 50% (25.2 Gy) isodose line, green line represents 42.84 Gy, and blue line represents 50.4 Gy. Red dots represent maximum point doses on each view. (b) Plan summations on axial (upper left), frontal (lower left), and sagittal (lower right) views and DVH graph (upper right) of intensity-modulated radiation therapy plan. Outer red line of plan summations represents 50% (25.2 Gy) isodose line, green line represents 42.84 Gy, and blue line represents 50.4 Gy. Red dots represent maximum point doses on each view. (c) Plan summations on axial (upper left), frontal (lower left), and sagittal (lower right) views and DVH graph (upper right) of volumetric modulated arc therapy plan. Outer red line of plan summations represents 50% (25.2 Gy) isodose line, green line represents 42.84 Gy, and blue line represents 50.4 Gy. Red dots represent maximum point doses on each view.

Table 1: Comparison of treatment plans.

	PTV			Spinal cord	Lung			Esophagus		Monitor unit (MU)
	D50 (cGy)	D98 (cGy)	D2 (cGy)	D2 (cGy)	V20 (%)	V5 (%)	Mean (cGy)	33% (cGy)	Mean (cGy)	
3D	5370	5090	5468	5437	1.7	12.5	230	839	562	455
IMRT (5 field)	5182	5067	5302	5226	2	10	190	385	255	1353
ARC	5200	4950	5333	5220	1	12	207	540	326	1060

3D: conformal three-dimensional; IMRT: intensity-modified radiation therapy; ARC: volumetric modulated arc therapy; PTV: planning target volume; D95: dose covering 95% of the PTV; D50: median dose, D98: near-minimum dose, D2: near-maximum dose; cGy: centigray; V20: lung volume that received a dose of 20 Gy or more; V5: lung volume that received a dose of 5 Gy or more; 33%: dose received by 33% of esophagus.

Table 2: Liu classification for localization of spinal SFTs [13].

Type	Subtype
Type 1: extradural	IA, intracanal type IB, intra- and extracanal type
Type II: intradural	IIA, extramedullary type IIB, intramedullary invasion type
Type III: intra- to extradural and paravertebral type	

group IIA in the classification of Liu et al. [13] (Table 2). The majority of type IIA spinal SFTs arise at the thoracic spine [12]. Table 3 summarizes the cases present in the PUBMED database.

Due to their rareness, SFTs are not on the top of the differential diagnoses list when the clinician is faced with a lesion in the spinal cord [14]. MRI is the preferred modality to delineate the tumor and evaluate for invasion, but the imaging findings are variable and nonspecific [15]. Nevertheless, the diagnosis is less of a challenge with the advances in knowledge in pathological markers. CD34, although not specific, is deemed to be the histological hallmark of SFTs and has been found to be expressed in 79% of cases [16, 17]. A retrospective study with 16 SFTs located in the spinal cord confirmed this finding with 100% SFTs being positive for CD34 and negative for EMA, GFAP, and MBP staining. S-100 positivity varied with 5 of the patients staining positive [18]. Lately, STAT6 and GRIA2 are proposed to be distinguishing markers for SFTs [19, 20]. STAT6 expression is driven by NAB2-STAT6 gene fusion, and STAT6 has lately been sought to be a specific marker for SFT [19, 21, 22]. STAT6 positivity in SFTs and HPCs is considered as finding that supports the abolishment of the thin boundary between these 2 entities in late 1990s [3, 23, 24].

Achieving complete surgical resection is the main goal in extrathoracic SFTs, and it is associated with improved local control and survival. Routine long-term follow-ups must be ensured for the early detection of recurrence [25]. Although there are no standardized follow-up routines for these patients. The anatomical location of the tumor may not allow the total resection in some cases [4]. The role of radiotherapy is under debate in SFTs. There are studies advocating that RT is not strictly indicated after complete resection due to close follow-up and low recurrence rate [4] and that adjuvant radiotherapy can be considered in the case of subtotal resection [26–28] or if we are facing a high grade SFT [29]. There are studies advocating adjuvant radiotherapy be standard of treatment [18, 30]. Complete resection, low-grade tumor and young age were reported to be factors that led the clinicians to omit radiotherapy [31]. Krengli et al. revised 151 extrathoracic SFT patients while Wang et al. reviewed 16 spinal SFT patients in terms of the effect of GTR vs. GTR+RT on local recurrence (LC), disease-free survival (DFS), and overall survival (OS), and they both came up with the same conclusion: addition of adjuvant RT improved LS and DFS while GTR was the main predictor of OS [18, 32]. While a retrospective review reveals that the median radiation dose for extracranial SFTs is 60 Gy [32], this dose seems to be unachievable in the spinal SFTs due to dose constraints of the spinal cord, which is 45-50 Gy. Retrospective single center study of Wang et al. reported a median dose of 40 Gy in patients with spinal SFT [18]. The treatment plan must be tailored according to location and extent of the tumor. Radiation doses may vary in between patients if the plan cannot limit spinal cord doses in the desired limits.

Herein, we present a case of IDEM SFT who had STR 27 months prior to presentation to our clinic with bilateral pain over the arms and legs and newly developed radiological evidence of recurrence. Radiotherapy was the treatment of choice for this patient due to the location of the tumor. To our knowledge, we present the 5th case of a recurrent SFT treated with radiotherapy [18, 33–35].

Table 3: Reported cases of spinal intradural extramedullary solitary fibrous tumor/hemangiopericytoma.

Case report, year	Age/sex	Chief complaint at presentation	Level	T1-W	T2-W	Contrast enhancement	Treatment	RT regimen (if performed)	Outcome	Treatment of recurrence
Pitlyk et al., 1965 [36]	39/M	Total paraplegia	T8	N/A	N/A	N/A	GTR	N/A	Tumor recurred 4 times in 8 years	Reoperation
Pitlyk et al., 1965 [36]	60/M	Paresthesia and weakness of RL	C4	N/A	N/A	N/A	GTR	N/A	N/A	
Pitlyk et al., 1965 [36]	49/F	Left-sided weakness and paresthesias	C3	N/A	N/A	N/A	GTR	N/A	10 years NED	—
Kitanaka et al., 1993 [37]	59/F	Gait disturbance	T6	Isointense	N/A	HomE	EBR	N/A	16 months NED	
Malek et al., 1997 [38]	33/M	Back pain Progressive myelopathy LE dysesthesias	T7-T8	—	Hypointense	Mild enhancement	Resection, NS	N/A	N/A	
Kanahara et al., 1998 [39]	62/M	Sensory disturbance of bilateral lower extremity	C6-C7	Hypointense	Hypointense	Marginal enhancement	GTR	N/A	N/A	
Brunori et al., 1999 [40]	46/F	Left sciatalgia	T12-L1	T1 görüntü	NS	HomE	GTR	N/A	4 months NED	
Vorster et al., 2000 [41]	51/M	Burning sensation and numbness in both thighs weakness in the LLE	T2-T3	Well-circumscribed mass at T2–3, which enhanced homogeneously on T1-weighted MR imaging with gadolinium	NS	HomE	GTR	N/A	7 months NED	
Kurtkaya et al. 2001 [42]	70/F	RL weakness	T3	Irregular isointensity	Irregular hypointensity	E	CR	N/A	No recurrence until the report	
Dufour et al., 2001 [43]	45/M	Paraparesis	Cervical (not specified)	N/A	N/A	N/A	CR	N/A	2 years NED	
Dufour et al., 2001 [43]	18/F	Dorsalgia	Thoracal (not specified)	NM	N/A	N/A	STR + RT	40 Gy	Alive after 4.6 years of f/u	
Dufour et al., 2001 [43]	43/F	Intercostal neuralgia	Thoracal (not specified)	NM	N/A	N/A	CR	N/A	4.1 years NED	

TABLE 3: Continued.

Case report, year	Age/ sex	Chief complaint at presentation	Level	T1-W	T2-W	Contrast enhancement	Treatment	RT regimen (if performed)	Outcome	Treatment of recurrence
Dufour et al., 2001 [43]	38/ M	Intercostal neuralgia	Thoracic (NS)	N/A	N/A	N/A	CR + RT	40 Gy	12.8 years NED	
Betchen et al., 2002 [44]	31/ M	B/L leg paresthesia LE cramping and fatigue	L4	Intermediate signal	Increased signal	Diffuse enhancement	EBR	N/A	No recurrence at the time	
Pizzolitto et al., 2004 [45]	36/ M	Paresthesias of right foot LE weakness Urinary loss and rectal incontinence	T7/T8	NS	NS	HomE	CR	N/A	12 months NED	
Bohinski et al., 2004 [46]	49/F	Neck pain and stiffness	C4	Isointense	Hypointense	HomE	EBR	NA	10 months NED	
Piana et al., 2004 [47]	67/ M	Lumbar pain Weakness in RLE	L1-L2	NS	NS	HetE	GTR	—	—	—
Ogawa et al., 2005 [48]	63/F	Sensory disturbance of LE	T11	Mildly hypointense	Hypointense	HomE	GTR	—	18 months NED	—
Pakasa et al., 2005 [49]	27/ M	Back pain	T5-T7	—	—	—	STR	—	Recurrence after 14 years	Surgery
Munoz et al., 2008 [33]	35/ M	Hypoesthesia	Sacral	—	—	—	CR	—	Pulmonary mets at 4th year	Observation
									New nodules and lumbosacral recurrence at the 6th year	Palliative RT
									New metastatic lesions in lungs and liver at the 7th year	Chemotherapy
Fitzpatrick et al., 2009 [50]	54/ M	Left paraspinal, buttock, and anterolateral thigh pain radiating down the anterior shin and left foot	L4-L5	Soft tissue signal intensity	Soft tissue signal intensity	NS	GTR + RT	NS	N/A	

Table 3: Continued.

Case report, year	Age/sex	Chief complaint at presentation	Level	T1-W	T2-W	Contrast enhancement	Treatment	RT regimen (if performed)	Outcome	Treatment of recurrence
Arantes et al., 2009 [22]	22/M	Dorsal pain associated with B/L hypoesthesia and weakness of the LE	T1-T2	Isointense	Isointense	HomE	GTR	—	18 months NED	
Moscovici et al., 2011 [51]	20/M	Mild thoracic back pain radiating to the LL progressive paraparesis fecal and urinary incontinence	T9-T10	Isointense	Isointense	HomE	GTR Patient was referred to RT but declined and went with imaging and clinical follow-up	Patient declined the treatment	2 years NED	
Ackerman et al. 2011 [52]	58/M	Acute weakness of the LE bladder and bowel incontinence	T10	Isodense	Hyperdense	E	EBR	—	N/A	
Kirkbride et al., 2011 [53]	72/M	Acute urinary retention	C3	NS	Moderately hyperintense	HomE	CR	—	—	—
Bisceglia et al. [54]	47/M	Weakness in RLE	T3-T4	NS	NS	—	GTR	—	11.6 years NED	—
Brigui et al., 2012 [55]	56/M	Neuropathic pain of the RLE LL pain and gait difficulties	T6-T7	Isointense	Isointense	HomE	GTR	—	29 months NED	
Mariniella et al., 2012 [56]	67/M	Pain dysesthesia and weakness in left arm and leg	C4-7	Isointense	Hypointense	HomE	GTR	—	1 year NED	
Shirzadi et al., 2013 [31]	49/M	Patient with a history of SFT presented with left LE weakness and B/L radicular pain	T9-T12	NS	NS	E	Debulking	—	Recurred in postoperative month 4 with multiple metastases	No intervention
Shirzadi et al., 2013 [31]	57/M	Lower back pain	T9-T10	NS	NS	E	Preoperative embolization followed by microdissection + adjuvant RT	(IMRT of 5580 cGy over 48 elapsed days) to his resection cavity	3 years NED	
Shirzadi et al., 2013 [31]	56/M	Neck discomfort radiating into head and both shoulders	C1-C3	NS	NS	E	GTR	Radiosurgery was performed on recurrence (month 6- T2-3 level)	3 years NED	

Table 3: Continued.

Case report, year	Age/sex	Chief complaint at presentation	Level	T1-W	T2-W	Contrast enhancement	Treatment	RT regimen (if performed)	Outcome	Treatment of recurrence
Drazin et al., 2013 [34]	56/M	Neck pain radiating to head and shoulders	C0-C4	NS	NS	E	CR	—	Metastasis at T2-T3 6 months postoperative	Radiosurgery
Lee et al., 2013 [57]	21/M	Neck pain B/L tingling sensation in both hands	C1-C2	Isointense	Hyperintense	HomE	CR	—	1 year NED	
Kobayashi et al., 2014 [58]	40/M	Gait disturbance and numbness in both hands	C4-C5	Hypointense	NS	HomE	Resection, NS	—	Recurrence after 17.7 years	STR
Sade et al., 2015 [59]	43/M	Weakness of LE		NS	Hypointense	HomE	Resection, NS	N/A	NM	
Das et al., 2015 [60]	50/M	Quadriparesis, numbness in B/L UE	C4-C5	NS	NS	E	GTR + adjuvant RT (EBRT) + adjuvant CT	NS	23 months NED	
Das et al., 2015 [60]	12/F	Paraparesis	T11-L1	NS	NS	E	GTR + RT	NS	9 months NED	
Kaur et al., 2015 [11]	16/M	Loss of strength in LE	T9	N/A	N/A	N/A	Excision, NS followed by RT	f 45 Gy in 25 fractions over a period of 5 weeks	5 years NED	
Basaran et al., 2015 [61]	67/M	Walking disability	L3	NS	Hypointense	HomE	Surgery, NS	—	12 months NED	
Biswas et al., 2017 [62]	35/F	Backache LE weakness	T10-T11	Hypointense	Hyperintense	NM	STR + metastasectomy	20 Gy in five fractions over 1 week to the primary residual site		
Chew et al., 2017 [63]	63/M	Back pain Paraparesis Sensory deficit of LE	T9	NS	NS	E	GTR	N/A	12 months NED	
Albert et al. 2017 [64]	10/M	RUE weakness	C1-C3	Hypointense	Hypointense	HomE	GTR	—	1 year NED	—
Tomamatsu et al., 2019 [65]	68/F	Incidental lesion on imaging	T9	Isointense	Hypointense	HetE	GTR	N/A	3 years NED	
Wang et al. 2019 [18]	21/M	Backache	T3-T4	NS	Slightly hyperintense	NS	GTR + RT	Not specified for the patient; median dose is	96 months NED	

Table 3: Continued.

Case report, year	Age/sex	Chief complaint at presentation	Level	T1-W	T2-W	Contrast enhancement	Treatment	RT regimen (if performed)	Outcome	Treatment of recurrence
								40 Gy (35-45 Gy)		
Wang et al. 2019 [18]	43/F	Backache	T8	NS	Slightly hyperintense	NS	GTR + RT	Not specified for the patient; median dose is 40 Gy (35-45 Gy)	Recurrence 49 month postoperatively	RT
Wang et al. 2019 [18]	35/F	Neck pain UE numbness	C4-C6	NS	Slightly hyperintense	NS	STR	N/A	Recurrence at month 32 postoperatively	No treatment
Wang et al. 2019 [18]	33/F	Backache	T9	NS	Slightly hyperintense	NS	GTR + RT	Not specified for the patient; median dose is 40 Gy (35-45 Gy)	70 months NED	
Wang et al. 2019 [18]	57/M	Backache	T3-T4	NS	Slightly hyperintense	NS	GTR	N/A	67 months NED	
Wang et al. 2019 [18]	37/F	Backache	T6	NS	Slightly hyperintense	NS	GTR	N/A	Recurrence at month 22 postoperatively	RT
Wang et al. 2019 [18]	40/F	Backache LE weakness	T11-t12	NS	Slightly hyperintense	NS	STR + RT	Not specified for the patient; median dose is 40 Gy (35-45 Gy)	42 months NED	
Wang et al. 2019 [18]	49/M	Backache	T4	NS	Slightly hyperintense	NS	GTR	N/A	35 months NED	
Wang et al. 2019 [18]	34/F	Neck discomfort	C6-c7	NS	Slightly hyperintense	NS	GTR	Not specified for the patient; median dose is 40 Gy (35-45 Gy)	24 months NED	
Murata et al., 2020 [35]	49/F	Chest pain	T6	İsointense	Hypointense	NS	GTR	—	Recurrence at 12 month postoperatively	Carbon ion radiotherapy-64 Gy
Kim et al., 2020 [66]	64/M	RL pain		Hypointense	Hypointense	HetE	Surgical removal, NS	N/A	1 year NED	
Glauser et al., 2020 [67]	72/M	LE weakness, pain and numbness	C5-C7	T1w hypointense (?)	NS	NS	GTR	N/A	N/A	

Table 3: Continued.

Case report, year	Age/ sex	Chief complaint at presentation	Level	T1-W	T2-W	Contrast enhancement	Treatment	RT regimen (if performed)	Outcome	Treatment of recurrence
Singla et al., 2020 [68]	50/ M	Quadriparesis, numbness in B/L UE	C4-C5	N/A	N/A	N/A	GTR + adjuvant RT + adjuvant CT	Not specified	Recurrence at 62 months postoperatively	
Singla et al., 2020 [68]	12/F	Acute conus cauda syndrome	T11-L1	N/A	N/A	N/A	GTR + adjuvant RT	NS	52 months NED	
Singla et al., 2020 [68]	38/ M	Spastic paraplegia bladder dysfunction	C7-T1	N/A	N/A	N/A	GTR	N/A	50 months NED	
Koduru et al., 2020 [69]	16/F	Weakness of RUE and RLE	C5-C7	Hypointense	Hyperintense	HomE	CR	N/A	N/A	
Dauleac et al., 2020 [70]	67/ M	Asthenia and weakness RLE	T8-T9	NS	Hyposignal	NS	CR	N/A	1 year NED	

Abbreviations are as follows: M: male; F: female; LE: lower extremity; RLE: right lower extremity; LLE: left lower extremity; UE: upper extremity; RUE: right upper extremity; LUE: left upper extremirt; LL: left leg; RL: right leg; B/L: bilateral; C: cervical; T: thoracal vertebra; L: lombar vertebra; HomE: homogenous enhancement; HetE: heterogenous enhancement; E: enhancement (not specified) GTR: gross total resection; STR: subtotal resection; CR: complete resection; EBR: en bloc resection; NS: not specified; RT: radiotherapy; CT: chemotherapy N/A: not applicable NED: no evidence of disease; Gy: gray.

4. Conclusion

Spinal type IIA SFT is a rare entity with less than 50 case reports in the literature. GTR is the required treatment option while the role of adjuvant radiotherapy and its indications is yet to be discussed. We contribute to the literature by presenting a rare case in which close follow-up ensued STR, and radiotherapy was performed when the lesion recurred. We believe that the increase in the number of cases in the literature will help and contribute to the embodiment of the therapeutic algorithm of the disease in question.

References

[1] S. C. Huang and H. Y. Huang, "Solitary fibrous tumor: an evolving and unifying entity with unsettled issues," *Histology and Histopathology*, vol. 34, no. 4, pp. 313–334, 2019.

[2] M. Zhanlong, S. Haibin, F. Xiangshan, S. Jiacheng, and N. Yicheng, "Variable solitary fibrous tumor Locations," *Medicine*, vol. 95, no. 13, article e3031, 2016.

[3] C. E. Yalcin and T. Tihan, "Solitary fibrous tumor/hemangiopericytoma dichotomy Revisited," *Advances in Anatomic Pathology*, vol. 23, no. 2, pp. 104–111, 2016.

[4] B. Davanzo, R. E. Emerson, M. Lisy, L. G. Koniaris, and J. K. Kays, "Solitary fibrous tumor," *Translational Gastroenterology and Hepatology*, vol. 3, p. 94, 2018.

[5] I. Djan, B. Petrovic, M. Erak, I. Nikolic, and S. Lucic, "Radiotherapy treatment planning: benefits of CT-MR image registration and fusion in tumor volume delineation," *Vojnosanitetski Pregled*, vol. 70, no. 8, pp. 735–739, 2013.

[6] F. M. Kong, T. Ritter, D. J. Quint et al., "Consideration of dose limits for organs at risk of thoracic radiotherapy: atlas for lung, proximal bronchial tree, esophagus, spinal cord, ribs, and brachial plexus," *International Journal of Radiation Oncology • Biology • Physics*, vol. 81, no. 5, pp. 1442–1457, 2011.

[7] J. P. Kirkpatrick, A. J. van der Kogel, and T. E. Schultheiss, "Radiation dose-volume effects in the spinal cord," *International Journal of Radiation Oncology • Biology • Physics*, vol. 76, no. 3, 3 Supplement, pp. S42–S49, 2010.

[8] S. M. Bentzen, L. S. Constine, J. O. Deasy et al., "Quantitative Analyses of Normal Tissue Effects in the Clinic (QUANTEC): an introduction to the scientific issues," *International Journal of Radiation Oncology • Biology • Physics*, vol. 76, no. 3, pp. S3–S9, 2010.

[9] K. Aghayev, F. Vrionis, and M. C. Chamberlain, "Adult intradural primary spinal cord tumors," *Journal of the National Comprehensive Cancer Network*, vol. 9, no. 4, pp. 434–447, 2011.

[10] S. Grimm and M. C. Chamberlain, "Adult primary spinal cord tumors," *Expert Review of Neurotherapeutics*, vol. 9, no. 10, pp. 1487–1495, 2009.

[11] J. Kaur, S. Pandit, M. C. Sharma, P. K. Julka, and G. K. Rath, "Intradural extra medullary hemangiopericytoma of dorsal spine," *Child's Nervous System*, vol. 31, no. 1, pp. 173–175, 2015.

[12] K. K. Koeller and R. Y. Shih, "Intradural extramedullary spinal neoplasms: radiologic-pathologic correlation," *Radiographics*, vol. 39, no. 2, pp. 468–490, 2019.

[13] H. G. Liu, A. C. Yang, N. Chen, J. Yang, X. G. Qiu, and J. G. Zhang, "Hemangiopericytomas in the Spine," *Neurosurgery*, vol. 72, no. 1, pp. 16–24, 2013.

[14] J. W. M. van Goethem, L. van den Hauwe, Ö. Özsarlak, A. M. A. de Schepper, and P. M. Parizel, "Spinal tumors," *European Journal of Radiology*, vol. 50, no. 2, pp. 159–176, 2004.

[15] A. R. Keraliya, S. H. Tirumani, A. B. Shinagare, A. Zaheer, and N. H. Ramaiya, "Solitary fibrous tumors: 2016 imaging update," *Radiologic Clinics of North America*, vol. 54, no. 3, pp. 565–579, 2016.

[16] B. Ghanim, S. Hess, P. Bertoglio et al., "Intrathoracic solitary fibrous tumor - an international multicenter study on clinical outcome and novel circulating biomarkers," *Scientific Reports*, vol. 7, no. 1, p. 12557, 2017.

[17] A. Flint and S. W. Weiss, "CD-34 and keratin expression distinguishes solitary fibrous tumor (fibrous mesothelioma) of pleura from desmoplastic mesothelioma," *Human Pathology*, vol. 26, no. 4, pp. 428–431, 1995.

[18] J. Wang, K. Zhao, L. Han et al., "Solitary fibrous tumor/ hemangiopericytoma of spinal cord: a retrospective single-center study of 16 cases," *World Neurosurgery*, vol. 123, pp. e629–e638, 2019.

[19] L. A. Doyle, M. Vivero, C. D. M. Fletcher, F. Mertens, and J. L. Hornick, "Nuclear expression of STAT6 distinguishes solitary fibrous tumor from histologic mimics," *Modern Pathology*, vol. 27, no. 3, pp. 390–395, 2014.

[20] M. Vivero, L. A. Doyle, C. D. M. Fletcher, F. Mertens, and J. L. Hornick, "GRIA2 is a novel diagnostic marker for solitary fibrous tumour identified through gene expression profiling," *Histopathology*, vol. 65, no. 1, pp. 71–80, 2014.

[21] S. C. Huang, C. F. Li, Y. C. Kao et al., "The clinicopathological significance ofNAB2-STAT6gene fusions in 52 cases of intrathoracic solitary fibrous tumors," *Cancer Medicine*, vol. 5, no. 2, pp. 159–168, 2016.

[22] M. Arantes, M. Honavar, A. R. Vaz, M. Resende, and J. R. Pereira, "Tumeur fibreuse solitaire du rachis dorsal," *Neurochirurgie*, vol. 55, no. 6, pp. 573–575, 2009.

[23] L. A. Doyle, "Sarcoma classification: an update based on the 2013 World Health Organization Classification of Tumors of Soft Tissue and Bone," *Cancer*, vol. 120, no. 12, pp. 1763–1774, 2014.

[24] C. D. Fletcher, "The evolving classification of soft tissue tumours - an update based on the new 2013 WHO classification," *Histopathology*, vol. 64, no. 1, pp. 2–11, 2014.

[25] B. Kayani, A. Sharma, M. D. Sewell et al., "A review of the surgical management of extrathoracic solitary fibrous tumors," *American Journal of Clinical Oncology*, vol. 41, no. 7, pp. 687–694, 2018.

[26] A. J. Bishop, G. K. Zagars, E. G. Demicco, W. L. Wang, B. W. Feig, and B. A. Guadagnolo, "Soft tissue solitary fibrous Tumor," *American Journal of Clinical Oncology*, vol. 41, no. 1, pp. 81–85, 2018.

[27] K. Nakahara, M. Yamada, S. Shimizu, and K. Fujii, "Stereotactic radiosurgery as adjuvant treatment for residual solitary fibrous tumor," *Journal of Neurosurgery*, vol. 105, no. 5, pp. 775-776, 2006.

[28] Y. Zhao and J. Z. Zhao, "Clinical and pathological characteristics of primary intraspinal hemangiopericytoma and choice of treatment," *Chinese Medical Journal*, vol. 120, no. 2, pp. 115–119, 2007.

[29] Y. Wang, J. Zhang, Q. Liu, F. Liu, X. Zhu, and J. Zhang, "Solitary fibrous tumor of the pineal region with delayed ectopic intracranial metastasis: a case report and review of the literature," *Medicine*, vol. 98, no. 21, article e15737, 2019.

[30] Q. Jia, Z. Zhou, D. Zhang et al., "Surgical management of spinal solitary fibrous tumor/hemangiopericytoma: a case series of 20 patients," *European Spine Journal*, vol. 27, no. 4, pp. 891–901, 2018.

[31] A. Shirzadi, D. Drazin, M. Gates et al., "Surgical management of primary spinal hemangiopericytomas: an institutional case series and review of the literature," *European Spine Journal*, vol. 22, Supplement 3, pp. 450–459, 2013.

[32] M. Krengli, T. Cena, T. Zilli et al., "Radiotherapy in the treatment of extracranial hemangiopericytoma/solitary fibrous tumor: study from the Rare Cancer Network," *Radiotherapy and Oncology*, vol. 144, pp. 114–120, 2020.

[33] E. Muñoz, A. Prat, B. Adamo, S. Peralta, S. Ramón y Cajal, and C. Valverde, "A rare case of malignant solitary fibrous tumor of the spinal cord," *Spine*, vol. 33, no. 12, pp. E397–E399, 2008.

[34] D. Drazin, J. P. Johnson, F. Shweikeh, and S. Bannykh, "Hemangiopericytoma invading the craniovertebral junction: first reported case and review of the literature," *Journal of Neurosurgery*, vol. 4, no. 1, pp. 32–34, 2013.

[35] K. Murata, K. Endo, T. Aihara et al., "Salvage carbon ion radiotherapy for recurrent solitary fibrous tumor: a case report and literature review," *Journal of Orthopaedic Surgery (Hong Kong)*, vol. 28, no. 1, 2020.

[36] P. J. Pitlyk, M. B. Dockery, and R. H. Miller, "Hemangiopericytoma of the spinal cord: report of three cases," *Neurology*, vol. 15, no. 7, pp. 649–653, 1965.

[37] C. Kitanaka, M. Kuwahara, and A. Teraoka, "Intradural, purely extramedullary hemangioblastoma of the spinal cord–case report," *Neurologia Medico-Chirurgica*, vol. 33, no. 6, pp. 377–380, 1993.

[38] A. M. Malek, S. J. Weller, D. L. Price Jr., and J. R. Madsen, "Solitary fibrous tumor presenting as a symptomatic intraspinal mass: case report," *Neurosurgery*, vol. 40, no. 4, pp. 844–847, 1997.

[39] T. Kanahara, M. Hirokawa, M. Shimizu et al., "Solitary fibrous tumor of the spinal Cord," *Acta Cytologica*, vol. 43, no. 3, pp. 425–428, 1999.

[40] A. Brunori, S. Cerasoli, R. Donati, F. Giangaspero, and F. Chiappetta, "Solitary fibrous tumor of the meninges: two new cases and review of the literature," *Surgical Neurology*, vol. 51, no. 6, pp. 636–640, 1999.

[41] S. J. Vorster, R. A. Prayson, and J. H. Lee, "Solitary fibrous tumor of the thoracic spine. Case report and review of the literature," *Journal of Neurosurgery*, vol. 92, no. 2, pp. 217–220, 2000.

[42] O. Kurtkaya, I. Elmaci, A. Sav, and M. N. Pamir, "Spinal solitary fibrous tumor: seventh reported case and review of the literature," *Spinal Cord*, vol. 39, no. 1, pp. 57–60, 2001.

[43] H. Dufour, P. Métellus, S. Fuentes et al., "Meningeal hemangiopericytoma: a retrospective study of 21 patients with special review of postoperative external radiotherapy," *Neurosurgery*, vol. 48, no. 4, pp. 756–763, 2001.

[44] S. Betchen, A. Schwartz, C. Black, and K. Post, "Intradural hemangiopericytoma of the lumbar spine: case report," *Neurosurgery*, vol. 50, no. 3, pp. 654–657, 2002.

[45] S. Pizzolitto, G. Falconieri, and G. Demaglio, "Solitary fibrous tumor of the spinal cord: a clinicopathologic study of two cases," *Annals of Diagnostic Pathology*, vol. 8, no. 5, pp. 268–275, 2004.

[46] R. J. Bohinski, E. Mendel, K. D. Aldape, and L. D. Rhines, "Intramedullary and extramedullary solitary fibrous tumor of the cervical spine," *Journal of Neurosurgery*, vol. 100, no. 4, pp. 358–363, 2004.

[47] S. Piana, I. Putrino, A. Cavazza, and E. Nigrisoli, "Solitary fibrous tumor of the spinal nerve rootlet: report of a case mimicking schwannoma," *Archives of Pathology & Laboratory Medicine*, vol. 128, no. 3, pp. 335–337, 2004.

[48] T. Ogawa, E. Moriyama, H. Beck, and H. Sonobe, "Solitary fibrous tumor of the thoracic spinal Cord-Case Report-," *Neurologia Medico-Chirurgica*, vol. 45, no. 7, pp. 371–374, 2005.

[49] N. M. Pakasa, B. Pasquier, M. L. Chambonnière et al., "Atypical presentations of solitary fibrous tumors of the central nervous system: an analysis of unusual clinicopathological and outcome patterns in three new cases with a review of the literature," *Virchows Archiv*, vol. 447, no. 1, pp. 81–86, 2005.

[50] D. Fitzpatrick, J. Mahajan, M. Lewkowitz, K. Black, A. Setton, and R. Woldenberg, "Intradural hemangiopericytoma of the lumbar spine: a rare entity," *American Journal of Neuroradiology*, vol. 30, no. 1, pp. 152–154, 2009.

[51] S. Moscovici, F. Ramirez-DeNoriega, Y. Fellig, G. Rosenthal, J. E. Cohen, and E. Itshayek, "Intradural extramedullary hemangiopericytoma of the thoracic spine infiltrating a nerve Root," *Spine*, vol. 36, no. 23, pp. E1534–E1539, 2011.

[52] P. D. Ackerman, A. Khaldi, and J. F. Shea, "Intradural hemangiopericytoma of the thoracic spine: a case report," *The Spine Journal*, vol. 11, no. 7, pp. e9–e14, 2011.

[53] M. Kirkbride, K. Heitman, and A. Szallasi, "Spinal solitary fibrous tumor mimicking hemangioma," *Clinical Neuropathology*, vol. 30, no. 5, pp. 149–151, 2011.

[54] M. Bisceglia, L. Dimitri, G. Giannatempo et al., "Solitary fibrous tumor of the central nervous System," *International Journal of Surgical Pathology*, vol. 19, no. 4, pp. 476–486, 2011.

[55] M. Brigui, S. Aldea, M. Bernier, S. Bennis, E. Mireau, and S. Gaillard, "Two patients with a solitary fibrous tumor of the thoracic spinal cord," *Journal of Clinical Neuroscience*, vol. 20, no. 2, pp. 317–319, 2013.

[56] G. Mariniello, M. Napoli, C. Russo et al., "MRI features of spinal solitary fibrous Tumors," *The Neuroradiology Journal*, vol. 25, no. 5, pp. 610–616, 2012.

[57] C. H. Lee, K. J. Kim, T. A. Jahng, and H. J. Kim, "Spinal hemangiopericytoma which needed intraoperative embolization due to unexpected bleeding," *Journal of Korean Neurosurgical Association*, vol. 54, no. 3, pp. 253–256, 2013.

[58] K. Kobayashi, S. Imagama, Z. Ito et al., "Recurrence of solitary fibrous tumor of the cervical spinal cord," *Nagoya Journal of Medical Science*, vol. 76, no. 1-2, pp. 217–223, 2014.

[59] R. Sade, M. Çakır, H. Ogul, Ç. Çalıkoğlu, and M. Kantarci, "Very rare reason of spinal cord compression: solitary fibrous tumor," *The Spine Journal*, vol. 15, no. 5, pp. 1158-1159, 2015.

[60] A. Das, P. K. Singh, V. Suri, M. N. Sable, and B. S. Sharma, "Spinal hemangiopericytoma: an institutional experience and review of literature," *European Spine Journal*, vol. 24, no. S4, pp. 606–613, 2015.

[61] R. Basaran, M. Kaksi, M. Onoz, E. Balkuv, and A. Sav, "Intradural solitary fibrous tumor of the lumbar spine: a distinctive case report," *Case Reports in Neurological Medicine*, vol. 2015, Article ID 708472, 5 pages, 2015.

[62] R. Biswas, A. Halder, P. P. Ramteke, and R. Pandey, "Malignant solitary fibrous tumor of thoracic spine with distant metastases: second reported case and review of the literature,"

Journal of Craniovertebral Junction & Spine, vol. 8, no. 1, pp. 79–81, 2017.

[63] L. S. Chew, X. J. Han, K. K. Tan, and M. M. Bundele, "Hemangiopericytoma of the thoracic spine: a case report," *Journal of Surgical Case Reports*, vol. 2017, no. 7, 2017.

[64] G. W. Albert and M. Gokden, "Solitary fibrous tumors of the spine: a pediatric case report with a comprehensive review of the literature," *Journal of Neurosurgery. Pediatrics*, vol. 19, no. 3, pp. 339–348, 2017.

[65] Y. Tomomatsu, Y. Iizuka, T. Mieda et al., "Intradural-extramedullary solitary fibrous tumor/hemangiopericytoma with a negative result on fluorodeoxyglucose-positron emission tomography/computed tomography," *Case Reports in Orthopedics*, vol. 2019, Article ID 3926903, 5 pages, 2019.

[66] B. J. Kim, E. Yoo, J. Choi, and S. Kim, "Intradural-extramedullary solitary fibrous tumor of the thoracic spine: a case report," *Radiology Case Reports*, vol. 15, no. 6, pp. 709–711, 2020.

[67] G. Glauser, N. Sharma, M. Kritikos, N. R. Malhotra, and O. Choudhri, "Cervical, intradural extramedullary solitary fibrous tumor of the spinal cord: a case report and review of the literature," *Asian Journal of Neurosurgery*, vol. 15, no. 1, pp. 204–209, 2020.

[68] R. Singla, P. K. Singh, G. Khanna et al., "An institutional review of 10 cases of spinal hemangiopericytoma/solitary fibrous tumor," *Neurology India*, vol. 68, no. 2, pp. 448–453, 2020.

[69] M. R. Koduru, S. Ail, J. Shetty, and V. Shetty, "Solitary fibrous tumour of cervical spinal cord," *Annals of African Medicine*, vol. 19, no. 2, pp. 144–146, 2020.

[70] C. Dauleac, A. Vasiljevic, and M. Berhouma, "How to differentiate spinal cord hemangiopericytoma from common spinal cord tumor?," *Neurochirurgie*, vol. 66, no. 1, pp. 53–55, 2020.

33

Management of Intracranial Metastases in EGFR-Mutated NSCLC: A Review of Literature following an Unusual Case Report

Víctor Albarrán, Javier Pozas, Juan José Soto, Jorge Esteban, Elena Corral, Yolanda Lage, Pablo Gajate, and Pilar Garrido

Thoracic Tumors Unit from Medical Oncology Department, Ramón Y Cajal University Hospital, Madrid, Spain

Correspondence should be addressed to Víctor Albarrán; vicalbarranfernandez@gmail.com

Academic Editor: Francesco A. Mauri

The arrival of subsequent generations of tyrosine-kinase inhibitors (TKIs) has significantly broaden the EGFR-mutated lung cancer therapeutic landscape. Results from the FLAURA clinical trial have pushed osimertinib to the first-line treatment for patients with advanced-stage disease, showing outstanding control rates of intracranial metastases, considerably higher than those of the first and second-generation EGFR TKIs. A progressively better knowledge of short and long-term neurocognitive side effects of radiotherapy, as well as the lack of evidence about the benefit of its combination with TKIs, has opened a debate about its indication at diagnosis of intracranial disease, at least before the response to targeted therapy has been evaluated. However, there is a small percentage of primarily resistant cases to osimertinib, mainly due to histologic transformation, acquired EGFR mutations and off-target genetic resistances that lead to a scenery of poor clinical prognosis in which radiotherapy may have a higher relevance for the management of brain metastases. We offer a review of the current recommendations for the management of intracranial metastases in EGFR-mutated NSCLC and the resistance mechanisms to third-generation TKIs, following the report of an unusual clinical case with a rapid progression to osimertinib.

1. Introduction

Lung cancer continues to be one of the first causes of cancer-related deaths around the world, being non-small-cell lung cancer (NSCLC) the most frequent histological subtype (85% of the cases) and presenting in over 80% of the patients at an advanced stage of disease (IIIB-IV).

Brain metastases are associated with a poor prognosis and significantly reduce overall survival (OS), being more prevalent in tumors that express somatic mutations of epidermal growth factor receptors (EGFR).

Over the last few years, the development of successful therapies against a wide spectrum of molecular targets, including the approval of multiple generations of EGFR tyrosine-kinase inhibitors (TKIs), has dramatically changed the therapeutic approach to NSCLC.

Due to the difficulty for conventional drugs to cross the blood-brain barrier, radiotherapy has been for years the preferred treatment strategy for NSCLC with brain metastatic disease, despite a significant rate of neurological toxicity resulting in a nonnegligible morbidity.

Promising data regarding TKI effectiveness, including their intracranial disease control rate, have led the international scientific community to discuss the current role of radiotherapy in this subpopulation of patients.

2. Case Presentation

Our patient is a 58-year-old nonsmoker woman with no relevant previous medical history, who was admitted to the hospital emergency department after an episode of disorientation following a complex partial seizure. She had been previously asymptomatic except for a several-weeks long minor headache, and physical examination only revealed mild bradypsychia and tangential speech, without any further focal neurological symptom.

Brain CT scan was performed, displaying a bulky lesion emerging from the parietal bone. This finding was later confirmed by brain MRI, showing a direct contact between the lesion and dura mater, as well as an intravascular tumor thrombus in the superior sagittal sinus (Figure 1).

An additional 18 mm intracranial lesion was identified in the left frontal lobe, associated with an incipient brain midline shift due to significant perilesional edema, together with at least four smaller brain metastases (<10 mm).

An extensive body workup was performed, revealing a 44 mm lung mass on the left lower lobe, as well as mediastinal, supraclavicular and axillary lymph nodes, metastatic lesions in the left kidney, left adrenal gland, and left iliac bone (stage cT2bN3M1c) (Figure 2).

A large-core needle biopsy of a supraclavicular lymph node was compatible with an EGFR-mutated lung adenocarcinoma (exon 19 deletion). Following current treatment guidelines, first-line therapy with third-generation EGFR inhibitor osimertinib was initiated, with an adequate tolerance and no immediate toxicity. Brain radiotherapy was deferred after the case was discussed in the multidisciplinary tumor board, given the molecular profile of the tumor and the possibility of using targeted therapy.

High-dose steroids (dexamethasone 4 mg/8 h) and anticonvulsant treatment with levetiracetam were initiated. Given the risk of dura mater external exposure, palliative excisional surgery was performed. The patient presented a favorable clinical outcome and was later discharged from the hospital. Partial response of the other intracranial lesions was confirmed by early brain CT scan reevaluation (Figure 3).

Nevertheless, three months after hospital discharge, the patient was admitted at the emergency department after a new episode of disorientation and decreased conscious level. A CT scan was performed, showing transtentorial and subfalcine herniation due to progressive intracranial disease with intense perilesional edema. After moderate clinical improvement with high-dose steroids, the patient received stereotactic body radiation therapy (SBRT) and initiated and a second-line treatment with platinum-based chemotherapy.

Progression to chemotherapy was confirmed after three months, and since further active treatment was contraindicated due to significant clinical deterioration, the patient settled in a palliative care center to receive the best supportive care, passing away soon afterwards.

3. Discussion

Nearly 25% of patients with EGFR-mutated NSCLC present intracranial metastasis at diagnosis, increasing to 45% after 3 years from debut [1]. Brain disease is a potential major complication that decreases median overall survival to 7-12 months and significantly impacts on global quality of life.

Over the past few years, therapeutic management of EGFR-mutated NSCLC has been profoundly transformed by successive generations of tyrosine-kinase inhibitors (TKIs). First-generation TKIs (erlotinib and gefitinib) entailed a significant survival improvement when compared to platinum-based chemotherapy, reaching response rates of 56-74% and a median progression-free survival (PFS) of 10-14 months [2].

However, most patients relapsed within the first two years of treatment due to acquired resistance mechanisms, being the most frequent one (50-60%) an additional mutation on EGFR (T790) that increases ATP affinity and triggers molecular pathways that decrease TKI effectiveness [3].

A new generation of irreversible TKIs (afatinib and dacomitinib), despite their promising results in preclinical models, attained response rates below 10% and PFS below 4 months in patients pretreated with first-generation TKIs, probably due to the difficulty of inhibiting T790M at a clinically tolerable dosage [4].

Third-generation TKIs began to arise in this context, with a powerful inhibitory activity over T790M and EGFR sensitivity mutations. In November 2015, osimertinib received FDA approval for the treatment of EGFR-T790M mutated NSCLC, according to data from phase II clinical trial AURA, which showed its efficacy after disease progression to first- and second-generation TKIs [5]. According to final phase III AURA3 overall OS analysis, no statistically significant benefit in OS was observed for osimertinib versus platinum-pemetrexed as a second-line treatment, although this possibly reflects a high crossover rate from chemotherapy to the TKI group [6].

Direct comparison of osimertinib vs. erlotinib and gefitinib in TKI-naïve patients (FLAURA trial) showed a significant clinical benefit with a PFS increase of 8.2 months (18.9 vs. 10.2) and an OS increase of 6.8 months (38.6 vs. 31.8, HR 0.799) [7]. These results allowed osimertinib to become a new *standard of care* in first-line treatment for patients with advanced EGFR-mutated NSCLC.

Erlotinib and gefitinib effectiveness on brain metastases reaches response rates around 36.5% and a median PFS of 11.2 months, with no reported case of complete radiological response in patients that received TKIs alone (without concomitant radiotherapy) [8].

Surprisingly, osimertinib has an outstanding efficacy on nervous central system, reaching intracranial response rates between 54% [9] and 70% [10], with several reported cases of complete remission in patients that never received radiotherapy and irrespective of the number of lesions.

Data from FLAURA trial, collected from 128 patients with brain metastases, showed a clear advantage for osimertinib, with a not reached median intracranial PFS at time of analysis (16.5 months) vs. 13.9 months for the control group with a first-generation TKI (HR 0.48).

Osimertinib had a global response rate of 91% in patients with brain metastases (versus 68% for erlotinib), and this benefit was observed irrespective of previous radiotherapy treatment. Furthermore, patients that received osimertinib as first-line treatment had a better intracranial response than those who received it after disease progression to first or second-generation TKIs.

Although radiotherapy has been the most effective approach to unresectable intracranial metastases for decades, its wide spectrum of toxicity is well known, entailing both acute neurological symptoms (somnolence, headache, or worsening of previous focal deficits), subacute encephalopathy secondary to diffuse demyelination, and late effects that generally appear after 6 months from treatment initiation,

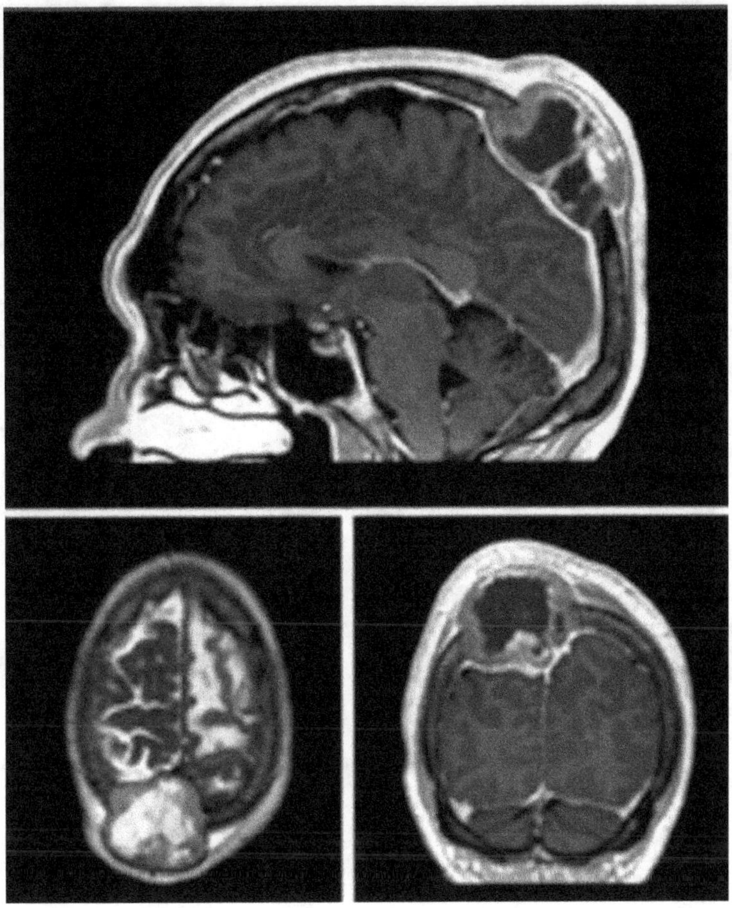

FIGURE 1: Images from brain MRI study at diagnosis.

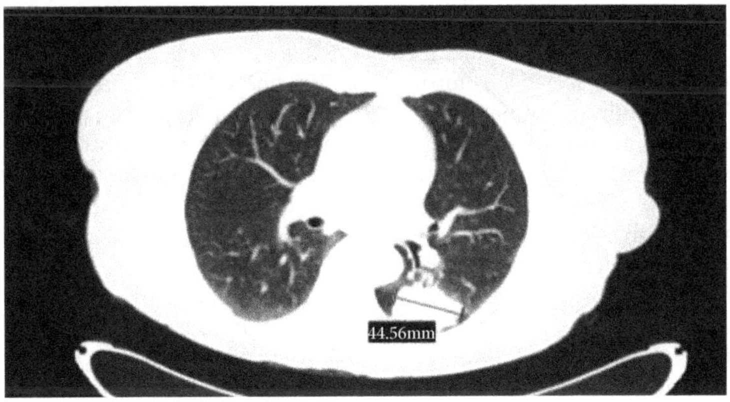

FIGURE 2: Lung mass on thoracic CT scan at diagnosis.

such as intracranial hypertension and severe neurocognitive decline.

Twenty-nine studies including 748 adults that received therapeutic cranial irradiation (TCI) and eighteen studies of prophylactic cranial irradiation (PCI) with 368 patients were reviewed in a meta-analysis, showing significant adverse outcomes in terms of cognitive and emotional functioning in 213 TCI patients (28.5%) and 100 PCI patients (27.2%) [11].

A better knowledge of brain radiation side effects and the rapid improvement of targeted therapies—reaching intracranial response rates that match or even surpass those of radiotherapy—have unavoidably led scientific community to reconsider its benefit for NSCLC with *driver* mutations.

Up to date, radiotherapy treatment prior to osimertinib initiation has not shown to increase response rates, PFS, or OS in patients with EGFR-mutated NSCLC [12].

Some authors have hypothesized that TKIs might lead to tumor radiosensitization and also that radiotherapy may facilitate TKIs arrival to the central nervous system through increasing the blood-brain barrier permeability. Meta-

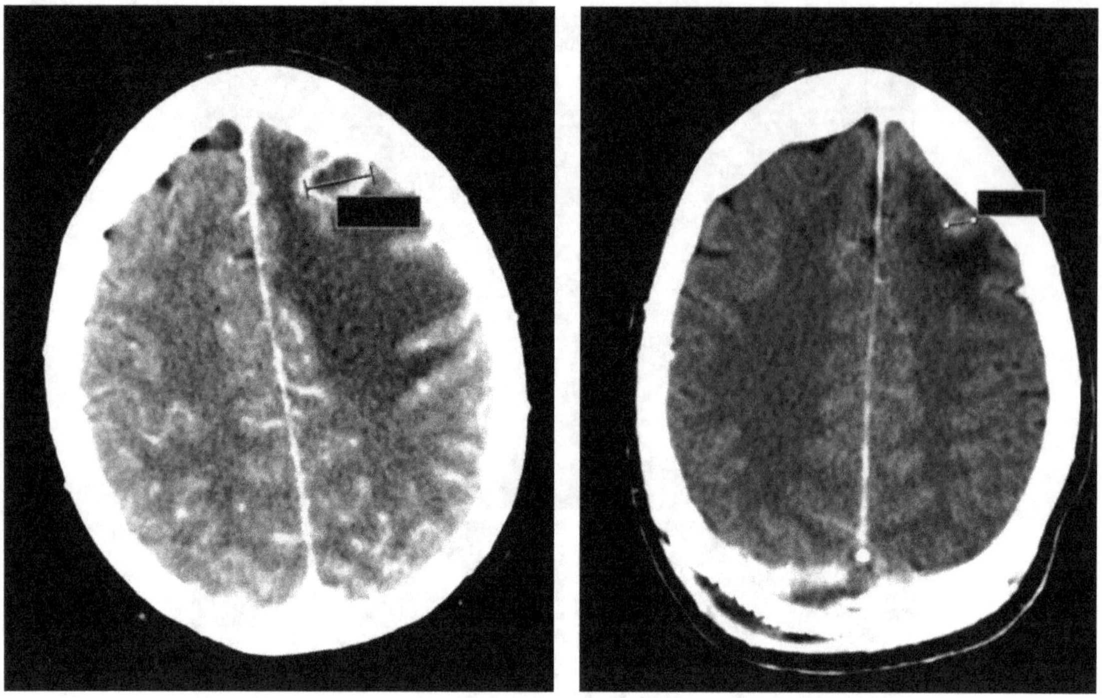

(a) (b)

Figure 3: Image of left frontal lobe lesion from CT scan at diagnosis (a) and reevaluation CT scan performed six weeks after the initiation of osimertinib (b), showing a partial response (from 18 mm to 8 mm).

analysis and retrospective studies performed so far have shown ambivalent results, being some of them favorable to the use of radiotherapy alone or combined with TKIs [13], whereas others support the use of TKIs in monotherapy [14, 15], perpetuating the discussion about the most appropriate strategy for this subgroup of patients. Nevertheless, it is worth commenting that the above-mentioned studies used only first- and second-generation TKIs as active comparators; hence, new studies with osimertinib are awaited in order to further address this topic.

To our knowledge, there is just one phase III trial (BRAIN [16]) that compares the efficacy and safety of EGFR-TKIs (icotinib) vs. radiotherapy (in combination with platinum-based chemotherapy), with a scarce benefit for the second group. Although direct comparison between radiotherapy and osimertinib alone has not been done yet, given its clear superiority to previous TKIs in terms of intracranial activity, a negligible or even insignificant clinical benefit is expected from combining radiotherapy to new-generation TKIs.

Taking into account the low incidence of intracranial disease progression in patients that receive osimertinib as first-line treatment, the rapid lesion shrinkage (median of 6 months in FLAURA experimental group), and the relevant late toxicity that radiotherapy may cause in patients with increasing survival rates, it seems reasonable to delay brain irradiation at least until initial response to osimertinib has been evaluated.

Every EGFR-mutated NSCLC eventually develops resistance to TKIs that can be essentially grouped into EGFR-dependent and EGFR-independent mechanisms. Data from AURA3 and FLAURA studies indicate different resistance patterns according to treatment line.

However, most of the available data on resistance mechanisms to osimertinib were obtained through plasma genotyping analysis that misses histological transformation rate and has a lower sensitivity for copy number changes and gene fusions [17].

Schoenfeld et al. showed that a small percentage of EGFR-mutated lung tumors are primarily resistant to osimertinib, with very short or even lacking disease response, mainly due to squamous histological transformation, acquired EGFR mutations (such as *G724S*) and off-target genetic resistance (MET amplifications, KRAS mutation, RET, or BRAF fusions) [18]. These emerging primary resistance mechanisms to osimertinib could explain the rapid disease progression in our patient and are associated with poor clinical outcomes, a context in which radiotherapy may have a higher relevance in the management of intracranial metastatic disease.

4. Conclusion

Third-generation TKI osimertinib has shown high response rates of intracranial metastases from EGFR-mutated NSCLC, what together with a better recognition of short- and long-term neurocognitive toxicity derived from radiotherapy has raised some doubts about the indication of early brain irradiation for this subgroup of patients. The existence of a significant percentage of tumors that are primarily resistant to EGFR-TKIs, usually entailing poor clinical outcomes, is an emerging matter of concern. Further research is needed for a better characterization of the mechanisms of resistance to osimertinib, the finding of predictive biomarkers of TKI failure, and the development of novel therapeutic strategies.

Consent

Informed consent was obtained from the patient for publication of this case report and any accompanying images.

Authors' Contributions

VAF and JP are responsible for the conception of the work, review of literature, and writing of the article. JSC and JEV contributed to the article writing. ECF, YLG, and PGB contributed to the review of the literature. PG supervised the work.

References

[1] H. Wei, M. Su, R. Lin, H. Li, and C. Zou, "Prognostic factors analysis in EGFR mutation-positive non-small cell lung cancer with brain metastases treated with whole brain-radiotherapy and EGFR-tyrosine kinase inhibitors," *Oncology Letters*, vol. 11, no. 3, pp. 2249–2254, 2016.

[2] C. Zhou, Y. L. Wu, G. Chen et al., "Erlotinib versus chemotherapy as first-line treatment for patients with advanced _EGFR_ mutation-positive non-small-cell lung cancer (OPTIMAL, CTONG-0802): a multicentre, open-label, randomised, phase 3 study," *The Lancet Oncology*, vol. 12, no. 8, pp. 735–742, 2011.

[3] C. H. Yun, K. E. Mengwasser, A. V. Toms et al., "The T790M mutation in EGFR kinase causes drug resistance by increasing the affinity for ATP," *Proceedings of the National Academy of Sciences*, vol. 105, no. 6, pp. 2070–2075, 2008.

[4] J. C. Yang, J. Y. Shih, W. C. Su et al., "Afatinib for patients with lung adenocarcinoma and epidermal growth factor receptor mutations (LUX-lung 2): a phase 2 trial," *The Lancet Oncology*, vol. 13, no. 5, pp. 539–548, 2012.

[5] J. C. Yang, M. J. Ahn, D. W. Kim et al., "Osimertinib in pretreated T790M-positive advanced non-small-cell lung cancer: AURA study phase II extension component," *Journal of Clinical Oncology*, vol. 35, no. 12, pp. 1288–1296, 2017.

[6] V. A. Papadimitrakopoulou, T. S. Mok, J. Y. Han et al., "Osimertinib versus platinum-pemetrexed for patients with _EGFR_ T790M advanced NSCLC and progression on a prior EGFR-tyrosine kinase inhibitor: AURA3 overall survival analysis," *Annals of Oncology*, vol. 31, no. 11, pp. 1536–1544, 2020.

[7] J. C. Soria, Y. Ohe, J. Vansteenkiste et al., "Osimertinib in untreatedEGFR-mutated advanced non-small-cell lung cancer," *The New England Journal of Medicine*, vol. 378, no. 2, pp. 113–125, 2018.

[8] H. Bai, L. Xiong, and B. Han, "The effectiveness of EGFR-TKIs against brain metastases in EGFR mutation-positive non-small-cell lung cancer," *Oncotargets and Therapy*, vol. Volume 10, pp. 2335–2340, 2017.

[9] G. Goss, C. M. Tsai, F. A. Shepherd et al., "CNS response to osimertinib in patients with T790M-positive advanced NSCLC: pooled data from two phase II trials," *Annals of Oncology*, vol. 29, no. 3, pp. 687–693, 2018.

[10] Y. L. Wu, M. J. Ahn, M. C. Garassino et al., "CNS efficacy of osimertinib in patients with T790M-positive advanced non-small-cell lung cancer: data from a randomized phase III trial (AURA3)," *Journal of Clinical Oncology*, vol. 36, no. 26, pp. 2702–2709, 2018.

[11] J. R. Crossen, D. Garwood, E. Glatstein, and E. A. Neuwelt, "Neurobehavioral sequelae of cranial irradiation in adults: a review of radiation-induced encephalopathy," *Journal of Clinical Oncology*, vol. 12, no. 3, pp. 627–642, 1994.

[12] L. Xie, S. Nagpal, H. A. Wakelee, G. Li, S. G. Soltys, and J. W. Neal, "Osimertinib for EGFR-mutant lung cancer with brain metastases: results from a single-center retrospective study," *The Oncologist*, vol. 24, no. 6, pp. 836–843, 2019.

[13] Q. Zhu, Y. Sun, Y. Cui et al., "Clinical outcome of tyrosine kinase inhibitors alone or combined with radiotherapy for brain metastases from epidermal growth factor receptor (EGFR) mutant non small cell lung cancer (NSCLC)," *Oncotarget*, vol. 8, no. 8, pp. 13304–13311, 2017.

[14] T. Jiang, C. Su, X. Li et al., "EGFR TKIs plus WBRT demonstrated no survival benefit other than that of TKIs alone in patients with NSCLC and _EGFR_ mutation and brain metastases," *Journal of Thoracic Oncology*, vol. 11, no. 10, pp. 1718–1728, 2016.

[15] S. Byeon, J. S. Ham, J. M. Sun et al., "Analysis of the benefit of sequential cranial radiotherapy in patients with EGFR mutant non-small cell lung cancer and brain metastasis," *Medical Oncology*, vol. 33, no. 8, p. 97, 2016.

[16] J. J. Yang, C. Zhou, Y. Huang et al., "Icotinib versus whole-brain irradiation in patients with _EGFR_ -mutant non-small-cell lung cancer and multiple brain metastases (BRAIN): a multicentre, phase 3, open-label, parallel, randomised controlled trial," *The Lancet Respiratory Medicine*, vol. 5, no. 9, pp. 707–716, 2017.

[17] A. Leonetti, S. Sharma, R. Minari, P. Perego, E. Giovannetti, and M. Tiseo, "Resistance mechanisms to osimertinib in _EGFR_ -mutated non-small cell lung cancer," *British Journal of Cancer*, vol. 121, no. 9, pp. 725–737, 2019.

[18] A. J. Schoenfeld, J. M. Chan, D. Kubota et al., "Tumor analyses reveal squamous transformation and off-target alterations as early resistance mechanisms to first-line osimertinib inEGFR-mutant lung cancer," *Clinical Cancer Research*, vol. 26, no. 11, pp. 2654–2663, 2020.

34

Tocilizumab Controls Paraneoplastic Inflammatory Syndrome but does not Suppress Tumor Growth of Angiomatoid Fibrous Histiocytoma

Hideaki Sabe,[1] Akitomo Inoue,[1] Shigenori Nagata,[2] Yoshinori Imura,[1] Toru Wakamatsu,[1] Satoshi Takenaka,[1] and Hironari Tamiya[1,3]

[1]*Department of Orthopedic Surgery, Osaka International Cancer Institute, Osaka 541-8567, Japan*
[2]*Department of Diagnostic Pathology and Cytology, Osaka International Cancer Institute, Osaka 541-8567, Japan*
[3]*Department of Rehabilitation, Osaka International Cancer Institute, Osaka 541-8567, Japan*

Correspondence should be addressed to Hironari Tamiya; tamiya-hi@mc.pref.osaka.jp

Academic Editor: Ossama W. Tawfik

Angiomatoid fibrous histiocytoma (AFH) is a rare soft tissue tumor that rarely metastasizes but lacks effective systemic therapy once it propagates. In some reports, high interleukin-6 (IL-6) production promotes tumor growth by autocrine stimulation and tocilizumab, an IL-6 receptor antagonist, can control AFH growth. Here, we present a case report on a patient with local recurrence and distant lymph node metastasis of AFH treated with tocilizumab. As a result, the inhibition of the IL-6 signaling pathway controlled paraneoplastic inflammatory syndrome (PIS); however, the local recurrent tumor progressed. This case implied that IL-6 is not necessarily the cause of tumor growth in AFH. Therefore, physicians should bear in mind that watchful observation is needed whether tocilizumab can control tumor progression despite the amelioration of PIS associated with the attenuated effect of IL-6 on AFH.

1. Introduction

Angiomatoid fibrous histiocytoma (AFH) was initially described as angiomatoid malignant fibrous histiocytoma by Enzinger in the late 1970s [1]. AFH often presents in the subcutaneous region in the children and young adults' extremities, with an approximate mean age of 30 years (range: 2 months–71 years) [2]. The World Health Organization's (WHO's) classification categorized AFH as "intermediate tumors of uncertain differentiation [3]." Generally, AFH is nonfatal. However, approximately 15% of patients with AFH develop local recurrence [4]. Therefore, it is often radically resected with a wide margin [5]. Sometimes, unplanned surgery is performed in subcutaneous tumors, including AFH, which may cause local recurrence or distant metastasis [6, 7]. Few studies have reported on the effective treatment for metastatic or unresectable AFH. The occurrence of metastatic and aggressive lesions is usually associated with a fetal outcome. Therefore, a multidisciplinary approach, including surgery, chemotherapy, radiotherapy, and other medical agents, is warranted to control tumor progression in advanced AFH.

Recently, the importance of interleukin-6 (IL-6) in AFH has been highlighted. Some AFH tumors produce IL-6 continuously [8, 9], promoting tumor growth by autocrine stimulation. Tocilizumab, an IL-6 receptor antagonist, which blocks IL-6 binding to the IL-6 receptor, can control tumor progression [10, 11]. Here, we present a recurrent AFH case with nodal metastasis, which we attempted to control using tocilizumab but failed to inhibit tumor progression.

2. Case Presentation

A 29-year-old female noticed a small subcutaneous nodule in her right ankle region and underwent tumor resection in 2015. One year later, she recognized a tumor recurrence at the same region. She went to another hospital to undergo tumor resection, with pathological diagnosis of pigmented villonodular synovitis. After a while, she was referred to our hospital because of re-recurrence and came with an approximately 5 cm tumor with skin breakdown in the same region (Figure 1(a)). Magnetic resonance imaging (MRI) revealed a tumor in the ankle region's subcutaneous tissue presenting isointensity and high intensity in the inner cystic region on T1- and T2-weighted images, respectively (Figures 1(b) and 1(c)). Moreover, lymph node enlargement was detected in the right inguinal and external iliac regions (Figures 1(d) and 1(e)). In our institute, histological review revealed AFH. A proliferation of uniform spindle-shaped histiocytoid cells with blunt nuclear atypia and scattered mitoses, accompanying pseudoangiomatous spaces and a pericapsular lymphoplasmacytic rim, was seen with immunohistochemical negativity for S-100 protein, smooth muscle actin (SMA), CD31, and STAT6 (Figures 2(a)–2(e)). Moreover, a chimeric transcript EWSR1 exon 7/ATF1 exon 5 was detected using reverse transcription polymerase chain reaction (primers: EWSR1, forward 5′-TCCTACAGCCAAGCTCCAAGTC-3′ ; ATF1, reverse 5′-GCCTGGACTTGCCAACTGTAAG-3′). On the first visit to our hospital, the patient's blood test showed C-reactive protein (CRP), hemoglobin (Hb), and IL-6 of 9.84 mg/dl, 9.2 g/dl, and 51.5 pg/ml, respectively, indicating PIS with elevated inflammatory response and mild anemia associated with chronic inflammation (Table 1). The treatment plan was determined by conducting an open biopsy of the right inguinal lymph node swelling, resulting in the diagnosis of lymph node metastasis of AFH (Figure 2(f)). Three months after the first visit, the tumor had been growing rapidly with severe PIS deterioration (Table 1). Therefore, we performed an additional extensive resection of the recurrent tumor with flap reconstruction. The inflammatory response quickly regressed to normal levels following surgery. At 3 and 6 months postoperation, the pelvis lymph node metastasis remained in a stable size and the CRP level increased, respectively. Eight months postoperatively, MRI showed a local recurrence (Figure 3(a)). Because the CRP level increased along with tumor growth, prednisolone (30 mg/day) was initiated to reduce the inflammatory response. However, CRP remained positive and the tumor size continues to grow. Hence, we increased the prednisolone dose to 40 mg/day and considered administering tocilizumab.

After knowing the risks and benefits, the patient consented to off-label therapy using tocilizumab, an IL-6 receptor antagonist. She received the subcutaneous injection fortnightly at 162 mg/body. After the treatment started, laboratory parameters normalized within a few weeks, with improved PIS symptoms. Specifically, the CRP level, which was 1.62 mg/dl before the treatment, lowered to less than 0.01 mg/dl in a month and was kept normal. The prescribed prednisolone, which was tapered by 10 mg every 2 weeks in the first 2 months, was eventually discontinued in 3 months. Images showed that both the ankle tumor and external iliac lymph node metastasis retained their size 2 months following the start of tocilizumab treatment (Figure 3(b)). However, the tumor enlarged up to 51 mm 4 months after the first evaluation despite adequate PIS control using tocilizumab. It indicates that tocilizumab had no suppressive effect on AFH growth (Figure 3(c)). Figure 4 shows the tumor sizes and CRP levels according to the treatment course.

3. Discussion

IL-6 was originally identified in the 1970s. Subsequently, it was revealed that IL-6 plays a critical role in inflammatory diseases (e.g., rheumatoid arthritis). An anti-IL-6 receptor antibody, tocilizumab, blocks IL-6 receptor signaling cascade via IL-6 binding to the IL-6 receptor and is commonly used for chronic and acute inflammatory diseases [12]. As previously shown, IL-6 is highly expressed in cancers and a potential promising target but with no approved drugs for cancer therapy so far [13].

AFH is a rare soft tissue tumor, having low-grade malignancy, usually occurring in children and young adults' extremities [5]. Morphologically, it is a multinodular proliferation of bland spindle to ovoid eosinophilic cells, sometimes lining pseudoangiomatous spaces and covered with a thick fibrous pseudocapsule, featuring a pericapsular cuff of prominent lymphoplasmacytic infiltrates. Immunohistochemically, the most relevant finding is the expression of desmin in approximately 40% of cases, suggesting myogenic differentiation [14]. There are three types of characteristic translocation as a causative gene in AFH: t(2;22)(q33;q12) EWSR1-CREB1, t(12;22)(q13;q12) EWSR1-ATF1, and t(12;16)(q13;p11) FUS-ATF1 [8]. Translocations are the initial or early steps in tumor formation, resulting in gene fusions. It frequently leads to the formation of novel, tumor-specific chimeric transcription factors, which can cause gene expression dysregulation [15]. The EWSR1 protein, a member of the TET family, is characterized by a COOH-terminal RNA-binding domain, acting as an adapter between transcription and RNA processing. The CREB protein is a transcription factor regulating cell proliferation, differentiation, and survival [10]. The EWSR1-CREB1 fusion gene, being the most frequent, is constitutively active to promote CREB1 target gene transcription, including IL-6. The IL-6 promoter region includes the binding sites of nuclear factor-kappa B, CREB, CCAAT/enhancer binding protein, and activator protein 1. Whether the EWSR1-ATF1 transcript detected in this tumor can activate the IL-6 gene similarly is unknown. According to a study, an excessive production of IL-6 is detected in AFH with the EWSR1-ATF1 fusion gene, similar to this case [9]. IL-6 triggers STAT3 activation related to cell growth, antiapoptosis, and inflammatory reactions and acts as an autocrine growth factor in a malignant tumor, such as renal cell or prostate cancer [16, 17]. Similarly, IL-6 may also play pivotal roles in both PIS and AFH tumor growth [10]. Thus, patients with AFH may experience systemic symptoms (e.g., pyrexia, anemia, and malaise) due to tumor cytokine production, similar to this case [18]. Several reasons exist for choosing the aforementioned treatment for this case in our hospital. At the time of referral to our hospital by the previous doctor, the patient had an AFH local recurrence and an external iliac lymph node metastasis following resection surgery. Since the tumor was self-destructing, a local surgical intervention was required. Moreover, the tumor produced IL-6, caused

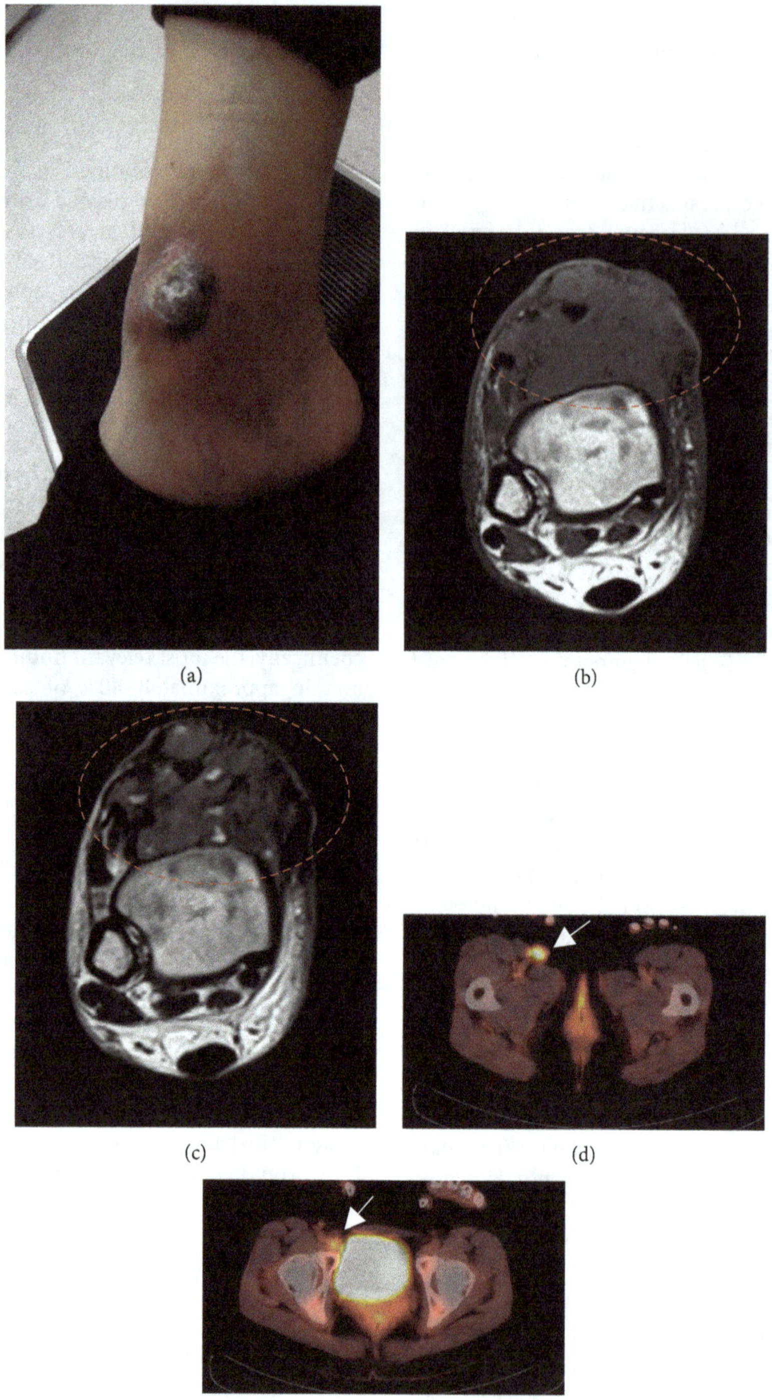

(a) (b) (c) (d) (e)

FIGURE 1: Local recurrence and lymph node metastasis at the initial visit. (a) Visual appearance of the ankle region during the patient's first visit to our hospital. (b) Axial image of the ankle region acquired using T1-weighted MRI. (c) Axial image of the ankle region acquired using T2-weighted MRI. (d) Axial image focused on the inguinal iliac lymph node acquired using positron emission tomography (PET). (e) Axial image focused on the external iliac lymph node acquired using PET.

inflammatory syndrome, and may be getting bigger, due to IL-6 autocrine stimulation. Considering the patient's general condition, we determined that causative primary tumor removal was necessary. For the lymph node metastasis, we determined that careful follow-up without resection is necessary. First, we hoped that the size will get smaller because of the normalized IL-6 production, owing to primary lesion resection. Second, radical metastasis treatment is difficult. We feared that lymphadenectomy would cause lymphedema, which could affect the patient's ability to perform daily living activity. Therefore, we decided to perform only additional wide resection of the primary tumor. Postoperatively, the

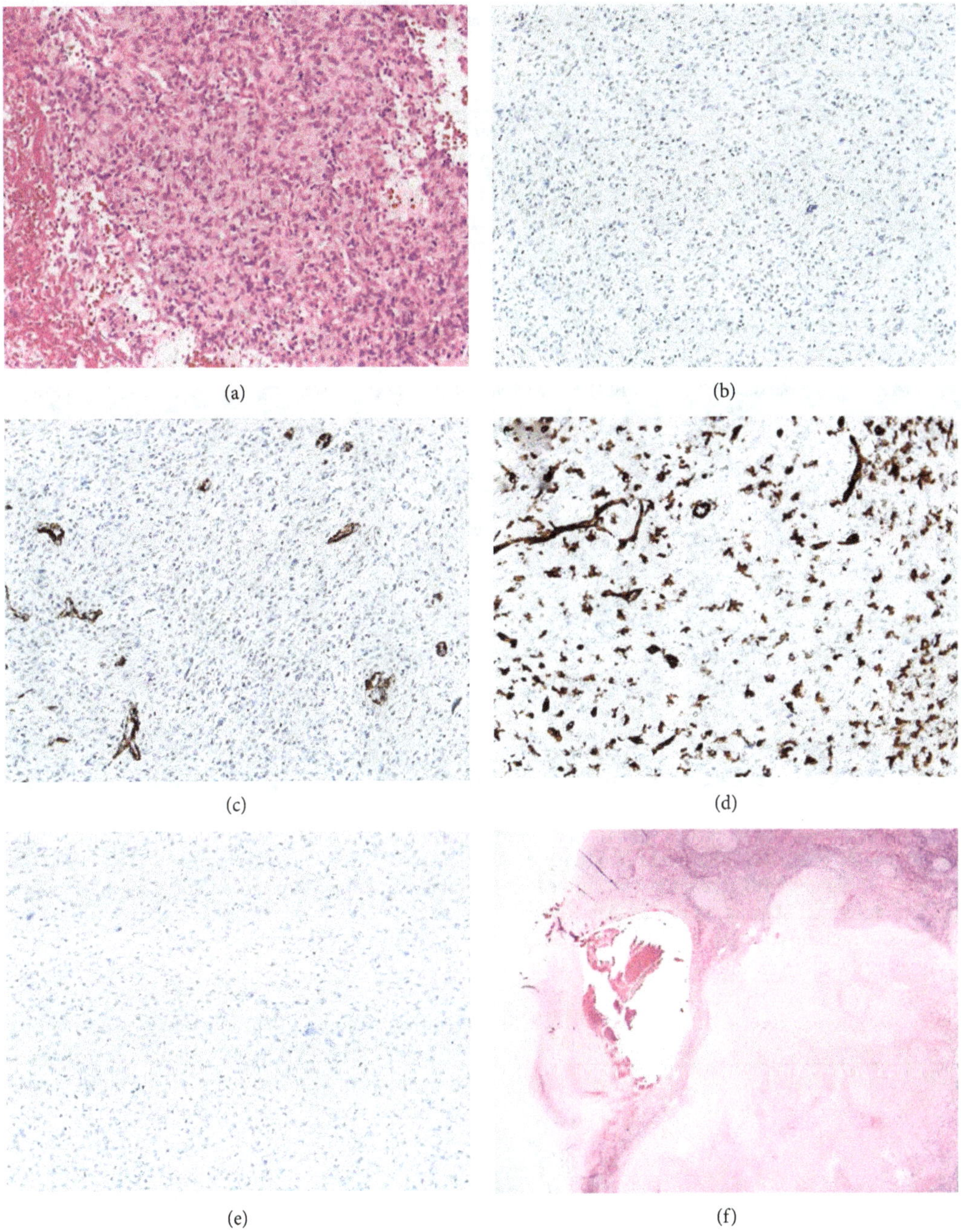

FIGURE 2: Photomicrographs of the angiomatoid fibrous histiocytoma. (a) Local recurrence featuring solid nodules of epithelioid to spindle cells arranged in a syncytial pattern with peripheral blood cells (hematoxylin and eosin (HE) stain, ×200). Tumor cells negative for (b) S-100 protein, (c) smooth muscle actin, (d) CD31, and (e) STAT6 (immunohistochemical stains, ×200). (f) Excisional biopsy revealing inguinal node metastasis of the tumor (HE, ×20).

CRP levels and IL-6 improved to normal ranges rapidly. The lymph metastasis remained at a stable size. Then, the patient had a tumor recurrence. However, we believe that the aforementioned treatment route was reasonable since we were able to treat the skin's self-destructive area, prevent lymphedema, and temporally improve PIS symptoms.

AFH's standard treatment is surgical resection [18]. Even so, for patients with distant metastasis or frequent local recurrence, similar to this case, radical whole tumor resection may be difficult. According to a study, chemotherapy (e.g., ifosfamide and doxorubicin) can effectively reduce the tumor size of local recurrence or lymph node metastases postoperatively [19]. Conversely, some studies have reported that chemotherapy is ineffective [5]. Until recently, there is little evidence for the efficacy of other treatment modalities on AFH, except for surgery. However, Villiger et al. have reported that tocilizumab may be effective to control AFH growth [11]. As described above, IL-6 is produced

Table 1: The transition of laboratory parameters (e.g., C-reactive protein (CRP), hemoglobin (Hb), albumin (Alb), and interleukin-6 (IL-6)) and the size of the tumor and lymph node in our hospital during the first visit.

	First visit	Before surgery	After surgery	Recurrence	Before tocilizumab	After tocilizumab
CRP (mg/dl)	9.8	18	0.05	2.21	1.89	0.25
Hb (g/dl)	9.2	7.5	12.1	11.3	11.4	10.4
Alb (mg/dl)	3.5	2.3	4	4.2	4.1	3.9
IL-6 (pg/dl)	51.5	N/A	0.935	N/A	12.4	N/A
Tumor size (mm)	49	55	0	19	23	51
Lymph node size (mm)	19	22	21	27	27	27

Before surgery: the primary tumor; after surgery: tumor recurrence; N/A: not applicable.

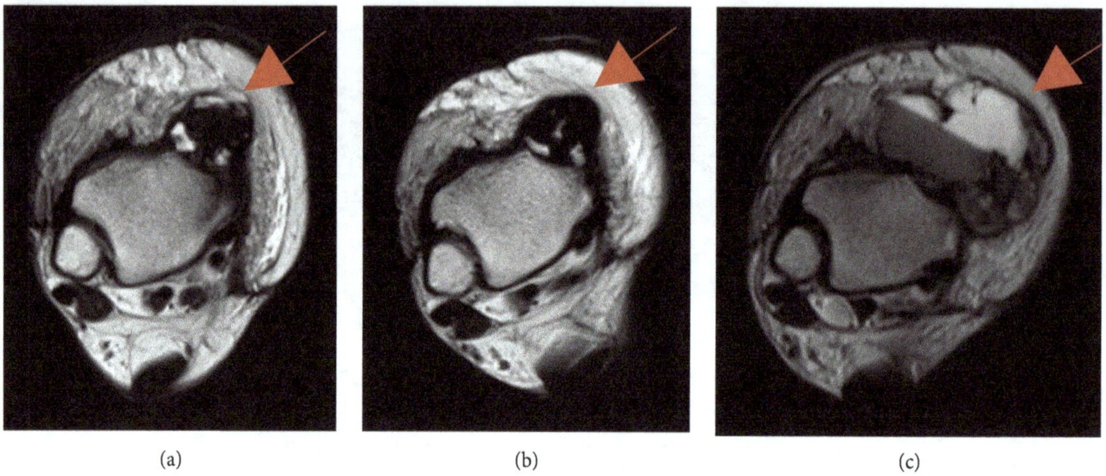

Figure 3: Tumor progression of the local recurrent tumor during tocilizumab treatment. (a) Axial image of the recurrence tumor in the ankle region acquired using T2-weighted MRI at the time of recurrence. (b) Axial image of the recurrence tumor in the ankle region acquired using T2-weighted MRI 2 months after starting on tocilizumab treatment. (c) Axial image of the recurrence tumor in the ankle region acquired using T2-weighted MRI 4 months after the first evaluation. The tumor is indicated by the arrows in red.

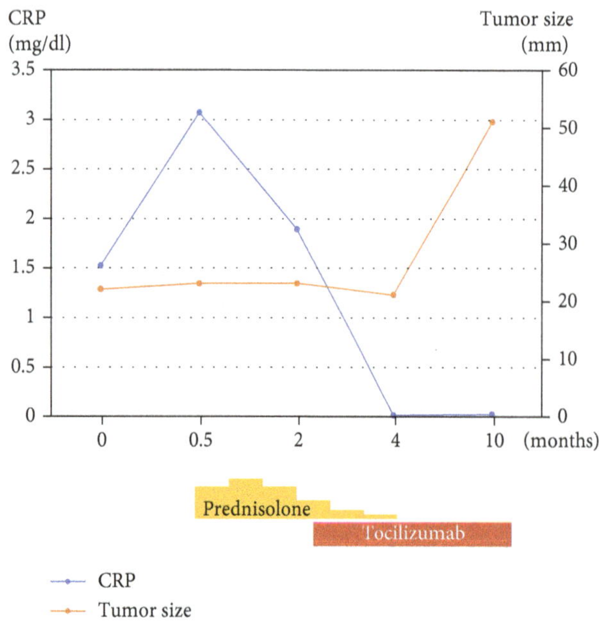

Figure 4: Scheme of the treatment indicating the tumor sizes and CRP levels. The time of tumor recurrence was regarded as time zero.

continuously in AFH, which may promote tumor growth by autocrine stimulation [10]. Hence, using tocilizumab to block the effects of IL-6 may control AFH growth [11, 20]. Based on these reports, we obtained the patient's consent to try this off-label therapy after explaining its risks and benefits. Tocilizumab was able to suppress tumor growth temporally. However, this effect did not last—eventually, the tumor progressed.

The role of IL-6 in AFH is unclear. However, this case report suggests that IL-6 is not necessarily critical for the AFH growth and controlling tumor growth with tocilizumab only is difficult. Following tocilizumab administration, the CRP level rapidly became normal and PIS symptoms, such as anemia or malaise, improved. In conclusion, tocilizumab can control PIS caused by inhibiting the effects of IL-6, although it does not always suppress tumor growth. In addition, moderate doses of prednisolone could suppress PIS. Considering the side effects of a moderate-dose steroid, tocilizumab was more suitable in suppressing PIS.

According to other studies, tocilizumab treatment for patients with AFH associated with EWSR1-ATF1 translocations did not suppress tumor progression [9]. A difference in tocilizumab's tumor suppression between EWSR1-ATF1 and EWSR1-CREB1 translocations possibly exists. Further investigation is warranted to clarify the difference in these fusion genes.

Consent

The patient provided consent to participate and for the publication of this case report.

Authors' Contributions

All authors reviewed and approved the final manuscript.

Acknowledgments

The paper was supported by JSPS KAKENHI (grant numbers 18K16639 and 21K16670).

References

[1] F. M. Enzinger, "Angiomatoid malignant fibrous histiocytoma. A distinct fibrohistiocytic tumor of children and young adults simulating a vascular neoplasm," *Cancer*, vol. 44, no. 6, pp. 2147–2157, 1979.

[2] K. Thway, "Angiomatoid fibrous histiocytoma: a review with recent genetic findings," *Archives of Pathology and Laboratory Medicine*, vol. 132, no. 2, pp. 273–277, 2008.

[3] WHO Classification of Tumours Editorial Board, "Soft tissue and bone tumours: WHO classification of tumors 5th edition," IARC Press, 2020.

[4] C. D. M. Fletcher, "The evolving classification of soft tissue tumours - an update based on the new 2013 WHO classification," *Histopathology*, vol. 64, no. 1, pp. 2–11, 2014.

[5] K. Saito, E. Kobayashi, A. Yoshida et al., "Angiomatoid fibrous histiocytoma: a series of seven cases including genetically confirmed aggressive cases and a literature review," *BMC Musculoskeletal Disorders*, vol. 18, no. 1, p. 31, 2017.

[6] K. Kikuta, R. Nakayama, S. Yamaguchi et al., "Wide-spread ignorance on the treatment of subcutaneous malignant tumors; a questionnaire-based study," *Japanese Journal of Clinical Oncology*, vol. 48, no. 2, pp. 130–134, 2018.

[7] K. Hashimoto, S. Nishimura, R. Kakinoki, and M. Akagi, "Treatment of angiomatoid fibrous histiocytoma after unplanned excision: a case report," *BMC Research Notes*, vol. 11, no. 1, p. 628, 2018.

[8] K. Thway and C. Fisher, "Tumors with EWSR1-CREB1 and EWSR1-ATF1 fusions," *The American Journal of Surgical Pathology*, vol. 36, no. 7, pp. e1–e11, 2012.

[9] L. Eberst, P. A. Cassier, M. Brahmi, F. Tirode, and J.-Y. Blay, "Tocilizumab for the treatment of paraneoplastic inflammatory syndrome associated with angiomatoid fibrous histiocytoma," *ESMO Open*, vol. 5, no. 3, article e000756, 2020.

[10] M. Akiyama, M. Yamaoka, Y. Mikami-Terao et al., "Paraneoplastic syndrome of angiomatoid fibrous histiocytoma may be caused by EWSR1-CREB1 fusion-induced excessive interleukin-6 production," *Journal of Pediatric Hematology/Oncology*, vol. 37, no. 7, pp. 554–559, 2015.

[11] P. M. Villiger, S. Cottier, M. Jonczy, V. H. Koelzer, P. Roux-Lombard, and S. Adler, "A simple Baker's cyst? Tocilizumab remits paraneoplastic signs and controls growth of IL-6-producing angiomatoid malignant fibrous histiocytoma," *Rheumatology*, vol. 53, no. 7, pp. 1350–1352, 2014.

[12] S. Kang, M. Narazaki, H. Metwally, and T. Kishimoto, "Historical overview of the interleukin-6 family cytokine," *Journal of Experimental Medicine*, vol. 217, no. 5, pp. 1–10, 2020.

[13] N. Kumari, B. S. Dwarakanath, A. Das, and A. N. Bhatt, "Role of interleukin-6 in cancer progression and therapeutic resistance," *Tumor Biology*, vol. 37, no. 9, pp. 11553–11572, 2016.

[14] S. Rossi, K. Szuhai, M. Ijszenga et al., "EWSR1-CREB1 and EWSR1-ATF1 fusion genes in angiomatoid fibrous histiocytoma," *Clinical Cancer Research*, vol. 13, no. 24, pp. 7322–7328, 2007.

[15] K. Thway and C. Fisher, "Angiomatoid fibrous histiocytoma: the current status of pathology and genetics," *Archives of Pathology & Laboratory Medicine*, vol. 139, no. 5, pp. 674–682, 2015.

[16] L. Alberti, M. C. Thomachot, T. Bachelot, C. Menetrier-Caux, I. Puisieux, and J. Y. Blay, "IL-6 as an intracrine growth factor for renal carcinoma cell lines," *International Journal of Cancer*, vol. 111, no. 5, pp. 653–661, 2004.

[17] W. Xiao, D. R. Hodge, L. Wang, X. Yang, X. Zhang, and W. L. Farrar, "Co-operative functions between nuclear factors NFκB and CCAT/enhancer-binding protein-β (C/EBP-β) regulate the IL-6 promoter in autocrine human prostate cancer cells," *The Prostate*, vol. 61, no. 4, pp. 354–370, 2004.

[18] A. Bauer, B. Jackson, E. Marner, and D. Gilbertson-Dahdal, "Angiomatoid fibrous Histiocytoma: a case report and review of the literature," *Journal of Radiology Case Reports*, vol. 6, no. 11, pp. 8–15, 2012.

[19] S. Ogden, S. Harave, J. McPartland et al., "Angiomatoid fibrous histiocytoma: a case of local recurrence and metastases to loco-regional lymph nodes that responded to chemotherapy," *Pediatric Blood & Cancer*, vol. 64, no. 6, article e26376, 2017.

[20] S. L. Potter, N. M. Quintanilla, D. K. Johnston, B. Naik-Mathuria, and R. Venkatramani, "Therapeutic response of metastatic angiomatoid fibrous histiocytoma carrying EWSR1-CREB1 fusion to the interleukin-6 receptor antibody tocilizumab," *Pediatric Blood & Cancer*, vol. 65, no. 10, article e27291, 2018.

35

An Unusual Association between Neurofibromatosis Type 1 and Diffuse B Cell Lymphoma

Anas Bizanti,[1] Ariege Bizanti,[2] Ahmad Al-abdouh,[1] Mohammed Mohammed,[1] and Maria Pardi[1]

[1]*Saint Agnes Hospital, Baltimore, MA, USA*
[2]*University of Central Florida, Orlando, FL, USA*

Correspondence should be addressed to Anas Bizanti; anasbiza@gmail.com

Academic Editor: Raffaele Palmirotta

Neurofibromatosis type 1 (NF-1) is known to be associated with increased risk of malignancy by at least fourfold. Malignant lymphomas are rare in adults with NF-1. Hereby, we present a 75-year-old male with NF-1 complaining of weakness, nausea, and vomiting associated with abdominal pain. Three months prior to presentation, he had suffered a motor vehicle accident (MVA) resulting in multiple rib fractures that was seen in chest X-ray. For the following three months, he had intermittent chest pain, but it was attributed to the recent rib fracture. During this admission, the severity of chest pain worsened and the associated vomiting inclined further investigation; including CT imaging and bone biopsy, it was revealed to be a rare case of diffuse B cell lymphoma in a patient with NF-1. However, we believe the recent MVA caused an anchoring bias in making a prompt diagnosis. In addition, the appearance of the neurofibroma, resulted in suboptimal physical examination, and hence, there was a delay in reaching the diagnosis. We will discuss here the presentation of this case, to highlight the rare association and to increase awareness of when encountering a challenging diagnosis.

1. Introduction

Neurofibromatosis type 1 (NF-1) or von Recklinghausen disease is known to be associated with increased risk of malignancy by at least fourfold [1]. Most commonly seen are nervous system tumors like optic gliomas, neurofibromyosarcomas, and leukemia [2]. Malignant lymphomas are rare in adults with NF-1 [3–5]. Hereby, we present a rare case of diffuse B cell lymphoma in a patient with NF-1 since childhood.

2. Case Presentation

A 75-year-old male with NF-1 presented generalized weakness, nausea, and vomiting for three months associated with intermittent epigastric abdominal pain, unspecified weight loss, anorexia, and progressive increase in the number of neurofibromas on the anterior and posterior trunks. His medical history was significant for atrial fibrillation on warfarin and a motor vehicle accident (MVA) that resulted in multiple rib fractures and a grade 1 liver laceration two months prior to presentation. Since the MVA, he has suffered from intermittent abdominal pain that required multiple urgent clinic visits; however, his complaints were attributed to the MVA and dismissed. Physical examination findings included a soft mass in the umbilical area that measured about 8×4 cm, was tender to palpation, and had well-defined margins. In addition, he had multiple, small-sized, flesh-colored, dome-shaped fibromas clustered on the trunk, abdomen, and upper extremities (Figure 1). Laboratory investigations demonstrated WBC count 20.0 K/μl with predominant neutrophils, calcium 16.2 mg/dl, parathyroid hormone (PTH) 9.5 pg/ml, PTH-related protein 2.6 pmol/ml, and vitamin D level 15.9 ng/ml. A computed tomography (CT) scan of the abdomen showed a dominant, oval-shaped, soft tissue density in the middle of the upper abdomen, superficial to the abdominal aorta and multiple paraesophageal lymphadenopathy, the largest measuring $8 \times 4 \times 6$ cm (Figure 2). Pathology

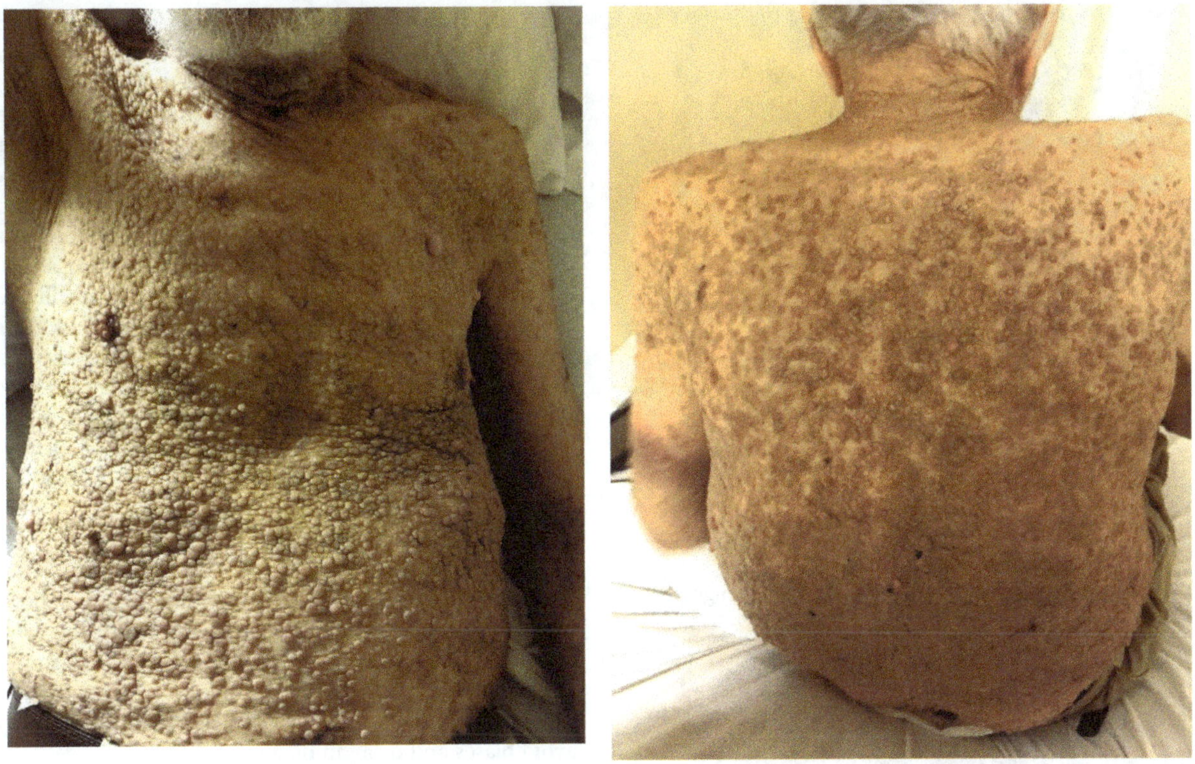

(a) (b)

FIGURE 1: (a, b) The classic neurofibromas of neurofibromatosis type 1 covering the entire surface of the upper extremities and trunk.

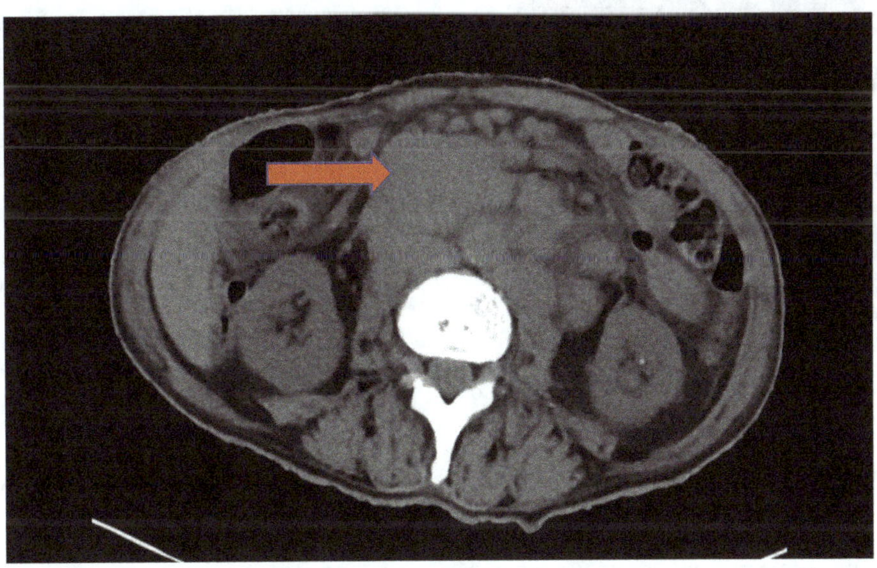

FIGURE 2: CT of the abdomen, axial view, showing a soft tissue mass anterior to the abdominal aorta and posterior to the body of the pancreas measuring 8 × 6 × 4 cm (red arrow) representing lymphadenopathy from the diffuse B cell lymphoma.

from a CT-guided biopsy of a retroperitoneal lymph node was consistent with diffuse large B cell lymphoma (DLBCL) (Figures 3 and 4). Bone marrow aspirates did not show atypical cells. Hypercalcemia was managed medically. Subsequently, he was started on treatment with chemotherapy (CHOP). He tolerated the first cycle well with no major side effects and was discharged to a rehabilitation program.

3. Discussion

NF-1 is known to be a significant risk factor for malignancy, mainly the peripheral nerve sheath tumors, gliomas, and leukemia. Various studies have estimated the frequency of malignancy in NF-1 patients to be between 5% and 29% [6]. Overall, diffuse B cell lymphoma were reported to be

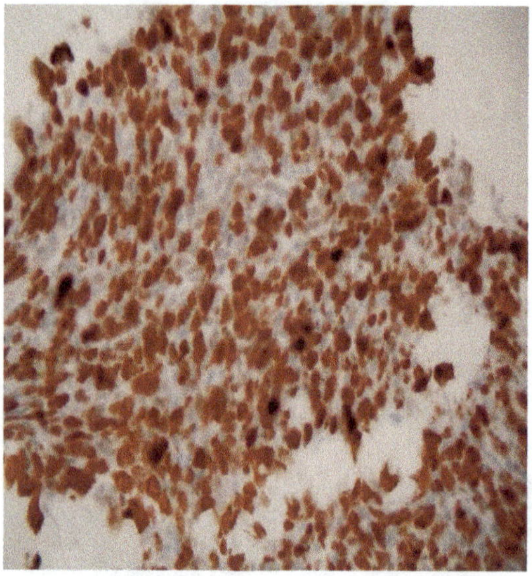

Figure 3: The soft tissue biopsy under H&E stain and high power: no atypia or malignancy noted.

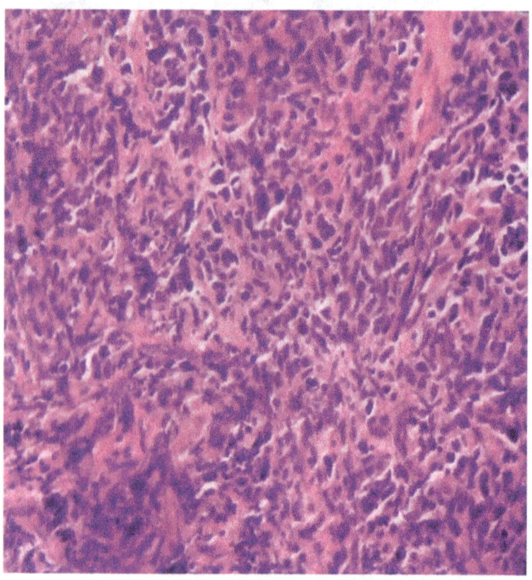

Figure 4: Immunohistochemical stains show that the majority of cells in the specimen are CD20-positive B cells. There is background smaller CD3-positive T-cells. Overall, the findings are most consistent with a diffuse large B cell lymphoma.

uncommon in association with NF-1. This further contributes to the complexity of clinical heterogeneity associated with NF-1 and the need of a greater understanding of the association between NF-1 and associated malignancies. We performed a literature review through the National library of Medicine (PubMed) searching for case reports of NF-1 associated with lymphoma. Only 29 cases of malignant lymphoma were reported in NF-1 patients [7–9], and only three of them were DLBCL [10–12]. It is worth mentioning that unlike our case, most of the cases reported in previous studies had a history of multiple health conditions that might be confounding variables. Moreover, the American College of Medical Genetics and Genomics (ACMG) has laid a surveillance guideline for adults with NF-1 [13], yet there is no recommendation for imaging nor biomarker surveillance at this point for DLBCL due to it rarity, and thus reporting such cases is a key for physician awareness and to establish surveillance guideline for NF-1 adults' population. Furthermore, the physical presence of the neurofibromas can interfere with the clinician's ability to perform an adequate examination, either due to their anatomical interference during palpation or the unease lesions of this sort might trigger. Another aspect to be highlighted is how the MVA had caused an anchoring bias in the differential diagnosis of abdominal pain which led to a delay in the diagnosis of the lymphoma. Thus, the case presented here should increase clinician's awareness to reach a correct diagnosis when presented with similar case to prevent the patient being denied timely and effective treatment.

4. Conclusion

This case emphasizes and enforce the importance of having a high index of suspicion for malignancies during follow-up of patients with a history of NF-1. Finally, physicians should be extremely cautious when examining patients that may impose a challenge on physical examination, in order to avoid biases and delay in diagnosis.

References

[1] R. A. Kallionpaa, E. Uusitalo, J. Leppävirta, M. Pöyhönen, S. Peltonen, and J. Peltonen, "Prevalence of neurofibromatosis type 1 in the Finnish population," *Genetics in Medicine*, vol. 20, no. 9, pp. 1082–1086, 2018.

[2] J. S. Guillamo, A. Creange, C. Kalifa et al., "Prognostic factors of CNS tumours in neurofibromatosis 1 (NF1): a retrospective study of 104 patients," *Brain*, vol. 126, no. 1, pp. 152–160, 2003.

[3] K. Jett and J. M. Friedman, "Clinical and genetic aspects of neurofibromatosis 1," *Genetics in Medicine*, vol. 12, no. 1, pp. 1–11, 2010.

[4] B. R. Korf, "Malignancy in neurofibromatosis type 1," *The Oncologist*, vol. 5, no. 6, pp. 477–485, 2000.

[5] L. Walker, D. Thompson, D. Easton et al., "A prospective study of neurofibromatosis type 1 cancer incidence in the UK," *British Journal of Cancer*, vol. 95, no. 2, pp. 233–238, 2006.

[6] R. D. Brasfield and T. K. Das Gupta, "Von Recklinghausen's disease: a clinicopathological study," *Annals of Surgery*, vol. 175, no. 1, pp. 86–104, 1972.

[7] B. W. Berman, R. A. Binder, and D. B. Cornfield, "Burkitt-lymphoma in a patient with neurofibromatosis and pheochromocytoma," *Jama-Journal of the American Medical Association*, vol. 237, no. 10, pp. 993-994, 1977.

[8] M. M. Cajaiba and M. Reyes-Mugica, "Gaucher or pseudo-Gaucher? The challenge of several diseases colliding in a pediatric patient," *Human Pathology*, vol. 40, no. 4, pp. 594–598, 2009.

[9] W. Wertelecki, K. Iinuma, and H. P. Bentley, "Non-neural malignancy complicating neurofibromatosis in two relatives," *Cancer Genetics and Cytogenetics*, vol. 18, no. 1, pp. 87–89, 1985.

[10] O. Dohi, M. Hatori, R. Ichinohasama, M. Hosaka, S. Hashimoto, and S. Kokubun, "Diffuse large B-cell lymphoma arising in a patient with neurofibromatosis type I and in a patient with neurofibromatosis type II," *The Tohoku Journal of Experimental Medicine*, vol. 208, no. 2, pp. 169–176, 2006.

[11] S. J. Kim, J. H. Seo, S. W. Lee et al., "A case of non-Hodgkin's lymphoma in a patient with neurofibromatosis type 1," *The Korean Journal of Internal Medicine*, vol. 18, no. 3, pp. 202–205, 2003.

[12] S. Lueangarun and C. U. Auewarakul, "Diffuse large B cell lymphoma presenting as Horner's syndrome in a patient diagnosed with neurofibromatosis type 1: a case report and review of the literature," *Journal of Medical Case Reports*, vol. 6, no. 1, 2012.

[13] D. R. Stewart, B. R. Korf, K. L. Nathanson, D. A. Stevenson, and K. Yohay, "Care of adults with neurofibromatosis type 1: a clinical practice resource of the American College of Medical Genetics and Genomics (ACMG)," *Genetics in Medicine*, vol. 20, no. 7, pp. 671–682, 2018.

36

A Rare Case of Pure Primary Large Cell Neuroendocrine Carcinoma of the Gallbladder

Rodney E. Shackelford,[1] Ekin Ozluk,[2] Jehan Abdulsattar,[2] Terry C. Lairmore,[3] Quyen Chu,[3] and Eric X. Wei[1]

[1]Department of Pathology, University of South Alabama Health, Mobile, Alabama 36617, USA
[2]Department of Pathology & Translational Pathobiology, LSU Health Sciences Center Shreveport, Shreveport, Louisiana 71130, USA
[3]Department of Surgery, Louisiana State University Health Shreveport, Louisiana 71130, USA

Correspondence should be addressed to Eric X. Wei; ericxwei@yahoo.com

Academic Editor: Ossama W. Tawfik

Primary large cell neuroendocrine carcinoma (LCNEC) of the gallbladder is a rare malignancy which is often associated with non-LCNEC histologic components. Histologically "pure" LCNECs of the gallbladder are exceedingly rare with only 15 cases reported in the medical literature. Clinically, LCNECs present with abdominal pain and jaundice and follow an aggressive course with patients surviving a median of 15 months following initial diagnosis. To our knowledge, we present the 16th case of a histologically pure LCNEC in a 62-year-old African American male who was successfully treated surgically. After discharge, he was subsequently lost to follow-up. Due to the extreme rarity of such disease entity, accurate diagnosis and proper management are essential for the best clinical outcome.

1. Introduction

The current World Health Organization (WHO) classification of neuroendocrine tumors of the gallbladder includes grade I and II neuroendocrine tumors, small cell neuroendocrine carcinoma, large cell neuroendocrine carcinoma (LCNEC), mixed adenoneuroendocrine carcinoma, goblet cell carcinoid, and tubular carcinoid tumors [1]. Histologically, neuroendocrine tumors frequently grow in trabecular or organoid patterns, often with rosettes and with "salt and pepper" nuclear patterns. The more poorly differentiated and clinically aggressive subtypes show a high mitotic index. Neuroendocrine tumors typically show immunoreactivity towards the neuroendocrine markers chromogranin, synaptophysin, CD56, Leu 7, and neuron-specific enolase [1–5]. LCNECs are composed of large cells that are usually two to three times larger than those of small cell neuroendocrine tumors and show brisk mitotic activity, with hyperchromatic nuclei and prominent nucleoli [1–5].

Primary neuroendocrine tumors of the gallbladder are rare, totaling only 0.5% of all neuroendocrine tumors and 2.1% of all gallbladder malignancies [2]. LCNECs were first described in 1991 when pulmonary cases were reported [3]. LCNECs of the gallbladder are extremely rare and are commonly composed of neuroendocrine cells with other associated histologies, including adenocarcinoma, adenosquamous carcinoma, and mucinous adenocarcinoma components [4]. LCNECs composed solely of enteroendocrine features ("pure" LCNECs) are exceptionally rare, with only 15 cases described in the medical literature [5]. Here, to our knowledge, we describe the 16th case of a primary gallbladder LCNEC composed solely of large neuroendocrine carcinoma cells.

2. Case Presentation

A 62-year-old African American male presented with a history of acute vomiting and right upper-quadrant and

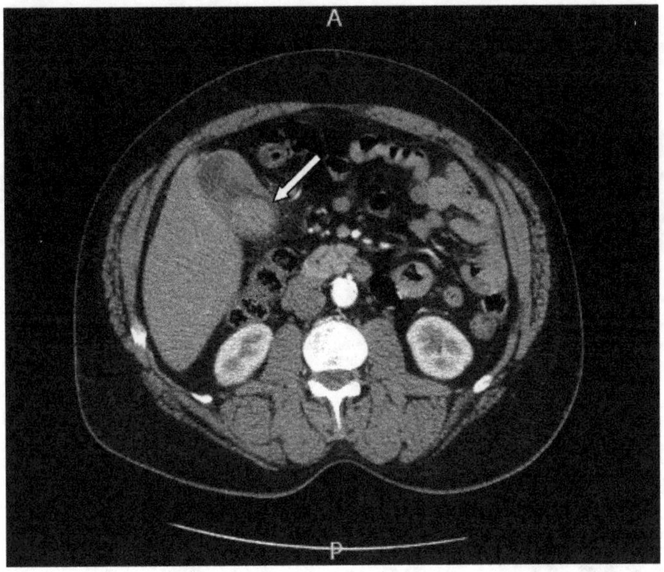

FIGURE 1: A noncontrast CT scan of the patient's abdomen revealing thickening of the gallbladder wall with a possible polyp (white arrow).

epigastric pain, one day before admission to the hospital. His pain had become so unbearable that he was prompted to call an ambulance. The patient's previous medical history included hypertension, hyperlipidemia, atherosclerosis, and type II diabetes, all of which were medically managed. He also had an extensive 40-year smoking history. The patient did not reveal any significant family medical history. His physical exam was significant for high blood pressure of 190/96 mmHg and guarding on palpation of the abdomen. His serum chromogranin or other neuroendocrine markers were not tested. Initial imaging studies were performed with ultrasound of the abdomen, which was significant for hepatomegaly and cholelithiasis, without evidence of cholecystitis. A noncontrast abdominal CT scan was performed where stones, a possible gallbladder polyp, and thickening of the gallbladder wall were identified, which were concerning for malignancy (Figure 1). A laparoscopic cholecystectomy was performed, and the gallbladder was found to be grossly distended, partially filled with multiple multifaceted calculi, containing a central polypoid mass roughly 3.0 cm in size and exhibiting focal thickening of the gallbladder wall. An attached gallbladder lymph node partially involved by metastatic tumor cells was also identified. Histologically, the tumor showed extensive necrosis and large cells with salt and pepper nuclei, prominent nucleoli, and a trabecular growth pattern (Figures 2(a)–2(c)). Immunohistochemical staining for AE1/AE3, chromogranin, synaptophysin, CD20, CD56, DOG-1, Ki-67, MART-1, S-100, SOX-10, TTF-1, neuron-specific enolase (NSE), and c-kit were performed on the polypoid mass. The tumor cells were immunoreactive to CD56 (membranous), AE1/AE3, c-kit, and NSE (cytoplasmic) (Figures 2(d)–2(g)) and negative for CD20, chromogranin, synaptophysin, DOG-1, S-100, and other markers performed, consistent with a LCNEC [1–5]. The Ki-67 immunostaining revealed a brisk miotic index with over 95% immunopositivity (Figure 2(h)). The tumor was staged as pT3, pN1. After the sixth day of hospitalization postoperatively, the patient recovered without further complications and was sent home with scheduled follow-up. His medications included treatment regimens for his hypertension, hyperlipidemia, and diabetes without further chemotherapy. After the discharge, the patient was subsequently lost to follow-up.

3. Discussion

Here, we presented a 62-year-old African American male with pure LCNEC of the gallbladder. The histological features and positive immunostainings for AE1/AE3, CD56, c-kit, and NSE and high proliferation index at 95% would support the diagnosis of LCNEC. Negative synaptophysin and chromogranin expression is unusual and may suggest poor differentiation of the tumor. Negative S-100 expression excludes a high-grade peripheral nerve sheath tumor. Although the tumor cells express c-kit, negative DOG-1 staining rules out an epithelioid gastrointestinal stomal tumor (GIST). The expression of c-kit in tumor cells may indicate tumor origin from undifferentiated stem cells. The fact that the tumor cells are negative for CD20 also removes the consideration of a large B cell lymphoma. Neuroendocrine tumors of the gallbladder are rare with LCNEC tumors of this organ being very uncommon [1, 5]. "Pure" gallbladder LCNECs containing only the large cell neuroendocrine histology are exceedingly rare, with only 15 cases recorded in the medical literature [5]. Neuroendocrine cells are not normally found in the gallbladder, which is a likely reason why these tumors are so rare in this organ [6–8]. How these tumors arise in the gallbladder is unknown; however, it has been hypothesized that these malignancies may arise from undifferentiated stem cells or from chronic inflammation such as cholecystitis leading to intestinal or gastric metaplasia and neuroendocrine cell formation with later malignant transformation [5–7]. LCNECs have presented in patients between the ages of 55 to 76 years, usually with symptoms similar to the more common gallbladder malignancies,

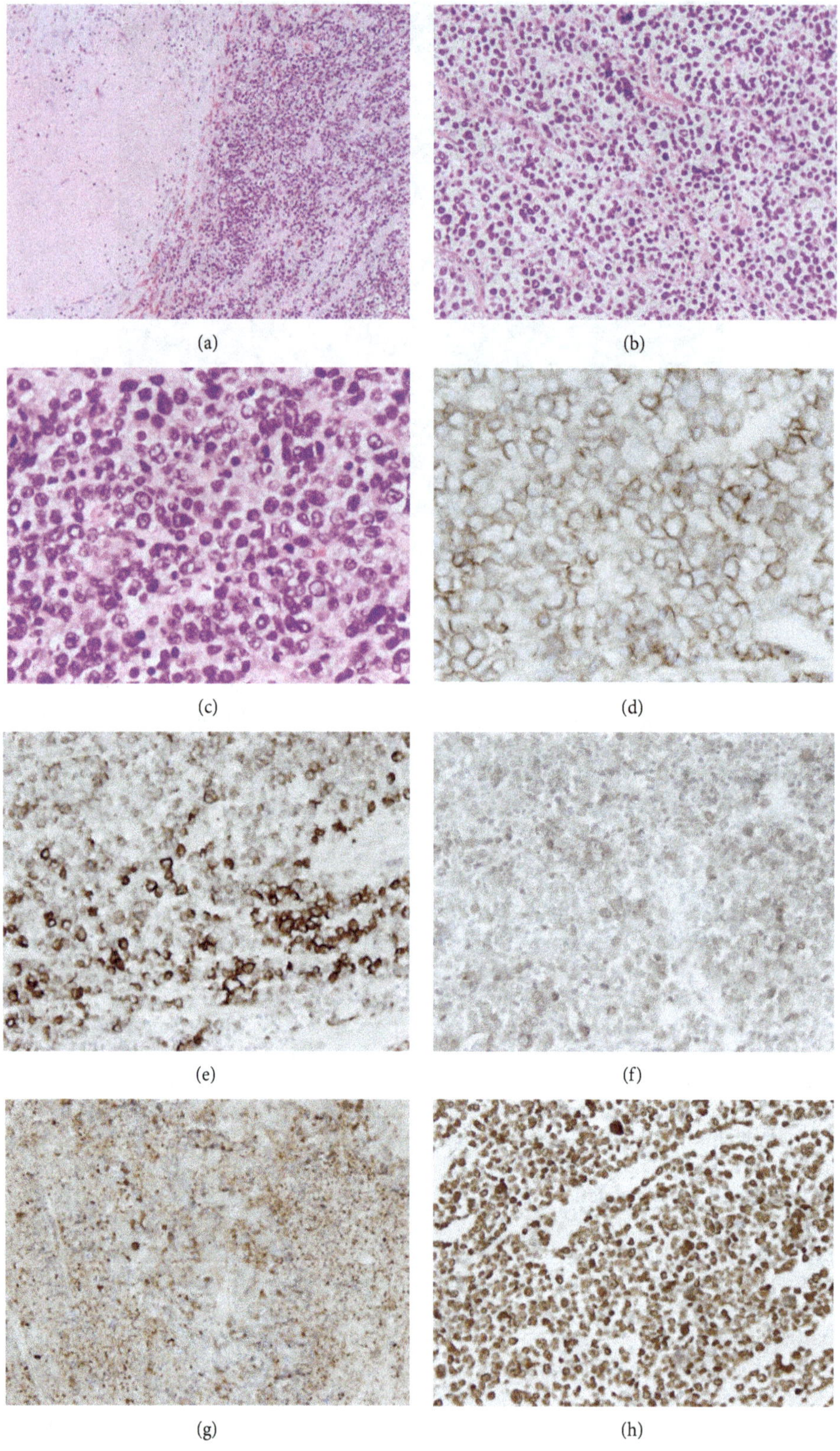

Figure 2: Representative H&E sections of the gallbladder LCNEC and some of the immunostains performed. Very low-power H&E view (20x) of the LCNEC showing necrosis and tumor cells (a), low-power H&E section (40x) showing the trabecular growth pattern (b), and a middle-power view (200x) showing the neuroendocrine features of the LCNEC (c). Sections (d–h) show the CD56, AE1/AE3, c-kit, neuron-specific enolase, and Ki-67 immunostains, respectively.

including jaundice and abdominal pain/discomfort [5]. Common radiological findings include a mass in place of the gallbladder, focal or diffuse gallbladder wall thickening, and direct invasion of the tumor into the liver or metastasis to the surrounding lymph nodes [1]. LCNECs are typically very aggressive, with a median survival time of 15 months and with a range of 21 days to 69 months [5]. For qualifying patients, optimal treatment for these tumors is complete surgical resection with surrounding lymph node clearance and hepatic lobectomy, with recurrences being very common [5]. In the event of an unresectable tumor, systemic chemotherapy is the next treatment option, which employs the same platinum-based chemotherapy regimen, often with radiation therapy, as is used for small cell neuroendocrine carcinoma treatment [5, 8]. The efficacy of traditional chemotherapy with additional radiotherapy remains unclear due to insensitivity of general neuroendocrine tumors to radiotherapy; however, this is a treatment option for patients with multiple metastases or an unresectable tumor [9]. Recently, immunotherapy with ipilimumab and nivolumab has shown some promise in a small phase II clinical trial treating LCNECs [10]. Due to the rarity of these tumors, especially of pure LCNECs of the gallbladder, there is much that is unknown about how these extremely rare tumors should be treated [8, 10]. An accurate diagnosis of LCNEC is also essential as the treatment for these tumors is different than that used for the more common adenocarcinomas of the gallbladder [5, 8, 11]. In conclusion, histologically pure LCNEC tumors of the gallbladder are exceedingly rare [5, 11]. The unique nature of this tumor requires that further studies be utilized to optimize its treatment. In particular, immune and DNA sequence analyses, multimodal treatment regimes, and immune therapies will likely play an important role in the future treatment of these rare malignancies [5, 11].

References

[1] K. M. Eltawil, B. I. Gustafsson, M. Kidd, and I. M. Modlin, "Neuroendocrine tumors of the gallbladder," *Journal of Clinical Gastroenterology*, vol. 44, no. 10, pp. 687–695, 2010.

[2] M. Papotti, P. Cassoni, A. Sapino, G. Passarino, J. E. Krueger, and J. Albores-Saavedra, "Large cell neuroendocrine carcinoma of the gallbladder: report of two cases," *The American Journal of Surgical Pathology*, vol. 24, no. 10, pp. 1424–1428, 2000.

[3] W. D. Travis, R. I. Linnoila, M. G. Tsokos et al., "Neuroendocrine tumors of the lung with proposed criteria for large-cell neuroendocrine carcinoma. An ultrastructural, immunohistochemical, and flow cytometric study of 35 cases," *The American Journal of Surgical Pathology*, vol. 15, no. 6, pp. 529–553, 1991.

[4] W. Liu, L. Wang, X. D. He, C. Feng, X. Y. Chang, and Z. H. Lu, "Mixed large cell neuroendocrine carcinoma and adenocarcinoma of the gallbladder: a case report and brief review of the literature," *World Journal of Surgical Oncology*, vol. 13, no. 1, p. 114, 2015.

[5] A. Tidjane, N. Boudjenan, A. Bengueddach et al., "Pure large cell neuroendocrine carcinoma of the gallbladder, is surgical relentlessness beneficial? A case report and literature review," *International Cancer Conference Journal*, vol. 10, no. 2, pp. 127–133, 2021.

[6] M. Murakami, K. Katayama, S. Kato et al., "Large-cell neuroendocrine carcinoma of the common bile duct: a case report and a review of literature," *Surgical Case Reports*, vol. 2, no. 1, p. 141, 2016.

[7] S. B. Park, S. B. Moon, Y. J. Ryu et al., "Primary large cell neuroendocrine carcinoma in the common bile duct: first Asian case report," *World Journal of Gastroenterology*, vol. 20, no. 47, pp. 18048–18052, 2014.

[8] A. Iyoda, T. Makino, S. Koezuka, H. Otsuka, and Y. Hata, "Treatment options for patients with large cell neuroendocrine carcinoma of the lung," *General Thoracic and Cardiovascular Surgery*, vol. 62, no. 6, pp. 351–356, 2014.

[9] I. M. Modlin, M. Kidd, I. Drozdov, Z. L. Siddique, and B. I. Gustafsson, "Pharmacotherapy of neuroendocrine cancers," *Expert Opinion Pharmacotherapy*, vol. 9, no. 15, pp. 2617–2626, 2008.

[10] S. Patel, "A phase II basket trial of nivolumab and ipilimumab in rare tumors (NET cohort)," *American Association of Cancer Research*, vol. 79, 2019.

[11] S. Buscemi, E. Orlando, G. Damiano et al., ""Pure" large cell neuroendocrine carcinoma of the gallbladder. Report of a case and review of the literature," *International Journal of Surgery*, vol. 28, Supplement 1, pp. S128–S132, 2016.

37

A Rare Case of Large-Vessel Vasculitis following Checkpoint Inhibitor Therapy and Pegfilgrastim

Joseph Mort,[1] **Shipra Maheshwari**,[1] **Nayanika Basu**,[2] **Patrick Dillon**,[2] **Kevin Brady**,[2] **Harry Bear**,[3] **and Trish Millard**[2]

[1]*Department of Medicine, University of Virginia Health System, 1215 Lee Street, Charlottesville, VA 22908, USA*
[2]*Emily Couric Cancer Center, University of Virginia Health System, 1240 Lee Street, Charlottesville, VA 22903, USA*
[3]*Massey Cancer Center and Department of Surgery, Virginia Commonwealth University and VCU Health, Box 980011, Richmond, VA 23298-0011, USA*

Correspondence should be addressed to Joseph Mort; jfm6en@hscmail.mcc.virginia.edu

Academic Editor: Mauro Cives

Checkpoint inhibitors (CPIs) and pegfilgrastim, a long-acting growth factor agent, are vital components of current cancer treatments. Immune-related adverse events (irAEs) such as colitis and pneumonitis are well-established toxicities associated with CPI therapy. However, large-vessel vasculitis secondary to CPI utilization is reported only in rare case reports and case series. Interestingly, large-vessel vasculitis has also been reported as a rare complication of pegfilgrastim use. We present a 59-year-old female with left stage IIA (cT2N0M0) triple-negative breast cancer receiving neoadjuvant decitabine and pembrolizumab prior to neoadjuvant chemotherapy (NAC). NAC included standard-of-care dose dense doxorubicin and cyclophosphamide (ddAC) supported with pegfilgrastim use followed by weekly carboplatin and paclitaxel. After receiving her second cycle of ddAC with pegfilgrastim, the patient reported five days of left shoulder and arm pain. Subsequent CT imaging demonstrated wall thickening and inflammatory changes surrounding the left subclavian artery, aortic arch, left carotid artery, proximal innominate arteries, and the mid internal carotid arteries and its branching vessels. These findings were extremely concerning for large-vessel vasculitis. Excluding CPI therapy and pegfilgrastim use, no additional inciting event or medication that the patient was exposed to was noted to be associated with large-vessel vasculitis. We present this case to report on this rare but severe complication from commonly utilized agents in cancer treatment. We also extend the possibility of large-vessel vasculitis development in relation to the COVID-19 vaccine due to shared ingredients found in both the vaccine and pegfilgrastim. It is important to outline the treatment used for such a complication as no standardized treatment has been established for large-vessel vasculitis caused by CPI therapy or pegfilgrastim use.

1. Introduction

CPIs as a component of cancer treatment have revolutionized patient outcomes. However, these medications must be used with caution as they carry substantial risk for causing autoimmune side effects or irAEs because of stimulation of the immune system. IrAEs have been reported to affect nearly every organ system in the body, most frequently affecting the gastrointestinal, hepatic, pulmonary, cutaneous, and endocrine systems [1, 2]. The most frequent rheumatologic irAEs that occur due to CPI therapy are arthralgias and myalgias (11.0% and 7.3%, respectively) [3]. Vasculitis is a rare rheumatologic irAE of CPI therapy that has only been specifically described in case reports and case series [4]. Of the CPI-vasculitis cases reported in the literature, large-vessel vasculitis is the most common subtype [5].

Cases of large-vessel vasculitis induced by granulocyte colony-stimulating factors (G-CSFs) have also been reported [6–13]. In a large observational study of 102,014 subjects with malignant neoplasms in Japan, 0.47% of subjects treated with G-CSF developed aortitis compared to only 0.01% in subjects who did not receive G-CSF [9]. Although exposure to either pegylated or nonpegylated G-CSF was evaluated in this study, more patients developed aortitis after receiving pegylated G-CSF utilization [6–9]. Pegfilgrastim is a form of G-CSF with an attached polyethylene glycol (PEG) moiety that extends duration of action to allow for less frequent administrations compared to nonpegylated G-CSF which is injected daily. Pegylated G-CSF has demonstrated greater efficacy in prevention of severe neutropenia, dose reductions, and treatment delays when administering dose-dense chemotherapy in breast cancer [14, 15]. However, the addition of this PEG moiety could theoretically lead to an immunostimulatory effect causing the immune cells to target native vessels in the body. In one case of large-vessel vasculitis after pegfilgrastim administration, the patient was transitioned to nonpegylated G-CSF with additional cycles of chemotherapy without relapse of vasculitis [16].

Given the rare nature of CPI and G-CSF-induced vasculitis, standardized treatment of this adverse effect has not yet been established. Herein, we present a rare case of large-vessel vasculitis possibly induced by either CPI or G-CSF and the treatment that followed resulting in rapid resolution of symptoms.

2. Case Presentation

A 59-year-old female with left stage IIA (cT2N0M0) triple-negative breast cancer was treated on a clinical trial with neoadjuvant chemoimmunotherapy [17]. The investigational portion of treatment included decitabine (4 doses) administered on days 1–5 and pembrolizumab administered on days 8 and 22, prior to starting neoadjuvant chemotherapy (investigational use of an FDA approved agent). The patient then received standard-of-care chemotherapy with four cycles of ddAC and pegfilgrastim support followed by twelve weekly doses of carboplatin and paclitaxel. After receiving her second cycle of ddAC with pegfilgrastim, the patient reported 5 days of worsening left shoulder and arm pain. The pain started in the left scapula and radiated down the left arm to the back and under the left breast. It was pleuritic and severe in nature. The pain worsened with active but not passive range of motion. She denied chest pain, dyspnea, or fevers but also reported a pruritic, papular rash over her chest and back that started two weeks before the onset of arm pain. An X-ray of the left humerus showed no fracture. Given the pleuritic nature of her pain, the patient underwent a contrasted chest CT to assess for pulmonary embolism. This showed wall thickening and inflammatory changes surrounding the left subclavian artery extending into the aortic arch with involvement of the left carotid artery and proximal innominate arteries (Figure 1). These imaging findings were concerning for large-vessel vasculitis, and the patient was admitted to the hospital for work up and management.

Vital signs were within normal limits. Basic labs revealed a neutrophilic predominant leukocytosis and mild normocytic anemia. Her kidney function was normal and urinalysis showed trace protein and blood; the urine protein-to-creatinine ratio was mildly elevated at 0.21. Liver function tests were within normal limits. Her troponin and BNP were in the normal ranges. ECG on admission was normal and a transthoracic echocardiogram showed a normal ejection fraction, cavity size, and wall thickness. Inflammatory markers revealed a normal sedimentation rate, but C-reactive protein was elevated to 847 mmol/L (normal < 48 mmol/L). Rheumatology was consulted to assist with the work up of her large-vessel vasculitis. Serologic testing demonstrated a negative antinuclear antibody, rheumatoid factor, myeloperoxidase antibody, proteinase 3 antibody, and normal C4 complement level. Hepatitis serologies revealed a nonreactive hepatitis C antibody and evidence of prior immunization to hepatitis B. Creatine kinase was ordered to rule out myositis and was normal. Blood cultures were obtained to assess for infection and no microbial growth was identified. Further vascular imaging was acquired to assess for involvement of other organs. CT of the head and neck with contrast revealed that the wall thickening of the common carotid arteries extended cranially to the level of the midinternal carotid arteries but there was no significant stenosis or involvement of the intracranial vessels. The vessels in the abdomen and pelvis were without inflammatory changes.

After the above workup, the differential diagnosis for this patient's large-vessel vasculitis included CPI-induced vasculitis due to pembrolizumab- or pegfilgrastim-induced vasculitis. As part of the clinical trial for triple-negative breast cancer, she received two doses of pembrolizumab 45 and 31 days prior to onset of her left arm pain. Two doses of pegfilgrastim with ddAC were given 22 and 8 days prior to onset of her symptoms. Of note, she also received the two-dose Pfizer COVID-19 vaccine series prior to starting therapy for her breast cancer with doses administered two and three months prior to symptom onset. After being started on systemic steroids (prednisone 1 mg/kg) for treatment in the hospital, the patient demonstrated rapid improvement in her symptoms. The patient was discharged with plans to continue on a slow steroid taper.

She had continued improvement in her left arm pain and reported only mild residual weakness at follow-up 2 weeks after discharge. She did note a change in the character of her vision and was referred to ophthalmology for further evaluation with no findings of ocular inflammation seen on eye exam. Repeat inflammatory markers two weeks after discharge were normal, and repeat imaging 8 weeks later showed marked improvement in vasculitis (Figure 1). She completed a slow steroid taper over 12 weeks with no recurrence of symptoms.

The patient did not receive additional immunotherapy after onset of symptoms as she had already completed all doses per the clinical trial. The frequency of subsequent chemotherapy doses was decreased and carboplatin eventually discontinued to allow for avoidance of additional G-CSF doses and prevention of large-vessel vasculitis recurrence.

3. Discussion

While CPIs have significantly improved outcomes for patients with a variety of cancers, management of the associated irAEs requires prompt treatment and close monitoring by the treatment team. One rare irAE is vasculitis. One series

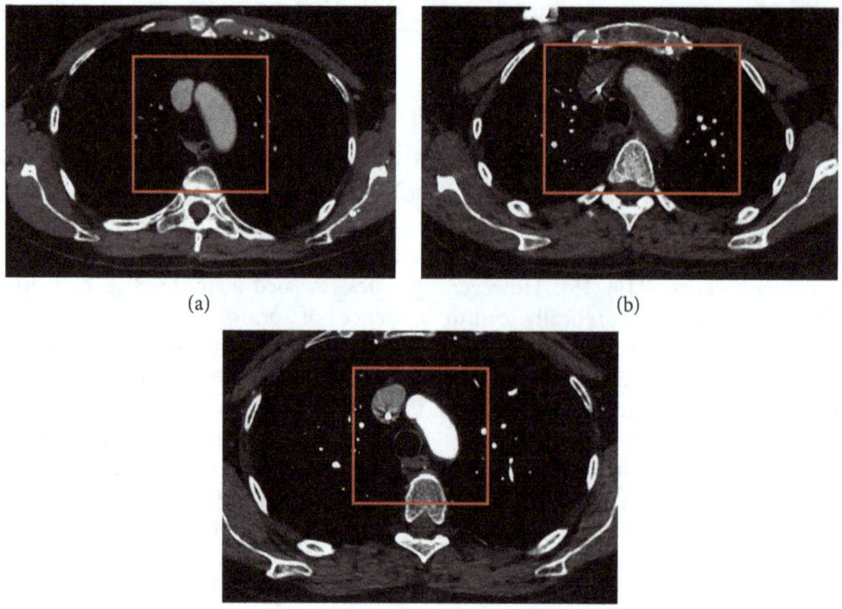

(a) (b) (c)

FIGURE 1: (a) CT chest with contrast of the patient on 2/11/21. (b) CT chest with contrast of the patient on 5/03/21. (c) CT chest with contrast of the patient on 7/01/21. Between February and March 2021, this patient received both pembrolizumab and pegfilgrastim. Her May CT was significant for wall thickening and inflammatory changes surrounding the left subclavian artery extending into the aortic arch with involvement of the left carotid artery and proximal innominate arteries, new findings as compared to her February CT. After the initiation of a long steroid taper in May, the patient's CT chest in July showed marked improvement of the wall thickening and inflammatory changes of the aortic arch and arch vessels, most compatible with resolving vasculitis.

of 20 cases of CPI-induced vasculitis revealed that large-vessel vasculitis (6 cases) was the most commonly reported type of vasculitis but medium vessel, small vessel, and single-organ vasculitis were also observed. Cases of large-vessel vasculitis included giant cell arteritis (GCA) and aortitis/periaortitis. Median time to onset after CPI therapy was 3 months but ranged from 1.2 to 6 months [5]. The case of large-vessel vasculitis we present above occurred after 2 doses of pembrolizumab that were given one and a half and one month prior to onset of her symptoms. Although this is a shorter duration of symptom onset after CPI therapy than the median onset of 3 months, it still lies within the reported range. Involvement of the aortic arch and major branches fits with the previously reported location of vessel involvement. It was also important to investigate irAEs involving other organ systems. The patient received a thorough workup to rule out concomitant organ involvement. Of note, special care was devoted to ensuring that the patient had no symptoms of GCA given its high prevalence in CPI-vasculitis and she was referred to ophthalmology in the outpatient setting after discharge.

In this case, it was imperative to consider all possible etiologies of vasculitis. Although this patient's case fits with CPI-induced vasculitis, cases of G-CSF-induced large-vessel vasculitis and aortitis have also been reported [6–13]. G-CSF aids the differentiation and maturation of neutrophils as well as stimulates inflammatory cytokine production. For these reasons, G-CSF may trigger vasculitis [11]. Interestingly, one case report suggests a higher incidence of G-CSF-related vasculitis in advanced cancer compared to earlier stage disease [11]. Our patient received pegfilgrastim with her first two cycles of ddAC 22 and 8 days prior to onset of her symptoms. The time to onset of symptoms after administration of G-CSF was 1–13 days in a review of seventeen cases and in a separate review of 5 cases in Japan as well as median onset of 8 days in a case series of 6 patients in Finland with breast cancer who developed large-vessel vasculitis [6, 7, 12]. The timeline of development of our patient's large-vessel vasculitis fits with the timeline in the cases previously reported. As mentioned above, pegfilgrastim was more commonly associated with large-vessel vasculitis compared to nonpegylated G-CSF [6–9]. In one case of large-vessel vasculitis after pegfilgrastim administration, the patient was transitioned to nonpegylated G-CSF with additional cycles of chemotherapy administered without relapse of vasculitis [16]. Still, other case reports indicate that both pegylated and nonpegylated G-CSF can be associated with the development of aortitis [10]. One case report suggested that those who received pegylated G-CSF required steroids and those who received nonpegylated G-CSF had resolution of vasculitis without steroids [13]. Given the potential for recurrent vasculitis with either pegylated or nonpegylated G-CSF, as well as patient's general chemotherapy tolerance to date, our patient's ddAC was switched to every three weeks of dosing so that growth factor support was no longer preemptively required; her symptoms did not recur. She was also treated with a prolonged steroid taper as would be typical for irAE from CPI. It should be noted that there is limited available data on the safety of CPI given with G-CSF; thus, it is hypothesized that exposure to both agents may increase one's risk for vasculitis.

Other possible contributing factors in this case were the patient's COVID-19 vaccination and her chemotherapy. Two months prior to starting chemotherapy, our patient received the mRNA COVID-19 vaccine. At the time of this patient's presentation, there were no reported cases of vasculitis secondary to the COVID-19 vaccine but both of the mRNA vaccines (Pfizer-BioNTech and Moderna) contain PEG as an ingredient [18]. Although it is unclear to what degree (if any) vaccination contributed to this patient's presentation, it is possible that immune stimulation associated with the vaccine in the presence of PEG made the patient more sensitive to subsequent exposure to PEG in the form of pegfilgrastim when she initiated chemotherapy. It will be important to monitor for additional cases of vasculitis associated with pegfilgrastim as more individuals receive the COVID-19 vaccine. The patient's prior dose of decitabine was also queried as a contributory factor, but the experience with this agent and the timeline suggest against it playing a role in vasculitis.

Since both CPI-vasculitis and pegfilgrastim-/G-CSF-induced vasculitis are rare conditions, standardized treatment does not exist. However, in the cases of CPI-vasculitis reported, discontinuation of the CPI therapy and initiation of high-dose glucocorticoids resulted in resolution of symptoms. Glucocorticoid regimens included high-dose oral prednisone (1–2 mg/kg daily) or several days of IV methylprednisolone followed by slow taper of oral glucocorticoids [5]. Disease-modifying antirheumatic drugs have been used to treat rheumatologic irAEs in patients with symptoms refractory to glucocorticoids or as steroid-sparing agents, including in two cases of CPI-vasculitis [3, 19, 20]. Use of tumor necrosis factor inhibitors (predominantly infliximab) and the interleukin-6 inhibitor tocilizumab has also been used with success for rheumatologic irAEs, but to our knowledge, they have not been used for CPI-vasculitis [3]. Our patient's symptoms and imaging findings are resolved with high-dose oral prednisone and a subsequent prolonged taper along with stopping pegfilgrastim. Her CPI therapy had previously been completed prior to onset of symptoms. Some cases of spontaneous resolution of symptoms and imaging findings of G-CSF vasculitis without steroid treatment have been reported. Hoshina and Takei reported 10 cases of G-CSF vasculitis and state that there was no difference in time to remission of aortitis with or without steroids [11]. Yukawa et al. reported 5 cases and differentiated treatment between pegylated G-CSF vasculitis and nonpegylated G-CSF vasculitis, stating that the patients who received pegylated G-CSF required steroids for resolution while those treated with nonpegylated G-CSF did not require steroids [13]. In cases such as these, repeat exposure to CPI and/or growth factors such as G-CSF requires careful assessment of risk to benefit ratio and open discussion with the patient on the uncertainty of safety with repeat exposure.

4. Conclusion

The case of therapy-associated large-vessel vasculitis that we present is unique in that it contains several possible etiologies: CPI-induced vasculitis, pegfilgrastim/G-CSF induced vasculitis, or a combination with a potential immunostimulatory contribution of the PEG-containing mRNA COVID-19 vaccine. Although large-vessel vasculitis is a rare adverse event in both of these lifesaving cancer therapies and should not preclude providers from utilizing them in the care of patients, oncologists should consider large-vessel vasculitis as a potential complication of immunotherapy and pegfilgrastim going forward with particular attention to when these medications are used in combination. They should be aware of such a complication when evaluating patients who have received the above agents and present with symptoms of unclear etiology.

Consent

No written consent has been obtained from the patient as there is no patient identifiable data included in this case report.

Acknowledgments

This research did not receive specific funding but was performed under the Emily Couric Cancer Center at the University of Virginia Health System.

References

[1] F. Martins, L. Sofiya, G. P. Sykiotis et al., "Adverse effects of immune-checkpoint inhibitors: epidemiology, management and surveillance," *Nature Reviews. Clinical Oncology*, vol. 16, no. 9, pp. 563–580, 2019.

[2] J. R. Brahmer, C. Lacchetti, B. J. Schneider et al., "Management of immune-related adverse events in patients treated with immune checkpoint inhibitor therapy: American Society of Clinical Oncology clinical practice guideline," *Journal of Clinical Oncology*, vol. 36, no. 17, pp. 1714–1768, 2018.

[3] M. Kostine, A. Finckh, C. O. Bingham et al., "EULAR points to consider for the diagnosis and management of rheumatic immune-related adverse events due to cancer immunotherapy with checkpoint inhibitors," *Annals of Rheumatic Diseases*, vol. 80, no. 1, pp. 36–48, 2021.

[4] T. M. Crout, D. S. Lennep, S. Kishore, and V. Majithia, "Systemic Vasculitis associated with immune check point inhibition: analysis and review," *Current Rheumatology Reports*, vol. 21, no. 6, p. 28, 2019.

[5] A. Daxini, K. Cronin, and A. G. Sreih, "Vasculitis associated with immune checkpoint inhibitors-a systematic review," *Clinical Rheumatology*, vol. 37, no. 9, pp. 2579–2584, 2018.

[6] J. Nakamura, T. M. Nishi, S. Yamashita et al., "Pegfilgrastim-associated large-vessel vasculitis developed during adjuvant chemotherapy for breast cancer: a case report and review of the literature," *Journal of Oncology Pharmacy Practice*, vol. 26, no. 7, pp. 1785–1790, 2020.

[7] K. Taimen, S. Heino, I. Kohonen, H. Relas, R. Huovinen, and A. Hänninen, "Granulocyte colony-stimulating factor- and chemotherapy-induced large-vessel vasculitis: six patient cases and a systematic literature review," *Rheumatology Advances Practice*, vol. 4, no. 1, 2020.

[8] A. Lardieri, L. McCulley, S. Christopher Jones, and

D. Woronow, "Granulocyte colony-stimulating factors and aortitis: a rare adverse event," *American Journal of Hematology*, vol. 93, no. 10, pp. E333–E336, 2018.

[9] Y. Oshima, S. Takahashi, K. Tani, and A. Tojo, "Granulocyte colony-stimulating factor-associated aortitis in the Japanese adverse drug event report database," *Cytokine*, vol. 119, pp. 47–51, 2019.

[10] J. J. Soto Castillo, J. Loarce-Martos, and J. M. Blanc-Molina, "Large vessel vasculitis secondary to granulocyte-colony stimulating factor," *VASA*, vol. 49, no. 6, pp. 509–513, 2020.

[11] H. Hoshina and H. Takei, "Granulocyte-colony stimulating factor-associated aortitis in a woman with advanced breast cancer: a case report and review of the literature," *BMC Cancer*, vol. 19, no. 1, p. 1217, 2019.

[12] K. Sasaki, M. Miyauchi, M. Ogura et al., "Arteritis after administration of granulocyte colony-stimulating factor: a case series," *International Journal of Hematology*, vol. 110, no. 3, pp. 370–374, 2019.

[13] K. Yukawa, S. Mokuda, Y. Yoshida, S. Hirata, and E. Sugiyama, "Large-vessel vasculitis associated with PEGylated granulocyte-colony stimulating factor," *The Netherlands Journal of Medicine*, vol. 77, no. 6, pp. 224–226, 2019.

[14] G. Molineux, "The design and development of pegfilgrastim (PEG-rmetHuG-CSF, Neulasta)," *Current Pharmaceutical Design*, vol. 10, no. 11, pp. 1235–1244, 2004.

[15] G. Kourlaba, M. A. Dimopoulos, D. Pectasides et al., "Comparison of filgrastim and pegfilgrastim to prevent neutropenia and maintain dose intensity of adjuvant chemotherapy in patients with breast cancer," *Supportive Care in Cancer*, vol. 23, no. 7, pp. 2045–2051, 2015.

[16] T. Chino, T. Oba, K. Yamamoto et al., "A case of arteritis that developed after pegfilgrastim administration during chemotherapy for breast cancer," *Gan to Kagaku Ryoho*, vol. 45, no. 12, pp. 1771–1774, 2018.

[17] *Neoadjuvant pembrolizumab + decitabine followed by Std neoadj chemo for locally advanced HER2-breast Ca*, https://clinicaltrials.gov/ct2/show/NCT02957968?term=Harry+Bear%2C+pembrolizumab&cond=Breast+cancer&cntry=US&state=US%3AVA&city=Richmond&draw=2&rank=1.

[18] Centers for Disease Control and Prevention, *COVID-19 vaccines for people with allergies*https://www.cdc.gov/coronavirus/2019-ncov/vaccines/recommendations/specific-groups/allergies.html.

[19] A. Tomelleri, C. Campochiaro, G. De Luca, G. Cavalli, and L. Dagna, "Anti-PD1 therapy-associated cutaneous leucocytoclastic vasculitis: a case series," *European Journal of Internal Medicine*, vol. 57, pp. e11–e12, 2018.

[20] R. R. Van den Brom, W. H. Abdulahad, A. Rutgers, B. J. Kroesen, C. Roozendaal, and D. J. Groot, "Rapid granulomatosis with polyangiitis induced by immune checkpoint inhibition," *Rheumatology (Oxford, England)*, vol. 55, no. 6, pp. 1143–1145, 2016.

38

A Pulmonary Zebra: Adult Primary Pulmonary Synovial Sarcoma

Sheffield Sandra, Nwachukwu Chidi, and Ashby Tracy

Department of Medicine, UF College of Medicine – Jacksonville, 653-1 West 8th Street, L20 4th Floor, LRC Jacksonville, FL 32209, USA

Correspondence should be addressed to Sheffield Sandra; sandrash@pcom.edu

Academic Editor: Ossama W. Tawfik

Primary pulmonary synovial sarcoma (PPSS) is an extremely rare tumor, with approximately 50 cases being reported in the English literature (Golota et al., 2018). Difficulties are often encountered in the diagnosis of PPSS as it can be confused with other spindle or round cell tumors, such as fibrosarcoma, hemangiopericytoma, mesothelioma, sarcomatoid carcinoma, or metastatic sarcomas. PPSS was first described by Zeren et al. in 1995. We present a case of PPSS in a 41-year-old woman, who complained of progressive dyspnea and left-sided chest pain.

1. Introduction

Sarcomas are a diverse group of malignant tumors. Sarcomas predominantly arise from the embryonic mesoderm [1]. More than 100 sarcoma subtypes have been identified with distinctive pathology, molecular characteristics, and clinical presentations. Sarcomas represent <1% of adult cancers and account for approximately 21% of pediatric malignancies [2]. There are two main categories of sarcomas: (1) tumors arising from the soft tissues (e.g., muscle, tendons, and blood vessels) and (2) those arising from the bone (e.g., osteosarcoma and Ewing's sarcoma). Approximately 80% arise from soft tissue and 20% originate from the bone. The World Health Organization has defined approximately 50 soft tissue sarcoma histologic subtypes [1]. Soft tissue sarcomas include angiosarcoma, liposarcoma, leiomyosarcoma, neurofibrosarcoma, schwannoma, Kaposi's sarcoma, rhabdomyosarcoma, vascular sarcoma, fibrosarcoma, mesenchymomas, myxofibrosarcoma, gastrointestinal stromal tumor, and synovial sarcomas.

Synovial sarcomas (SS) are one of the most common soft tissue tumors in adolescents and young adults, and it accounts for approximately 5–10% of all soft tissue sarcomas [3]. About one-third of cases occur in the first two decades of life with an average age of 30 years at diagnosis. The origin of synovial sarcoma is unclear. However, SS is associated with a recurrent reciprocal translocation between chromosomes X and 18, t(X; 18) (p11.2; q11.2), which leads to the expression of several different SS18:SSX fusion proteins. The fusion proteins SYT-SSX1 and SYT-SSX2 are believed to function as aberrant transcriptional regulators, resulting in either activation of protooncogenes or inhibition of tumor suppressor genes [4].

Primary SS is most common in the large joint of the extremities. However, primary SS have been documented in most human tissues and organs including the neck, brain, prostate, tongue, kidney, larynx, mediastinum, esophagus, heart, abdomen wall, small intestine, mesentery, vessels, retroperitoneum, and lungs [5]. PPSS can originate from vessels, pulmonary stroma, and mesenchymal elements of the bronchial wall. PPSS accounts for 0.1% to 0.5% of all primary lung malignancies [6]. Most of the available literature concerning PPSS is limited to case reports and case series [7].

2. Case Report

A 41-year-old female of Indian descent with no significant past medical history presented to the emergency room with a 2-month history of progressive dyspnea on exertion and sharp, pleuritic, substernal chest pain. She also endorsed anxiety and chest palpitations, denied edema, nausea,

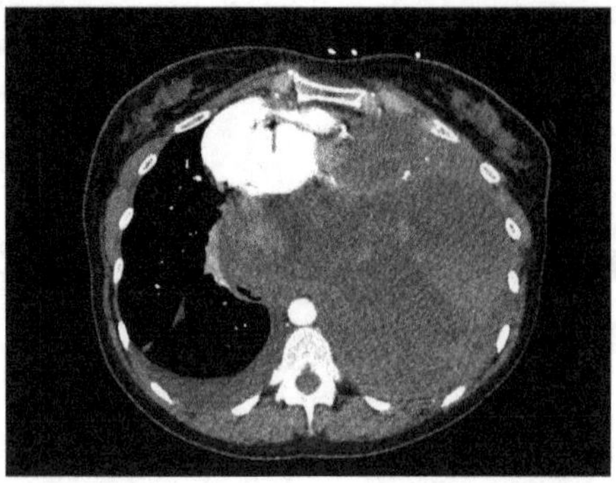

Figure 1: CT axial view arterial phase postcontrast large 17.9 × 17.6 × 18.3 cm heterogeneous mass centered within the left hemithorax, resulting in rightward mediastinal shift. An incidental right pleural effusion is present.

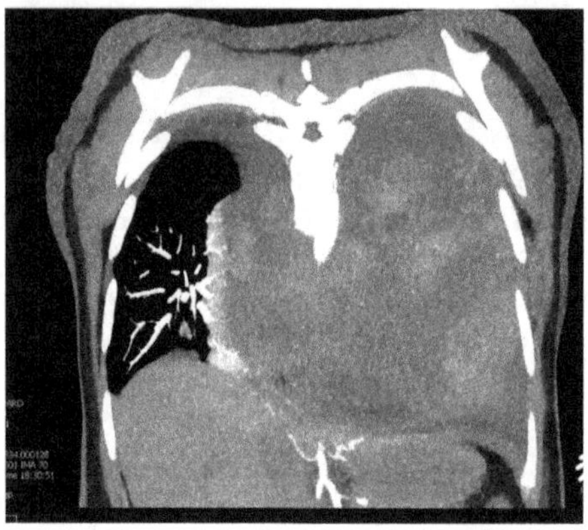

Figure 2: CT chest coronal MIP (maximum intensity projection) rightward mediastinal shift and partial right lung collapse secondary to left hemithoracic mass effect.

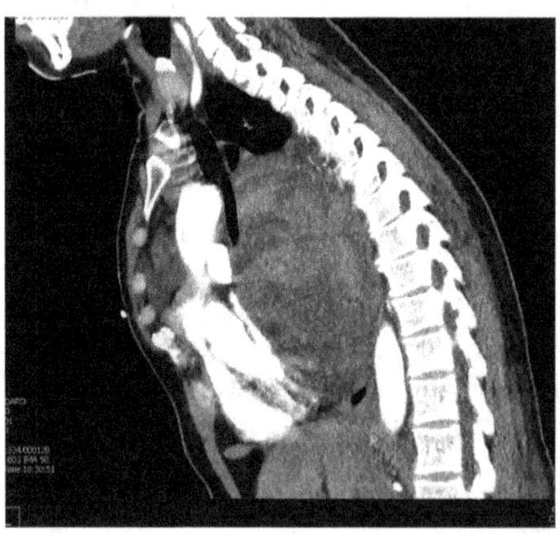

Figure 3: CT sagittal projection centered along the midline depicted anterior displacement of mediastinal structures secondary to larger left hemithoracic mass, which crosses the midline.

vomiting, fevers, and chills, and has no history of tobacco, alcohol, or illicit drug use.

On physical examination, vital signs revealed a heart rate of 126 beats per minute and a respiratory rate of 32 breaths per minute. She was pale with decreased respiratory movement on the left supraclavicular and infraclavicular areas. There was no cervical lymphadenopathy or clubbing.

Initial blood gas analysis was pH 7.2/CO2 47.9/HCO3 28/PO2 of 70. An electrocardiogram revealed sinus tachycardia. Cardiac biomarkers were negative. Complete hemogram revealed normocytic anemia with a hemoglobin level of 11.5 g/dl (reference [8]-16 g/dl), and a complete metabolic panel revealed a bicarb level of 35 (reference 21-29 mmol/l). A chest radiograph revealed opacification of the left hemithorax with a mass effect on the mediastinal structures. A chest computer tomography (CT) revealed a large mixed attenuated mass involving the left chest and mediastinum measuring 17.9 × 17.6 × 18.3 cm in dimension (Figures 1, 2, and 3). Furthermore, a video-assisted thoracoscopic biopsy from the lung mass showed an infiltrating spindle cell neoplasm. The immunohistochemistry of the tissue sample revealed cells expressing epithelial membrane antigen (EMA), CD99, BCL-2, and calponin. The cells were immune-negative for cytokeratin and S-100.

3. Case Discussion

PPSS is a rare and highly aggressive type of SS, usually occurring in young adults. It generally presents as a large, circumscribed mass. Metastatic SS from extremities is common in the pulmonary parenchyma and pleura. Patients with PPSS often present with chest wall pain, cough, dyspnea, hemoptysis, and ipsilateral pleural effusions. There may be a slight male predilection, but there is no relation to smoking status [9]. Toxic substances and radiation have been noted as risks factors. Furthermore, reciprocal translocations between chromosomes X and 18 and infectious pathogens have been noted to have an impact on the origin of PPSS.

The diagnosis of PPSS requires clinical, pathological, and immunohistochemical investigations and radiological findings to exclude alternative primary lung tumors and metastatic sarcomas [9, 10]. Primary pulmonary synovial sarcomas are composed of two morphologically different cell types: (1) epithelial cells or (2) fibroblast-like spindle cells [11]. Histopathologically, there are four subtypes of PPSS, monophasic fibrous cell and biphasic; less common subtypes include monophasic epithelial and poorly differentiated (round cell) tumors [12]. Immunohistochemically, PPSS is positive for markers such as CD99, Bcl-2, vimentin, desmin, actin, cytokeratin, and EMA [2]. Based on radiologic imaging alone, manifestations of PPSS are indistinguishable from other common pulmonary and pleural neoplasms [6]. Typical CT imaging findings are large, heterogeneous tumors with internal necrosis. Radiologic findings are useful for delineating the extent of tumor involvement, determining the potential for surgical resection, and monitoring the effects of chemotherapy or radiation therapy. Our case was characterized by a well-defined heterogeneous enhancing mass of the left hemithorax with the presence of spindle cell sarcoma on histopathological examination and the expression of positive tumor markers for EMA, CD99, BCL-2, and calponin.

Currently, there is no standardized therapy for patients with PPSS. Treatment options include surgery, chemotherapy, radiation, and recently adoptive immunotherapy using tumor-infiltrating lymphocytes [13]. The preferred modality of treatment for PPSS is complete surgical resection. The standard surgical strategy of PPSS includes lobectomy and pneumonectomy. According to Golota et al., the treatment of choice for PPSS is anatomical resection of lung tissue with a tumor-free margin. Male patients and those with tumors larger than 5 cm have worse prognoses. Golota et al. also reported higher overall survival in patients who underwent nonanatomical resections versus those who underwent anatomical resections.

For unresectable tumors, chemotherapy, radiotherapy, and immunotherapy can be considered [3, 6, 12]. PPSS is considered relatively chemosensitive to chemotherapy agents such as ifosfamide, doxorubicin, and dacarbazine [14]. Robbins et al. tested the effectiveness of adoptive immunotherapy with genetically engineered lymphocytes that targeted the NY-ESO-1 antigen expressed in patients with advance synovial cell sarcomas, demonstrating that treatment with engineered lymphocytes mediates tumor regression in patients with metastatic synovial cell sarcomas [13]. The overall survival of patients with PPSS is poor, with a 5-year survival rate of 50%. Future studies are needed to identify ideal therapeutic agents for the treatment of PPSS.

4. Conclusion

PPSS is a very rare and aggressive tumor that should be included on the differential for lung and pleural masses. Due to poor prognosis, prompt diagnosis and treatment is imperative.

References

[1] L. Guy, A. Lazar, and D. Lev, "Sarcoma epidemiology and etiology: potential environmental and genetic factors," *Surgical Clinics of North America*, vol. 88, no. 3, p. 451, 2008.

[2] B. Jenna, R. D. Ballim, S. Kimani et al., "Managing sarcoma: where have we come from and where are we going," *Therapeutic Advances in Medical Oncology*, vol. 9, no. 10, pp. 637–659, 2017.

[3] J. Golota, K. Osowiecka, and T. Orłowski, "Primary pulmonary sarcoma - long-term treatment outcomes and prognostic factors," *Polish Journal of Cardio-Thoracic Surgery*, vol. 15, no. 3, pp. 162–169, 2018.

[4] N. Naka, S. Takenaka, N. Araki et al., "Synovial sarcoma is a stem cell malignancy," *Stem Cells*, vol. 28, no. 7, pp. 1119–1131, 2010.

[5] H. Zeren, C. A. Moran, S. Suster, N. F. Fishback, and M. N. Koss, "Primary pulmonary sarcomas with features of monophasic synovial sarcoma: a clinicopathological, immunohistochemical, and ultrastructural study of 25 cases," *Human Pathology*, vol. 26, no. 5, pp. 474–480, 1995.

[6] G. H. Kim, M. Y. Kim, H. J. Koo, J. S. Song, and C.-M. Choi, "Primary pulmonary synovial sarcoma in a tertiary referral center: clinical characteristics, CT, and 18F-FDG PET findings, with pathologic correlations," *Medicine*, vol. 94, no. 34, p. e1392, 2015.

[7] D. J. Boulter, M. L. Rosado-de-Christenson, R. Stevens, and S. Suster, "Primary synovial sarcoma of the lung," *Radiology Case Reports*, vol. 2, no. 4, p. 82, 2007.

[8] P. Robbins, R. A. Morgan, S. A. Feldman et al., "Tumor regression in patients with metastatic synovial cell sarcoma and melanoma using genetically engineered lymphocytes reactive with NY-ESO-1," *Journal OF Clinical Oncology*, vol. 29, no. 7, pp. 917–924, 2011.

[9] A. Das, A. Sarkar, A. K. Dwari, S. Datta, and P. P. Roy, "A primary synovial sarcoma of lung," *North American Journal of Medical Sciences*, vol. 4, no. 5, pp. 241–243, 2012.

[10] P. H. Hartel, J. C. Fanburg-Smith, A. A. Frazier et al., "Primary pulmonary and mediastinal synovial sarcoma: a clinicopathologic study of 60 cases and comparison with five prior series," *Modern Pathology*, vol. 20, no. 7, pp. 760–769, 2007.

[11] D. Bhattacharya, S. Datta, A. Das, K. C. Halder, and S. Chattopadhyay, "Primary pulmonary synovial sarcoma: a case report and review of literature," *International Journal of Applied and Basic Medical Research*, vol. 6, no. 1, pp. 63–65, 2016.

[12] S. Okamoto, M. Hisaoka, T. Daa, K. Hatakeyama, T. Iwamasa, and H. Hashimoto, "Primary pulmonary synovial sarcoma: a clinicopathologic, immunohistochemical, and molecular study of 11 cases," *Human Pathology*, vol. 35, no. 7, pp. 850–856, 2004.

[13] L. Rajeev, R. Patidar, G. Babu, M. C. Suresh Babu, K. N. Lokesh, and G. V. Patil Okaly, "A rare case of primary synovial sarcoma of lung," *Lung India*, vol. 34, no. 6, p. 545, 2017.

[14] M. Panigrahi, G. Pradhan, N. Sahoo, P. Mishra, S. Patra, and P. R. Mohapatra, "Primary pulmonary synovial sarcoma: a reappraisal," *Journal of Cancer Research and Therapies*, vol. 14, no. 3, pp. 481–489, 2018.

Permissions

All chapters in this book were first published by Hindawi Publishing Corporation; hereby published with permission under the Creative Commons Attribution License or equivalent. Every chapter published in this book has been scrutinized by our experts. Their significance has been extensively debated. The topics covered herein carry significant findings which will fuel the growth of the discipline. They may even be implemented as practical applications or may be referred to as a beginning point for another development.

The contributors of this book come from diverse backgrounds, making this book a truly international effort. This book will bring forth new frontiers with its revolutionizing research information and detailed analysis of the nascent developments around the world.

We would like to thank all the contributing authors for lending their expertise to make the book truly unique. They have played a crucial role in the development of this book. Without their invaluable contributions this book wouldn't have been possible. They have made vital efforts to compile up to date information on the varied aspects of this subject to make this book a valuable addition to the collection of many professionals and students.

This book was conceptualized with the vision of imparting up-to-date information and advanced data in this field. To ensure the same, a matchless editorial board was set up. Every individual on the board went through rigorous rounds of assessment to prove their worth. After which they invested a large part of their time researching and compiling the most relevant data for our readers.

The editorial board has been involved in producing this book since its inception. They have spent rigorous hours researching and exploring the diverse topics which have resulted in the successful publishing of this book. They have passed on their knowledge of decades through this book. To expedite this challenging task, the publisher supported the team at every step. A small team of assistant editors was also appointed to further simplify the editing procedure and attain best results for the readers.

Apart from the editorial board, the designing team has also invested a significant amount of their time in understanding the subject and creating the most relevant covers. They scrutinized every image to scout for the most suitable representation of the subject and create an appropriate cover for the book.

The publishing team has been an ardent support to the editorial, designing and production team. Their endless efforts to recruit the best for this project, has resulted in the accomplishment of this book. They are a veteran in the field of academics and their pool of knowledge is as vast as their experience in printing. Their expertise and guidance has proved useful at every step. Their uncompromising quality standards have made this book an exceptional effort. Their encouragement from time to time has been an inspiration for everyone.

The publisher and the editorial board hope that this book will prove to be a valuable piece of knowledge for researchers, students, practitioners and scholars across the globe.

List of Contributors

Marta Peri, Antonino Grassadonia, Laura Iezzi, Michele De Tursi, Clara Natoli and Nicola Tinari
Medical Oncology Unit, Department of Medical, Oral and Biotechnological Sciences, University "G. D'Annunzio", Chieti, Italy

Patrizia Vici
Division of Medical Oncology 2, IRCCS Regina Elena National Cancer Institute, Rome, Italy

Marinella Zilli
Medical Oncology Unit, SS Annunziata Hospital, Chieti, Italy

Sophia Z. Shalhout and David M. Miller
Division of Hematology/Oncology, Department of Medicine, and Department of Dermatology, Massachusetts General Hospital, Harvard Medical School, Boston, MA 02114, USA

Kevin S. Emerick
Department of Otolaryngology, Massachusetts Eye and Ear Infirmary, Harvard Medical School, Boston, MA 02114, USA

Peter M. Sadow
Department of Pathology, Massachusetts General Hospital, Harvard Medical School, Boston, MA 02114, USA

Jenny J. Linnoila
Department of Neurology, Massachusetts General Hospital, Harvard Medical School, Boston, MA 02114, USA

Hung Van Nguyen, Long Thanh Nguyen and Hien Xuan Nguyen
Department of Oncology, Hanoi Medical University, Hanoi, Vietnam

Nga Quynh Pham, Hau Xuan Nguyen, Hieu Van Nguyen and Vuong Thi Nguyen
Department of Oncology, Hanoi Medical University, Hanoi, Vietnam
Department of Oncology and Palliative Care, Hanoi Medical University Hospital, Hanoi, Vietnam

Dmytro E. Makhmudov, Olena O. Kolesnik and Maryna O. Volk
Oncocoloproctology Department, National Cancer Institute, Lomonosova str. 33/43, Kyiv 03022, Ukraine

Natalia N. Lagoda
Department of Pathomorphology, National Cancer Institute, Lomonosova str. 33/43, Kyiv 03022, Ukraine

Tomoo Kakimoto, Mamoru Sasaki, Ko Lee, Shingo Nakayama and Naoto Minematsu
Department of Internal Medicine Hino Municipal Hospital, Hino-shi, Tokyo, Japan

Tatsuya Yamamoto and Arifumi Iwamaru
Department of Surgery, Federation of National Public Service Personnel Mutual Aid Associations, Tachikawa Hospital, Tachikawashi, Tokyo, Japan

Kentaro Ogata
Department of Pathology, Federation of National Public Service Personnel Mutual Aid Associations, Tachikawa Hospital, Tachikawa-shi, Tokyo, Japan

Prashanth Ashok Kumar and Shweta Paulraj
Department of Internal Medicine, SUNY Upstate Medical University, Syracuse, NY 13210, USA

Kanish Mirchia
Department of Pathology, SUNY Upstate Medical University, Syracuse, NY 13210, USA

Seung Shin Hahn
Department of Radiation Oncology, SUNY Upstate Medical University, Syracuse, NY 13210, USA

Abirami Sivapiragasam
Department of Hematology-Oncology, SUNY Upstate Medical University, Syracuse, NY 13210, USA

Christopher Larrimore and Annmarie Jaghab
Nova Southeastern University Dr. Kiran C. Patel College of Osteopathic Medicine, USA

Babak Baseri, Bachar Samra, Eric Tam and Edwin Chiu
Department of Hematology/Oncology, State University of New York Downstate Medical Center, Brooklyn, New York, USA

Andrea Leaf
Department of Hematology/Oncology, State University of New York Downstate Medical Center, Brooklyn, New York, USA
Department of Hematology/Oncology, Veterans Affairs New York Harbor Healthcare System, Brooklyn Campus, New York, USA

Essa M. AlGhunaim and Derar S. AlShehab
Thoracic and Foregut Surgery Unit, Chest Diseases Hospital, Kuwait

Hafsa AlNajem
General Surgery Department, Mubarak Al-Kabeer Hospital, Kuwait

Néstor Llinás-Quintero, Andrés Yepes and Javier Cuello-López
Clinical Oncology Group, Fundación Colombiana de Cancerología-Clínica Vida, Medellín, Colombia

David González-Hoyos
School of Medicine, CES University, Medellín, Colombia

Diego A. Herrera, Sebastián Peláez-Arroyave and Carlos Caicedo-Zamudio
Diagnostic Imaging Group, CEDIMED, Medellín, Colombia

Erick Blanco-Daza
School of Medicine, UPB University, Medellín, Colombia

Michael J. Harvey
University of Missouri Kansas City School of Medicine, Kansas City, MO, USA

Howard G. Rosenthal
University of Kansas, Sarcoma Center, Overland Park, KS, USA

Gabriel S. Makar and Kathryn Bush
Cooper Medical School of Rowan University, 401 Broadway Ave, Camden, NJ 08103, USA

Michael Makar
Robert Wood Johnson University Hospital, 1 Robert Wood Johnson Pl, New Brunswick, NJ 08901, USA

Joanna Ghobrial
AT Still University School of Osteopathic Medicine, 5850 E Still Cir, Mesa, AZ 85206, USA

Ryan Allen Gruner
Cooper University Hospital, Department of Surgery, 1 Cooper Plaza, Camden, NJ 08103, USA

Thomas Holdbrook
Cooper University Hospital, Department of Pathology, 1 Cooper Plaza, Camden, NJ 08103, USA

Antonio Maffuz-Aziz, Gabriel Garnica, Silvia López-Hernández and Patricia López-Jiménez
Department of Surgical Oncology, American British Cowdray Medical Center, Mexico City, Mexico

Javier Baquera-Heredia and Janet Pineda-Diaz
Department of Surgical and Molecular Pathology, American British Cowdray Medical Center, Mexico City, Mexico

Rajat N. Moman and Julie M. Rogers
Department of Anesthesiology and Perioperative Medicine, Mayo Clinic, Rochester, MN, USA

Thomas P. Pittelkow
Division of Pain Medicine, Department of Anesthesiology and Perioperative Medicine, Mayo Clinic, Rochester, MN, USA

Hajime Nakamura, Kohichi Takada, Kazuyuki Murase, Hiroki Sakamoto, Naotaka Hayasaka, Kazuma Ishikawa, Yuki Ikeda, Makoto Yoshida, Junji Kato and Koji Miyanishi
Department of Medical Oncology, Sapporo Medical University School of Medicine, Japan

Satoshi Iyama and Masayoshi Kobune
Department of Hematology, Sapporo Medical University School of Medicine, Japan

Ko Kobayashi, Tetsuya Shindo and Naoya Masumori
Department of Urology, Sapporo Medical University School of Medicine, Japan

Shintaro Sugita
Department of Surgical Pathology, Sapporo Medical University School of Medicine, Japan

Ashish Gupta and Elizabeth Guevara
Internal Medicine, The Brooklyn Hospital Center, Brooklyn, New York, NY, USA

Aung Tun and Katy Ticona
Hematology Oncology, The Brooklyn Hospital Center, Brooklyn, New York, NY, USA

Aam Baqui
Pathology, The Brooklyn Hospital Center, Brooklyn, New York, NY, USA

Amanda Wiggins, Zhaohui Arter and Tamie Kerns
Tripler Army Medical Center, 1 Jarrett White Road, DHCK-DM, Honolulu, HI 96859, USA

Tetsuro Kawagoe, Go Ikeda, Yu Oshiro, Yuta Maruki, Keiko Kaneko and Katsuhiko Iwakiri
Division of Gastroenterology, Department of Internal Medicine, Nippon Medical School, Japan

Piotr Młodożeniec and Mateusz Zasadny
Clinical Department of Urology and Urological Oncology, Municipal Hospital in Rzeszow, Poland

Krzysztof Balawender
Clinical Department of Urology and Urological Oncology, Municipal Hospital in Rzeszow, Poland
Morphological Sciences Department, Institute of Medical Sciences, Medical College of Rzeszow University, Poland

Kazumori Arai, Tomohiro Iwasaki and Chinatsu Tsuchiya
Department of Pathology, Shizuoka General Hospital, 4-27-1 Kitaando, Aoi-ku, Shizuoka 420-0881, Japan

Akihiro Sonoda
Department of Clinical Research, Shizuoka General Hospital, Japan

Takuji Seo, Emi Noguchi, Maki Tanioka, Kazuki Sudo, Akihiko Shimomura, Kan Yonemori, Yasuhiro Fujiwara and Kenji Tamura
Department of Breast and Medical Oncology, National Cancer Center Hospital, 5-1-1, Tsukiji, Chuo-ku, Tokyo 104-0045, Japan

Masayuki Yoshida and Taisuke Mori
Department of Pathology and Clinical Laboratories, National Cancer Center Hospital, 5 1-1, Tsukiji, Chuo-ku, Tokyo 104-0045, Japan

Cosphiadi Irawan and Rahmat Cahyanur
Division of Hematology-Medical Oncology, Department of Internal Medicine, Faculty of Medicine Universitas Indonesia, Dr. Cipto Mangunkusumo General Hospital, Jakarta, Indonesia

Reyhan Eddy Yunus
Department of Radiology, Faculty of Medicine Universitas Indonesia, Dr. Cipto Mangunkusumo General Hospital, Jakarta, Indonesia

Deepti Kantamani, Sai S. Bandaru, Jennifer L. Miatech and M. Patrick Stagg
Baton Rouge General Medical Center-Bluebonnet, Internal Medicine Residency Program, Baton Rouge, LA, USA 70809-3679

Áurea Lima
Medical Oncology Service, Centro Hospitalar de Entre o Douro e Vouga, EPE, Unit of Santa Maria da Feira, R. Dr. Cândido Pinho 5,4520-211 Santa Maria da Feira, Portugal
Molecular Oncology and Viral Pathology Group, Research Center of Portuguese Institute of Oncology of Porto, Portuguese Institute of Oncology of Porto Francisco Gentil, EPE, Rua Dr. António Bernardino de Almeida, 4200-072 Porto, Portugal
CESPU, Institute for Research and Advanced Training in Health Sciences and Technologies, Cancer Research Group, R. Central da Gandra, 1317 Gandra, Portugal

Isa Peixoto
Medical Oncology Service, Centro Hospitalar Universitário do Porto, EPE, Largo Prof. Abel Salazar 4099-001 Porto, Portugal

Susana Sarandão and Helena Pereira
External Radiotherapy Service, Portuguese Institute of Oncology of Porto Francisco Gentil, EPE, Rua Dr. António Bernardino de Almeida, 4200-072 Porto, Portugal

Daniel Melo
Pathologic Anatomy Service, Centro Hospitalar Universitário de São João, Alameda Prof. Hernâni Monteiro 4200-319 Porto, Portugal

Ângelo Rodrigues
Pathologic Anatomy Service, Portuguese Institute of Oncology of Porto Francisco Gentil, EPE, Rua Dr. António Bernardino de Almeida, 4200-072 Porto, Portugal

Joey El Khoury, Maher Abdessater, Rami Halabi, Johnny Boustany, Anthony Kanbar, Charbel El Hachem and Raghid El Khoury
Faculty of Medicine and Medical Sciences, Holy Spirit University of Kaslik (USEK), Jounieh, Lebanon
Department of Urology, University Hospital Center-Notre Dame des Secours, Byblos, Lebanon

Fadi Nasr
Faculty of Medicine and Medical Sciences, Holy Spirit University of Kaslik (USEK), Jounieh, Lebanon
Department of Oncology, University Hospital Center-Notre Dame des Secours, Byblos, Lebanon

Amanda Ramos
Division of Gynecologic Oncology, Department of Obstetrics and Gynecology, Hartford Healthcare, Hartford, CT 06102, USA

Marcela del Carmen
Division of Gynecologic Oncology, Vincent Obstetrics and Gynecology, Harvard Medical School, Boston, MA 02114, USA

Oladapo Yeku
Gynecologic Cancers Program, Massachusetts General Hospital, Harvard Medical School, Boston, MA 02114, USA

Anwar Chammout
Department of Oncology, University of Aleppo, Faculty of Medicine, Aleppo, Syria

Mike Ghabally, Christina Masri, Nour Tantak and Fadi Ward
University of Aleppo, Faculty of Medicine, Aleppo, Syria

Ghefar Omar
Department of Pathology, University of Aleppo, Faculty of Medicine, Aleppo, Syria

Arthur A. Parsee, Kerry L. Thomas, Jennifer Sweeney, Daniel Jeong and Abraham Ahmed
Department of Radiology, Moffitt Cancer Center, Tampa, Florida, USA

Masoumeh Ghayouri
Department of Pathology, Moffitt Cancer Center, Tampa, Florida, USA

Rutika Mehta
Department of Gastrointestinal Oncology, Moffitt Cancer Center, Tampa, Florida, USA

Kujtim Latifi
Department of Radiation Oncology, Moffitt Cancer Center, Tampa, Florida, USA

Christopher Le, Adam Jacob, Devarajan Iyengar, John Dedousis and Antonios Tsompanidis
Department of Graduate Medical Education, CarePoint Health Bayonne Medical Center, 29 E. 29th Street, Bayonne, NJ 07002, USA

Yi Xin Li
Duke-NUS Medical School, Singapore

Mihir Gudi
Department of Pathology and Laboratory Medicine, KK Women's and Children's Hospital, Singapore

Zhiyan Yan
Breast Department, KK Women's and Children's Hospital, Singapore

Alexandra Grubnik and Barend Van der Bergh
Netcare Breast Care Centre of Excellence, Milpark Hospital, 9 Guild Road Parktown, South Africa

Yastira Ramdas
Netcare Breast Care Centre of Excellence, Milpark Hospital, 9 Guild Road Parktown, South Africa
Department of Immunology, Faculty of Health Sciences, University of Pretoria, Corner Doctor Savage Road and Bophelo Road, Pretoria 0002, South Africa

Simon Nayler
Netcare Breast Care Centre of Excellence, Milpark Hospital, 9 Guild Road Parktown, South Africa
Drs Gritzman & Thatcher Inc. Laboratories, 4 Main Street, Bordeaux, Randburg, Johannesburg 2194, South Africa
University of the Witwatersrand, Donald Gordon Medical Centre, 21 Eton Road, Parktown Johannesburg, 2193, South Africa

Carol-Ann Benn
Netcare Breast Care Centre of Excellence, Milpark Hospital, 9 Guild Road Parktown, South Africa
Helen Joseph Hospital Breast Care Clinic, Department of Surgery, Faculty of Health Sciences, University of the Witwatersrand, 1 Perth Road, Auckland Park, Johannesburg, 2092 Gauteng, South Africa

Bernardo L. Rapoport
Netcare Breast Care Centre of Excellence, Milpark Hospital, 9 Guild Road Parktown, South Africa
Department of Immunology, Faculty of Health Sciences, University of Pretoria, Corner Doctor Savage Road and Bophelo Road, Pretoria 0002, South Africa
The Medical Oncology Centre of Rosebank, 129 Oxford Road, Johannesburg 2196, South Africa

Neris Dincer, Melisa Bagci, Metin Figen and Esengul Kocak Uzel
Department of Radiation Oncology, Şişli Etfal Teaching and Research Hospital, Istanbul, Turkey

Adem Yilmaz
Department of Neurosurgery, Şişli Etfal Teaching and Research Hospital, Istanbul, Turkey

Ahmet Mesrur Halefoglu
Department of Radiology, Şişli Etfal Teaching and Research Hospital, Istanbul, Turkey

Canan Tanik
Department of Pathology, Şişli Etfal Teaching and Research Hospital, Istanbul, Turkey

Víctor Albarrán, Javier Pozas, Juan José Soto, Jorge Esteban, Elena Corral, Yolanda Lage, Pablo Gajate and Pilar Garrido
Thoracic Tumors Unit from Medical Oncology Department, Ramón Y Cajal University Hospital, Madrid, Spain

Hideaki Sabe, Akitomo Inoue, Yoshinori Imura, Toru Wakamatsu and Satoshi Takenaka
Department of Orthopedic Surgery, Osaka International Cancer Institute, Osaka 541-8567, Japan

Shigenori Nagata
Department of Diagnostic Pathology and Cytology, Osaka International Cancer Institute, Osaka 541-8567, Japan

Hironari Tamiya
Department of Orthopedic Surgery, Osaka International Cancer Institute, Osaka 541-8567, Japan
Department of Rehabilitation, Osaka International Cancer Institute, Osaka 541-8567, Japan

Anas Bizanti, Ahmad Al-abdouh, Mohammed Mohammed and Maria Pardi
Saint Agnes Hospital, Baltimore, MA, USA

Ariege Bizanti
University of Central Florida, Orlando, FL, USA

Rodney E. Shackelford and Eric X. Wei
Department of Pathology, University of South Alabama Health, Mobile, Alabama 36617, USA

Ekin Ozluk and Jehan Abdulsattar
Department of Pathology & Translational Pathobiology, LSU Health Sciences Center Shreveport, Shreveport, Louisiana 71130, USA

Terry C. Lairmore and Quyen Chu
Department of Surgery, Louisiana State University Health Shreveport, Louisiana 71130, USA

Joseph Mort and Shipra Maheshwari
Department of Medicine, University of Virginia Health System, 1215 Lee Street, Charlottesville, VA 22908, USA

Nayanika Basu, Patrick Dillon, Kevin Brady and Trish Millard
Emily Couric Cancer Center, University of Virginia Health System, 1240 Lee Street, Charlottesville, VA 22903, USA

Harry Bear
Massey Cancer Center and Department of Surgery, Virginia Commonwealth University and VCU Health, Richmond, VA 23298-0011, USA

Sheffield Sandra, Nwachukwu Chidi and Ashby Tracy
Department of Medicine, UF College of Medicine – Jacksonville, 653-1 West 8th Street, L20 4th Floor, LRC Jacksonville, FL 32209, USA

Index